Pain Syndromes in Neurology

Butterworths International Medical Reviews

Neurology

Published titles

Pain Syndromes in Neurology

Edited by

Howard L. Fields, MD, PhD
Professor of Neurology and Physiology, University of California, San Francisco,
California, USA

Butterworths
London Boston Singapore Sydney Toronto Wellington

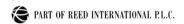 PART OF REED INTERNATIONAL P.L.C.

First published 1990

© **Butterworth & Co. (Publishers) Ltd, 1990**

British Library Cataloguing in Publication Data
Pain syndromes in neurology.
  1. Man. Nervous system. Pain
  I. Fields, Howard L.
  616.8'0472

  ISBN 0–407–01124–2

Library of Congress Cataloging-in-Publication Data

Pain syndromes in neurology/edited by Howard L. Fields.
     p. cm. – (Butterworths international medical reviews.
Neurology : 8)
  Includes bibliographical references.
  ISBN 0-407-01124-2
  1. Pain–Pathophysiology. 2. Nervous system–Pathophysiology.
I. Fields, Howard L. II. Series.
  [DNLM: 1. Nervous System–physiopathology. 2. Pain –
physiopathology. W1 BU98U/WL 704 P1473]
  RB 127.P35 1990
  616'.0472–dc20
  DNLM/DLC   89-22369
  for Library of Congress   CIP

Photoset by TecSet Ltd.
Printed and bound in Great Britain by Courier International Ltd, Tiptree, Essex.

Foreword

For almost a quarter of a century (1951–1975), subjects of topical interest were written about in the periodic volumes of our predecessor, *Modern Trends in Neurology*. Although both that series and its highly regarded editor, Dr Denis Williams, are now retired, the legacy continues in the present Butterworths series in Neurology. As was the case with *Modern Trends*, the current volumes are intended for use by physicians who grapple with the problems of neurological disorder on a daily basis, be they neurologists, neurologists in training, or those in related fields such as neurosurgery, internal medicine, psychiatry, and rehabilitation medicine.

Our purpose is to produce annually a monograph on a topic in clinical neurology in which progress through research has brought about new concepts of patient management. The subject of each monograph is selected by the Series Editors using two criteria: first, that there has been significant advance in knowledge in that area and, second, that such advances have been incorporated into new ways of managing patients with the disorders in question.

The present volume on Neuropathic Pain fits the criteria admirably. Dr Howard Fields has chosen his contributors well, and they have set forth clearly the current understanding of the pathophysiology of neuropathic pain and how best to manage it.

These two criteria have been the guiding spirit behind each volume, and we expect it to continue. In effect we emphasize research, both in the clinic and in the experimental laboratory, but principally to the extent that it changes our collective attitudes and practices in caring for those who are neurologically afflicted.

C. D. Marsden
A. K. Asbury
Series Editors

Preface

The diagnosis and treatment of painful conditions associated with dysfunction of the peripheral or central nervous system is an important part of neurologic practice. Although much progress has been made, these conditions are still incompletely understood and often unresponsive to treatment. This book is intended to address both of these problems by informing the reader about advances in three areas: first, the normal anatomy and physiology of pain, second, the pathophysiology of damaged sensory neurons and third, the diagnosis and treatment of patients with neuropathic pain.

This is an appropriate time for this book because there has been a great expansion of knowledge about the neurobiology of pain sensation. We now have a much more accurate and detailed idea of the normal sensory processing of the pain message. We have particularly detailed descriptions, in both humans and subhuman primates, of cutaneous primary afferents. Furthermore, extensive animal research has elucidated the neural circuitry of the spinal cord dorsal horn, the first central nervous system relay of input from primary afferent nociceptors. Progress has also been made in our knowledge of the central nervous system pathways that relay the pain message from the spinal cord to the thalamus and cortex.

It is clear that knowledge of the normal physiology of pain is critical to our understanding of clinical pain syndromes. Scientists and clinicians interested in pain have long been interested in the fascinating and troublesome paradox that damage to the segmental apparatus or central pathways for nociception can produce chronic, severe and intractable pain. The first attempt to provide a detailed explanation of this paradox based on our expanded knowledge of primary afferents and dorsal horn circuitry was Melzack and Wall's *Gate Control Hypothesis*, published in 1965. In the quarter century since that publication appeared our knowledge of dorsal horn circuitry has grown immensely and with it, the sophistication of our models of neuropathic pain. We are now aware that there are multiple factors other than intense stimuli that can generate a pain signal. These factors include sympathetic nervous system activity, crosstalk between damaged peripheral axons, hyperactivity in regenerating primary afferents or in deafferented central pain-transmission neurons.

It is obvious that better understanding and treatment of painful nervous system dysfunction will require accurate clinical description as well as animal research that is both innovative and clinically relevant. In this age of subspecialization, this means that scientists and clinicians must collaborate and communicate. Accordingly, this book has two major goals: first, to describe certain painful conditions that appear to result from dysfunction of the nervous system, and second, to review those recent advances in the neurobiology of pain that are directly relevant to understanding how such pain comes about. I am fortunate to have been able to recruit an outstanding group of neuroscientist and clinician contributors. I hope that their efforts will prove as informative and stimulating to the reader as they have been for me.

Howard L. Fields

Contributors

Arthur K. Asbury, MD
Van Meter Professor of Neurology, University of Pennsylvania, School of Medicine, Philadelphia, Pennsylvania, USA

Kim J. Burchiel, MD, FACS
Professor and Head, Division of Neurosurgery, The Oregon Health Sciences University, Oregon, USA.

James N. Campbell, MD
Associate Professor of Neurosurgery, Johns Hopkins University School of Medicine, Baltimore, Maryland, USA

Marshall Devor, PhD
Associate Professor and Chairman, Department of Zoology, Life Sciences Institute, Hebrew University of Jerusalem, Jerusalem, Israel.

Howard L. Fields, MD, PhD
Professor of Neurology and Physiology, Department of Neurology, School of Medicine, University of California, San Francisco, California, USA

Ronald C. Kramis, PhD
Senior Research Associate, Robert S. Dow Neurological Sciences Institute, Good Samaritan Hospital and Medical Center, Portland, Oregon, USA

Richard A. Meyer
Principal Professional Staff, Applied Physics Laboratory; Associate Professor of Surgery and Biomedical Engineering, Johns Hopkins University School of Medicine, Baltimore, Maryland, USA

Richard Payne, MD
Associate Professor of Neurology, University of Cincinnati Medical Center; Chief, Neurology Service, VA Medical Center, Cincinnati, Ohio, USA

Russell K. Portenoy, MD
Director of Analgesic Studies, Pain Service, Assistant Attending Neurologist, Department of Neurology, Memorial Sloan-Kettering Cancer Center; Assistant Professor of Neurology, Cornell University Medical College, New York, New York, USA

Srinivasa N. Raja, MD
Assistant Professor, Department of Anesthesiology and Critical Care Medicine, Johns Hopkins University School of Medicine, Baltimore, Maryland, USA

Z. Harry Rappaport, MD
Senior Lecturer in Neurosurgery, Hadassah University Hospital, Jerusalem, Israel

William J. Roberts, PhD
Senior Scientist and Chairman, Robert S. Dow Neurological Sciences Institute, Good Samaritan Hospital and Medical Center, Portland, Oregon, USA

Ronald R. Tasker, MD
Head, Division of Neurosurgery, Toronto General Hospital; Professor of Surgery, University of Toronto, Toronto, Ontario, Canada

C. Peter N. Watson, MD, FRCP(C)
Assistant Professor, Department of Medicine, University of Toronto, Toronto, Ontario, Canada

Contents

1
Introduction

H. L. Fields

INTRODUCTION

The major objective of this book is to present an overview of the clinical features, pathophysiology and treatment of certain painful conditions that neurologists are often called upon to see. The focus will be upon those syndromes for which there have been advances in treatment, clinical description, or relevant areas of basic research. Of particular importance are advances in understanding of the pain associated with dysfunction of the nervous system. These conditions (e.g. nerve entrapments and neuromas, postherpetic neuralgia, causalgia, thalamic syndrome) take a terrible toll on the patients afflicted by them because they are often severe, unremitting and refractory to treatment. Fortunately, over the past two decades significant progress has been made in unravelling the processes set in motion by neural injury. The search for effective treatments has also started. This chapter reviews neural mechanisms relevant to pain perception and ends with a brief review of neuropathic pain.

PAIN PATHWAYS

Three major processes underly sensory experiences that are produced by stimuli: transduction, transmission and perception. In this context *transduction* refers to the process by which a stimulus is converted to receptor membrane depolarization and then nerve impulses. In the somatosensory system this process normally occurs in the peripheral terminals of dorsal root ganglion cells (primary afferents). Primary afferents fall into distinct classes determined by the specific types of stimuli they respond to and the conduction velocity of their axons. Those that respond with increased discharge to stimuli that are tissue damaging or potentially tissue damaging are termed primary afferent nociceptors (PANs). Once impulses are generated in the PANs the process of *transmission* begins. Transmission includes the conduction of nerve impulses in PAN axons to the spinal cord (or trigeminal nucleus in the brain stem), synaptic activation by the PANs of second-order pain-transmission neurons (e.g. spinothalamic tract cells) and the conduction of impulses in these central pain-transmission neurons to the brain structures that underly subjective *perception*.

Primary afferent nociceptors

A peripheral nerve contains axons that differ widely in their cross-sectional diameter, degree of myelination and conduction velocity (CV). The axons of the primary afferents fall into three distinct groups: A-β (diameter 6–22 μm, heavily myelinated, CV 33–75 m/s), A-δ (diameter 2–5 μm, thinly myelinated, CV 5–30 m/s) and C fibers (diameter 0.3–3 μm, unmyelinated, CV 0.5–2 m/s) [1,2]. To which of these axonal groups classes do the primary afferent nociceptors belong?

At one level, there is a straightforward experimental approach to this question. One needs only to determine the response properties of an afferent and measure its conduction velocity. In fact, cutaneous nociceptors are defined by their character-istic discharge pattern. Using mechanical or thermal stimuli, PANs discharge when the stimulus intensity is at or above the level reported as painful when delivered to the normal skin of a human subject. Characteristically, PANs discharge with increasing frequency to stimuli of increasing intensity within the range reported as painful (Figure 1.1). Using these criteria most PANs fall into one of two groups of afferents: the unmyelinated C fibers and small-diameter myelinated or A-δ group (*see* Chapter 2 for details). Few, if any, belong to the A-β group.

The large myelinated primary afferents in the A-β group respond to low-intensity mechanical stimuli and show no increase in discharge frequency to more intense stimuli. Thus the A-β fibers cannot selectively signal the presence of potentially tissue-damaging stimuli. Consistent with this is the observation that in awake human subjects, electrical stimulation of A-β afferents elicits sensations that are not painful. In fact, there is evidence that selective activation of A-β afferents may actually inhibit nociceptive transmission at the spinal level [3,4].

Despite the evidence against a positive contribution of A-β afferents to pain perception, recent studies suggest that, under certain conditions, especially when there is nerve damage, activity in A-β afferents can elicit pain (e.g. *see* the discussions by Roberts and Kramis in Chapter 4 and by Raja, Meyer and Campbell in Chapter 2 in this book). Thus, although activity of PANs is sufficient to elicit the sensation of pain, it is likely that activity of PANs is not always required for a stimulus to evoke pain. This illustrates the crucial point that the term nociceptor refers to the type of stimuli to which a particular primary afferent responds, as opposed to the type of sensation it produces when it is active. Under normal conditions, nociceptors respond to intense stimuli and, when they are active, consistently elicit the sensation of pain. Under pathological conditions, activity in afferents that are not nociceptors can elicit pain.

The peripheral terminals of primary afferent nociceptors are sensitive to one or more of the following types of stimulus: thermal, mechanical or chemical. The most ubiquitous PAN can be activated by all three types of stimuli and is thus termed the polymodal nociceptor. Most polymodal nociceptors have axons that are unmyeli-nated. The other major classes of PAN respond only to relatively intense mechanical (high-threshold mechanoreceptors) or to both intense mechanical and thermal stimuli (mechanothermal nociceptors). The latter two classes of nociceptor usually have axons that are myelinated.

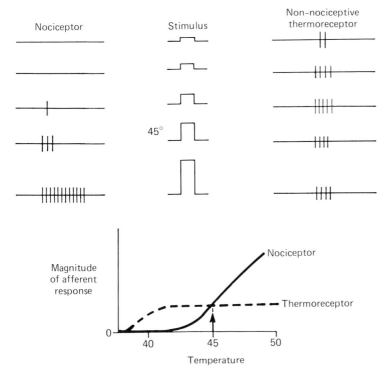

Figure 1.1 Comparison of response properties of thermal nociceptor and non-nociceptive thermoreceptor. At non-noxious temperatures, both types of receptors may fire. Then, as the temperature is raised into the noxious range, only the nociceptor continues to increase in discharge frequency. Both receptors can signal warming but only the nociceptor can transmit the message that the temperature is in the noxious range. (Adapted from Fields, H. L. *Pain*, McGraw-Hill, New York, p. 19 (1987) with permission)

Normally, PANs have no spontaneous activity in the absence of stimulation and do not discharge in response to stimuli that are innocuous when applied to normal skin [5]. However, the response properties of primary afferent nociceptors are dependent on previous stimuli. Most nociceptors become sensitized by tissue-damaging stimuli in the region of their terminals. This property of nociceptors is reviewed extensively in Chapter 2 of this book. Suffice it to say that, in a region of injury, some PANs undergo prolonged changes which result in a lowering of their threshold for activation (producing tenderness and hyperalgesia) and others become spontaneously active (producing continuous pain that outlasts the stimulus producing it).

Pain-producing substances

Most clinically significant pains have a time course of hours to days, far beyond the duration of the usual stimuli employed to study nociceptors in the experimental situation. In addition, clinical pains are accompanied by tenderness and, often, hypersensitivity. Tenderness and hyperalgesia simply mean that stimuli that are normally painful are even more painful. There are several contributors to tenderness and hyperalgesia. In part they reflect the sensitization of PANs (a shift to the left of the stimulus intensity–PAN discharge curve). It is likely that intense stimuli also elicit long-lasting changes in the central nervous system that enhance pain transmission [6]. In addition, tissue damage causes the release of a variety of chemical substances into the extracellular space around the receptor terminals (*see* Chapter 2 for a more complete discussion). These substances persist locally and can elicit pain and/or hypersensitivity. Table 1.1 lists the best-studied of the substances that appear in areas of tissue damage and that can either activate or sensitize PANs.

Table 1.1 Chemical intermediaries in nociceptive transduction

Substance	Source	Produces pain in man	Effect on primary afferents
Potassium	Damaged cells	+ +	Activates
Serotonin	Platelets	+ +	Activates
Bradykinin	Plasma kininogen	+ + +	Activates
Histamine	Mast cells	+	Activates
Prostaglandins	Arachidonic acid, damaged cells	±	Sensitizes
Leukotrienes	Arachidonic acid	±	Sensitizes
Substance P	Primary afferent	±	Sensitizes

From Fields, H. L. *Pain*, McGraw-Hill, New York, p. 134 (1987) with permission.

Bradykinin is one of the most potent pain-producing substances [7,8]. It is a 9-amino-acid peptide produced by cleavage of certain plasma proteins and is present in sites of injury, especially when there is visible inflammation. Bradykinin produces pain when injected into human skin. It activates polymodal nociceptors directly and causes them to become sensitized. Bradykinin could thus contribute to both the pain and tenderness of clinically significant injuries.

The prostaglandins and leukotrienes are among the most potent and ubiquitous of the inflammatory mediators. They are metabolic breakdown products of arachidonic acid. Prostaglandins sensitize, but do not activate, PANs and thus could have an important role in tenderness and hyperalgesia. It is currently assumed that the analgesic action of aspirin and non-steroidal anti-inflammatory drugs results from their inhibition of the enzyme cyclo-oxygenase, which is required for synthesis of prostaglandins from arachidonic acid [9,10].

Substances released from the peripheral terminals of primary afferent nociceptors: neurogenic inflammation

It is generally accepted that noxious stimuli can raise the level of pain-producing substances by damage to local tissues. It is not as well appreciated that substances contributing to nociception are present in the terminals of primary afferent nociceptors and that they can be released by those terminals when the nociceptor is active. The clearest evidence of this is from experiments in which the sensory axons are electrically stimulated near the spinal cord (*see* Figure 1.2). Impulses will propagate from the site of stimulation in both directions along the axon: toward the spinal cord (the normal, or orthodromic direction) and toward the peripheral terminals (opposite of normal, or antidromic direction). When the antidromic impulses arrive at the region of skin innervated by the activated PANs they produce neurogenic 'inflammation', which consists of reddening (vasodilatation), edema and hyperalgesia. Neurogenic inflammation is produced by a diffusible substance or substances released from the terminals of PANs [11,12].

It is by no means certain what these substances are. PANs contain a variety of neuropeptides including substances P and calcitonin gene-related peptide (CGRP). There is evidence that antidromic impulses cause the release of substance P from the peripheral terminals of primary afferents. Both substance P and CGRP are potent vasodilators. In addition, substance P has been shown to cause the release of histamine from mast cells. There is some evidence that histamine can also cause pain and/or sensitize PANs [12]. Thus the sensitizing effect of substance P on the PAN terminal may be indirect (via release of histamine). It is not clear whether other neuropeptides or non-peptide transmitters released from the PAN terminal are involved in neurogenic inflammation; however, it is clear that the PAN is not simply a passive messenger signalling the occurrence of a noxious stimulus but an active player in the peripheral events set in motion by tissue-damaging processes.

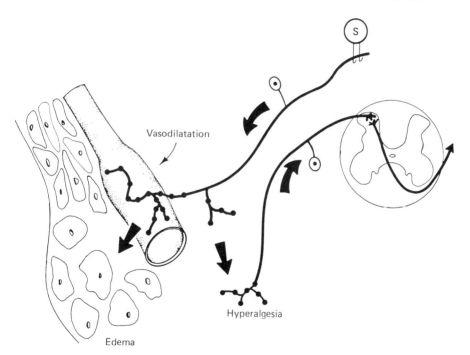

Figure 1.2 Effect of antidromic impulses in primary afferents. Stimulating the peripheral cut end of a primary afferent (S) results in impulses being conducted in an antidromic direction (opposite of normal, in this case outward toward the sensitive terminals). The antidromic impulses cause vasodilatation (flare), edema (wheal) and sensitize nociceptor terminals (hyperalgesia), presumably by the release of a chemical intermediary. (From Fields, H. L. *Pain*, McGraw-Hill, New York, p. 31 (1987) with permission)

Central pain pathways

Primary afferent nociceptors enter the spinal cord via the dorsal root, and synapse with second-order neurons, some of which project to supraspinal nuclei implicated in pain sensation, such as the ventrobasal nucleus of the thalamus. It is important to point out that the nociceptive message is not relayed unchanged to supraspinal sites but undergoes a significant transformation in the gray matter of the spinal cord.

All segmental primary afferents involved in somatic sensation have synaptic connections within the dorsal horn of the spinal gray and each central pain-transmission neuron receives input from many PANs. In addition, many central pain-transmission neurons also receive input from *non-nociceptive* primary afferents. In contrast to PANs, which are only excited by stimuli within their receptive fields, central neurons frequently have inhibitory inputs, presumably via interneurons. In addition to this massive direct and indirect input from primary afferents, the spinal pain-transmission neurons also receive significant inputs from supraspinal nuclei that provide a tonic control over their firing. Thus, the activity elicited in spinal neurons by PANs is modified by activity in other PANs, activity in non-nociceptive primary afferents, and activity in descending projections from supraspinal structures. The descending connections that control pain transmission can be activated under specific behavioral conditions such as stress and conditioning [13,14]. Understanding the anatomic and physiologic complexity of the neural systems underlying pain perception, and the changes that occur in it following injury to the nervous system, is crucial to improved understanding and care of the patient with chronic pain.

Dorsal horn lamination and pain-transmission neurons

The dorsal horn of the spinal cord (and trigeminal nucleus caudalis) has five or six anatomically distinct layers (Figure 1.3) [15]. This anatomic lamination is of physiologic significance in that the neuronal populations in the different layers have different physiologic properties. Of major importance for nociception are laminae I, II and V. Layer I, or the marginal zone, forms a cap over the top of the dorsal horn. It is a major termination site for the small myelinated or A-δ PANs. Most of the cells in lamina I are *nociceptive specific* (NS), so named because they only respond to stimuli in the noxious range. A smaller percentage of lamina I neurons are *wide dynamic range*, which means that they are excited by innocuous mechanical or thermal stimuli but then increase their discharge frequency as the stimulus intensity is increased into the noxious range. Wide-dynamic-range (WDR) neurons must have inputs from non-nociceptive primary afferents as well as PANs. A large proportion of both NS and WDR lamina I cells project to the contralateral mid-brain and thalamus and are considered to be prime candidates for mediating pain sensation [16,17].

Lamina II (also known as the substantia gelatinosa) is the major site of termination of the unmyelinated or C PANs. Few of the A-δ PANs terminate in lamina II. The neuronal population in lamina II differs from that in lamina I. Although there are many WDR and NS neurons in lamina II, a substantial number have response properties that do not fall into either group. Furthermore, very few lamina II neurons project to supraspinal sites. Most project within the spinal cord

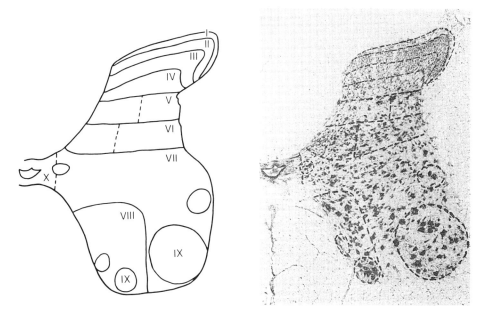

Figure 1.3 Rexed's Scheme for Lamination of the Spinal Gray. (From Rexed, B. A cytoarchitectonic atlas of the spinal cord in the cat. *Journal of Comparative Neurology*, **96**, 415–495 (1952), by permission) (a) Outline of 5th lumbar (L5) segment of the adult cat. In the segments that innervate the limbs (e.g. L5), the cytoarchitectural divisions of the ventral horn do not have an obvious laminar arrangement. (b) Photomicrograph of the L5 spinal segment that corresponds to the diagram of L5 in (a). This is a stain for cell bodies

and are thus local interneurons that modify the response properties of the projection neurons.

Lamina V receives some direct input from A-δ PANs. In contrast to lamina I it has a predominance of WDR neurons. The receptive fields of lamina V cells are larger than those in lamina I, suggesting greater convergence of afferent input. It is important to point out that many lamina V neurons have dendrites that extend dorsally into laminae I and II. Thus lamina V cells could receive both direct inputs from C and A-δ PANs and indirect inputs via interneurons in laminae I and II.

Cells in deeper layers of the spinal gray undoubtedly contribute to pain perception. These cells are more varied in their response properties and usually have very complex receptive fields with inputs from wide areas of skin as well as deep tissues [17]. Because of their variability and complexity it has been more difficult to assign them a definite role in nociception.

Segmental and distant afferent inhibition

In addition to their excitatory effects on dorsal horn neurons, primary afferents also have powerful inhibitory effects. The concept of afferent inhibition is important for understanding how injuries of peripheral nerves can result in pain and hyperalgesia because it can be used to explain how impaired sensation and hyper-reactivity to stimuli can coexist.

Experimental observations are quite clear on this matter. In human subjects, selective blockade of myelinated axons in a peripheral nerve results in an elevated threshold for stimuli to produce sensation. Pinpricks are dull, slight changes in temperature are not detected and stereognosis is completely lost. Nevertheless, if a stimulus is of sufficient strength to produce any sensation, that sensation is typically unpleasant or frankly painful. Even light, normally innocuous stimuli in the cutaneous distribution of the blocked nerve are felt as unpleasant and stimuli which would produce mild pain in normally innervated skin produce a severe, poorly localized pain with a burning, stinging quality [18–20]. Thus, although the block of myelinated axons produces an impairment of sensory function, there is also a paradoxical *increase* in the painfulness of all stimuli.

That myelinated afferents have a net inhibitory effect on pain transmission is supported by the observation that selective activation of myelinated afferents in a peripheral nerve has a pain-relieving effect, i.e. transcutaneous electrical stimulation of nerve (TENS) [20,21]. Furthermore, parallel studies in experimental animals reveal that the selective blockade of myelinated primary afferents results in a greatly enhanced response of pain-transmission cells in the dorsal horn to a constant afferent input over unmyelinated axons [22]. Thus, even though many dorsal horn neurons also have excitatory inputs from some myelinated primary afferents (both A-δ and/or A-β), the predominant effect of input from a large number of simultaneously active myelinated afferents is inhibition.

In addition to the inhibition exerted by these myelinated afferents upon nociceptive dorsal horn neurons, there is also an inhibitory effect produced by input from primary afferent nociceptors innervating distant parts of the body [23]. Thus a dorsal horn cell excited by noxious stimulation of the foot may be inhibited by noxious stimulation of the face (and vice versa). Although the physiologic function of this 'diffuse noxious inhibitory control' is unknown, it has been proposed to underly such phenomena as acupuncture and counter-irritation.

In summary, it is clear that in addition to activation of pain-transmission neurons in the spinal cord dorsal horn, primary afferents, particularly those with myelinated axons, exert significant inhibitory actions. When myelinated afferents are blocked, the responses of dorsal horn neurons to noxious stimuli are greatly exaggerated. In human subjects, the same maneuvers result in hyperalgesia.

Ascending pathways for pain

It is well established that the major ascending pathway for pain transmission is in the anterolateral white matter of the spinal cord. This fact is the basis for the well-known surgical procedure anterolateral chordotomy, which is commonly used for the treatment of intractable pain. Surgical interruption of the anterolateral quadrant results in a profound contralateral loss of pain sensation in areas innervated by spinal segments below the level of the lesion [24]. The analgesia is virtually complete for cutaneous stimuli and many patients will burn their feet after this operation because they are unaware of potentially injurious stimuli such as touching a hot surface. Loss of pain sensibility from deep structures is also profound, although usually incomplete. Over a period of months the majority of patients with damage of their spinothalamic tract experience a partial recovery of pain sensation: the upper level of the deficit drops and there is some return of pain sensitivity in more caudal segments. As functional regeneration does not occur in the spinal cord, the return of pain sensation must involve pathways outside the anterolateral quadrant.

Consistent with these clinical observations, many of the neurons in the spinal laminae implicated in pain transmission send their axons via the contralateral anterolateral quadrant to supraspinal targets. Many of these axons terminate in the contralateral thalamus. Lesions of this spinothalamic pathway anywhere along its trajectory through the brain stem impair pain sensation and electrical stimulation of it produces pain in conscious human subjects [24–26]. Thus, activity in spinothalamic tract neurons is both necessary and sufficient for *normal* pain sensation.

Brain-stem projections of spinal nociceptive neurons

In addition to their direct projection to the thalamus there are several brain-stem targets for axons of spinal nociceptive neurons. The two brain-stem areas that receive the most prominent input from spinal nociceptive neurons are the reticular formation of the rostral medulla (nucleus reticularis gigantocellularis) and the dorsolateral mid-brain (periaqueductal gray, nucleus cuneiformis and the parabrachial region). A significant part of the nociceptive spinal input to these brain-stem areas derives from collaterals of spinothalamic tract axons but much of the input terminates only in the brain stem [27,28]. Large numbers of neurons in both of these brain-stem areas project to the thalamus and there is reason to believe that they function, in part, as relay nuclei for pain transmission [17,29]. However, it should be pointed out that the significance of these brain-stem relays in *human* pain perception has not been established.

Thalamic nuclei and their cortical projections [29]

Four thalamic nuclei receive input from nociceptive spinal neurons: these are the ventrobasal, posterior, central lateral and submedius. The spinothalamic tract divides into a medial and lateral component as it approaches the thalamus. The medial component terminates in the central lateral and submedius nuclei, the lateral division in the ventrobasal and posterior nuclei (Figure 1.4).

The ventrobasal nucleus (VB) has the clearest role in pain transmission. Clinically, lesions of the VB cause analgesia and its electrical stimulation causes pain. Experimental studies have shown that the VB receives input from lamina I and V and both nociceptive-specific and wide-dynamic-range neurons similar to their spinal cord counterparts are found in VB. The VB projects to the somatosensory cortex where similar nociceptive neurons are found.

Although it seems likely that the other thalamic nuclei which receive input from spinothalamic tract neurons play a part, it is less clear what it is that they contribute to pain sensation. The nucleus submedius receives its input primarily from nociceptive neurons in lamina I of the spinal cord; however, it projects to the orbitofrontal cortex which does not have a clearly defined role in pain perception [30].

The central lateral nucleus (CL) receives its spinal input primarily from neurons in the deeper laminae of the spinal gray. These neurons have very large complex receptive fields and can often be excited by stimuli on both sides of the body. There

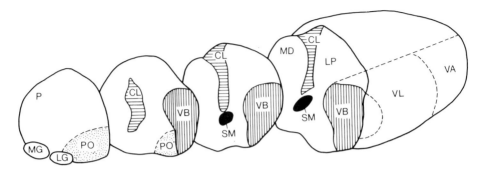

Figure 1.4 Conglomerate diagram of major thalamic nuclei that receive direct input from the spinal cord. These include the ventrobasal nucleus (VB) (striped), the posterior nuclear complex (PO) (stipple), the central lateral nucleus (CL) (crosshatch) and submedius (SM) (black). Adjacent nuclei [dorsomedial (MD), lateral posterior (LP), ventral lateral (VL), ventral anterior (VA), medial geniculate (MG), lateral geniculate (LG) and pulvinar (P)] do not receive significant direct spinal input. (From Fields, H. L. *Pain*, McGraw-Hill, New York, p. 66 (1987) with permission)

is also a major input to CL from that region of the medullary reticular formation which receives the largest nociceptive input from the cord. The CL projects to a variety of cortical areas, including frontal and somatosensory areas, but it is not certain to which area the nociceptive CL neurons project [31].

Sensory and affective components of pain

One way to make sense of the apparent multiplicity of pathways and thalamic and cortical targets for nociceptive input is to consider that there are multiple aspects to the experience of pain and that the different pathways contribute to these different aspects. In fact, Melzack and Casey [32] proposed that pain has two major components: the sensory and the affective. The sensory aspect has to do with quality (in other words the ability to *identify* the feeling as pain), intensity, location and time course. Pain threshold, for example, is a sensory measure. In contrast, affect relates to the characteristic emotional tone which is distinctly unpleasant. This unpleasantness is associated with a desire to terminate the sensation and/or to escape from the stimulus and, if this is not possible, anxiety.

There is some reason to believe that the sensory and affective aspects of pain are subserved in part by separate neural mechanisms. Clearly, the spinothalamic projection to the ventrobasal thalamus and its projection to the somatosensory cortex are required for the discriminative sensory aspects of pain. A lesion anywhere along that pathway impairs pain sensation. In contrast, the pathway which includes direct and indirect projections from spinal cord to medial thalamus and from medial thalamus to frontal cortex seems to have more to do with the affective aspects of pain. Supportive evidence for this comes from clinical studies of patients with severe pain who underwent frontal lobotomy as a treatment of last resort [33]. Interestingly, these patients usually obtained striking relief of their clinical pain problem but with *no impairment* in their ability to detect and identify noxious stimuli as painful. When asked about their pain they would say that it was of the same intensity as before the operation; however, they exhibited no 'appropriate' emotion and did not request pain medication. The suffering was apparently eliminated, with no effect on the 'purely sensory' aspect of their pain. These clinical observations not only support the neuro-anatomic separability of sensation and affect, they indicate that the affect is of greater importance to the patient.

Further clinical support for the separation of affective and sensory components of the experience of pain comes from recent studies by Berthier *et al.* [34] of patients with asymbolia for pain. They reported six patients who had minimal, if any, deficit in cutaneous pain threshold but a markedly reduced emotional response to intense, prolonged somatic stimuli. Interestingly, these patients had significantly elevated pain *tolerance* and were indifferent to verbal and visual threats. Computed tomography revealed that in all patients the area of damage involved the posterior insular cortex.

PAIN-MODULATING NETWORKS

It is now well established that there is a specific central nervous system network for pain control [35–37]. The analgesia produced by the action of this network is mediated by endogenous opioid substances which are synthesized by nerve cells and have pharmacologic properties nearly identical to those of narcotic analgesic drugs. The discovery of this network has provided a basis for improved understanding of the clinically well-known but scientifically puzzling variability of perceived pain.

The key observation leading to the discovery of the opioid-mediated analgesia system was of the phenomenon of stimulation-produced analgesia (SPA). First described in rats, SPA results when certain parts of the brain are electrically stimulated. The inhibition of pain that occurs during stimulation is strikingly selective. Although animals respond normally to innocuous stimuli, noxious stimuli do not produce the expected vocalization, biting and escape. Its selectivity for pain received crucial confirmation from observations of patients with intractable pain who had stimulating electrodes implanted at sites homologous to those from which SPA was elicited in animals [36–38]. Many patients with these electrodes report a gradual melting away of their pain. Although some report a feeling of warmth and/or sleepiness, no other effects are consistently associated with pain relief. Thus, the system activated appears to be specific for controlling pain.

Subsequent research has elucidated the anatomic, chemical and physiologic basis for this pain modulation. The pain-modulating system consists of a network of neurons running from the cortex and hypothalamus via the mid-brain periaqueductal gray, and rostral medulla to the dorsal horn [36–38] (*see* Figure 1.5). Although not tested in man, electrical stimulation at the medullary level in animals produces analgesia and inhibits nociceptive spinothalamic tract cells. Thus the selectivity of the pain-modulating network apparently derives from its selective inhibition of spinal cord pain-transmission cells.

Opiates

About the time that this pain-modulation network was being mapped anatomically, it became clear that it was involved in opioid analgesia. Structure–activity relations

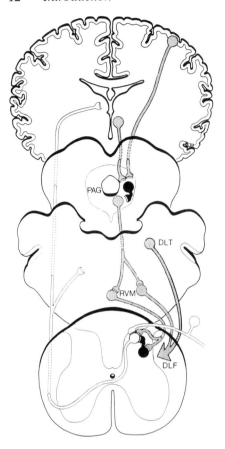

Figure 1.5 Diagram of the descending pain-modulating circuit. Four levels are shown: cortico-diencephalic, mid-brain, pontomedullary and spinal. Anatomic studies have confirmed large projections from frontal cortex and hypothalamus to the mid-brain periaqueductal gray (PAG), from PAG to the rostral ventromedial medulla (RVM) and from the RVM and dorsolateral pontine tegmentum (DLT) via the dorsolateral funiculus (DLF) of the spinal cord to the dorsal horn. At dorsal horn levels, this descending pathway modulates pain-transmission neurons. The solid black symbols represent enkephalin-containing interneurons. (Adapted from Basbaum and Fields [37])

for existing narcotic analgesics had already been well worked out and bioassays were available to assess new drugs of that class [39]. The analgesic potency of narcotic drugs was shown to correlate well with their binding affinity to certain membrane preparations from brain. This binding was shown to be stereospecific and to have a high affinity. In addition to the binding/potency relationship, the availability of a selective antagonist, naloxone, allowed these binding sites to be identified as opiate receptors.

It is now generally accepted that there are at least three distinct opiate receptors: μ, δ and κ. The μ binding site has characteristics consistent with a role in the clinical analgesic actions of opiates. There is some evidence, although less convincing, to suggest that the δ and κ sites also contribute to clinical analgesia.

In 1975, Hughes *et al.* [40] reported that two pentapeptides isolated from pig brain had a high affinity for the opiate receptor. These pentapeptides were active in bioassays and their action was blocked by the narcotic antagonist naloxone. These two pentapeptides, leucine and methionine enkephalin, were the first endogenous opioid peptides to be discovered. Many others have subsequently been found, including β-endorphin, a 31-amino-acid peptide that has powerful analgesic activity [41].

Many of the opioid-containing cells of the brain are anatomically associated with the analgesia networks described above. For example, the enkephalins are present in nerve cells at mid-brain, medullary and spinal loci implicated in pain modulation. Furthermore, there is a remarkably precise anatomic correlation between opiate receptor, enkephalin distribution and the nuclei from which analgesia can be elicited by electrical stimulation or microinjection of opiates. This evidence provides convincing support for the idea that there is a discrete network for pain modulation and that endogenous opioid peptides play a part in its operation.

Knowing that there are endogenous opioid peptides associated with pain-modulating networks leads to the prediction that drugs that enhance the action of opioid peptides would have analgesic efficacy. Enkephalins are inactivated by enzymes called enkephalinases and there are drugs that can, with reasonable selectivity, block these enzymes, leading to a build-up of enkephalins. Animal studies convincingly show that these enkephalinase inhibitors have analgesic actions [42,43].

In addition to providing both an anatomic and a chemical explanation for the phenomenon of stimulation-produced analgesia, the discovery of the opioid-mediated analgesia system has provided insights into how narcotic analgesics relieve pain. Thus, drugs like morphine, Demerol (pethidine or meperidine) and Percodan (oxycodone plus aspirin) presumably relieve pain by mimicking the action of endorphins at synapses in the pain-modulating networks.

Cytochemical studies of the pain-modulating networks have also revealed that, in addition to the endogenous opioid peptides, a variety of neurotransmitters are involved in controlling transmission of the pain message. For example, acetyl-choline, neurotensin, γ-aminobutyric acid (GABA), serotonin (5HT) and norepi-nephrine have all been implicated [37]. Each of these neurotransmitter links presents a possible opportunity for pharmacologic intervention.

The value of such an approach is suggested by experimental work with norepinephrine and 5HT. Both of these biogenic amine transmitters have an important role in pain modulation, especially in the connection between the brain stem and the spinal cord [44,45]. Both of these transmitters are present in brain-stem neurons and both inhibit spinal cord pain-transmission cells. These transmitters are of particular importance as they can be manipulated by a variety of pharmacologic agents, thus raising the possibility of new classes of centrally acting analgesic agents. In fact, there is evidence that the well-established value of tricyclic antidepressants in chronic pain management relates to their potency as blockers of the re-uptake of both norepinephrine and 5HT [46,47].

The use of antidepressants as analgesics opens up an entirely new approach to drug treatment for chronic pain. These drugs do not produce tolerance and dependence and their action is via a mechanism distinct from that of the opiates. Clinical trials have demonstrated their efficacy for headache [48,49], diabetic neuropathy, postherpetic neuralgia [50] and several other conditions.

Enhancement of pain transmission

Recent research has indicated that, in addition to the well-established pain-suppressing effect of the modulation system, there may also be a pain-enhancement function. Neurophysiologic studies of pain-modulating neurons in the brain stem have revealed that there are two types of nerve cells involved in pain control [51]. One cell type, the *off-cell*, is excited by morphine and its firing pattern indicates that it inhibits pain transmission; in other words, the off-cell produces analgesia.

Interestingly, there is another class of nerve cell, the firing pattern of which suggests that it can *enhance* pain transmission. These cells, called *on-cells*, are shut off by analgesic doses of morphine. Thus there is evidence of *bidirectional* control of pain transmission. With a constant noxious stimulus the brain may able to adjust the perceived pain intensity up or down! These results take on added significance in view of the finding that, under certain circumstances, awake primates can be trained to make their dorsal horn pain-transmission neurons fire in the absence of a noxious stimulus. For example, in primates that have learned that a cue light indicates that a noxious stimulus is about to occur, some dorsal horn nociceptive neurons begin to fire when the cue light comes on, long before the application of a noxious stimulus [14].

The presence of a network which has both excitatory and inhibitory actions on pain transmission raises interesting possibilities for the explanation of pain syndromes occurring with central nervous system injury. Hyperalgesia could result from either the loss of inhibition or the release of excitatory modulating neurons (on-cells) from inhibitory control.

Physiologic activation of the pain-modulating network

The pain-modulating network is activated by a variety of poorly understood environmental factors. In some patients, it can be activated by suggestion (placebo) in the setting of significant pain and stress [52]. It is also possible that certain physical methods for treating pain, such as heat, message, biofeedback and acupuncture, produce their analgesic effect, at least in part, via actions on the pain-modulating networks.

NEUROPATHIC PAIN

Fortunately, in the overwhelming majority of cases, pain is short-lived. It subsides within seconds or minutes if the stimulus has produced no irreversible damage. Even if there is damage which outlasts the insult that produced it (e.g. a bruise or burn), it heals within days in the overwhelming majority of people and the pain subsides. There are, however, circumstances in which pain, far from subsiding, persists or may even worsen with time. Such circumstances fall into three major categories: the tissue-damaging process persists (e.g. cancer, arthritis); there are psychological factors which play a part in either the genesis or perpetuation of the pain (e.g. somatization disorders, depression); the pain is due to disruption and/or abnormal activity of the nervous system (e.g. trigeminal neuralgia, postherpetic neuralgia, diabetic neuropathy). The first two categories of persisting pain are beyond the scope of this book, which is focused on pain due to neural abnormalities. In this chapter a brief overview of neuropathic pain is given.

The general term 'neuropathic' is used here to refer to pain due to abnormalities of nervous function. This avoids terms that imply mechanism (e.g. neurogenic or deafferentation pain) or particular clinical features (dysesthetic or causalgic pain). Despite the diversity of etiology and clinical findings, neuropathic pain syndromes do have certain characteristic features; these are listed in Table 1.2. Most of the

Table 1.2 Clinical features of neuropathic pain

Pain occurs in the absence of a detectable ongoing tissue-damaging process

Abnormal or unfamiliar unpleasant sensations (dysesthesiae) frequently having a burning and/or electrical quality

Delay in onset after precipitating injury

Pain is felt in a region of sensory deficit

Paroxysmal brief shooting or stabbing component

Mild stimuli painful (allodynia)

Pronounced summation and after-reaction with repetitive stimuli

---

From Fields, H. L. *Pain*, McGraw-Hill, New York, p. 134 (1987) with permission.

items in the Table are self-explanatory but a few need further description. Allodynia refers to the elicitation of pain by light mechanical stimuli that would be perceived as innocuous if applied to normal skin. Dramatic examples of this are the trigger points in patients with trigeminal neuralgia and the exquisite hypersensitivity of the affected skin areas in patients with causalgia. Allodynia is not quite the same as hyperalgesia, which refers to increased perceived intensity of a 'normally' noxious stimulus. Summation is defined as a progressive build up of perceived intensity (in this context, pain) with repeated application of an identical stimulus. Typically, patients with neuropathic pain will report that the first few pinpricks in a series are barely noticeable but, as they continue to be applied, they become increasingly painful, to the point of being unbearable. After-reaction simply refers to the persistence of sensation after the stimulus is withdrawn. Patients with neuropathic pain often report that the pain elicited by repeated stimuli is poorly localized and spreads spatially away from the locus of the stimulus.

If any of the listed features are present, the possibility that the patient's pain is neuropathic should be entertained. However, it should be stressed that patients rarely exhibit all of the features listed in the Table. For example, patients with diabetic neuropathy usually do not have a shooting component to their pain, whereas patients with trigeminal neuralgia characteristically have such a component but usually do not have a sensory deficit, nor summation (the build up of pain intensity with repeated cutaneous stimulation).

Because the clinical presentation of neuropathic pains is so diverse, it is likely that more than one mechanism is involved. Table 1.3 lists some of the possible mechanisms and the clinical pain syndromes they may account for. Each of these mechanisms is covered in detail in other chapters in this book.

As is evident on reading this book, this is a critical time in our understanding of neuropathic pains. Many of the questions about mechanisms of such pains have been defined and there is now an extensive body of knowledge based on experimental models. The challenge immediately before us is to relate these models to human disease and to translate laboratory advances into better patient management. It is hoped that this book will bring together scientists and clinicians for this worthwhile task.

Table 1.3 Possible mechanisms of neuropathic pain (*with clinical examples*)

Spontaneous hyperactivity of deafferented spinal pain-transmission neurons (brachial plexus avulsion)

Plasticity: development or activation of aberrant inputs to deafferented central pain-transmission neurons (stump neuroma, central pain syndromes)

Loss of afferent inhibition: nociceptive inputs produce an exaggerated response (entrapment neuropathies, postherpetic neuralgia)

Ectopic impulse generation in damaged nociceptive primary afferents: at the regenerating tip, near the dorsal root ganglion, or in demyelinated regions (tic douloureux, diabetic neuropathy)

Ephaptic transmission: to primary afferents from motor or sympathetic afferents or from other primary afferents

Sympathetic activation or facilitation of primary afferents (causalgia, reflex sympathetic dystrophy syndrome)

---

* Adapted from Fields, H. L. *Pain*, McGraw-Hill, New York, p. 155 (1987), with permission.

References

1. Burgess, P. R. and Perl, E. R. Cutaneous mechanoreceptors and nociceptors. In *Handbook of Sensory Physiology, Vol. II, Somatosensory System* (ed. A. Iggo), Springer-Verlag, Berlin, pp. 29–78 (1973)
2. Mountcastle, V. B. Sensory receptors and neural encoding: introduction to sensory processes. In *Medical Physiology*, 14th edn, Ch. 11 (ed. V. B. Mountcastle), Mosby, St Louis, pp. 327–347 (1980)
3. Woolf, C. J. Transcutaneous and implanted nerve stimulation. In *Textbook of Pain* (ed. P. D. Wall and R. Melzack) Ch. 3, Churchill Livingstone, Edinburgh, pp. 679–690 (1984)
4. Price, D. C., Hu, J. W., Dubner, R. and Gracely, R. H. Peripheral suppression of first pain and central summation of second pain evoked by noxious heat pulses. *Pain*, **3**, 57–68 (1977).
5. Perl, E. R. Sensitization of nociceptors and its relation to sensation. In *Advances in Pain Research and Therapy, Vol. 1* (ed. J. J. Bonica and E. Albe-Fessard), Raven Press, New York, pp. 17–28 (1976)
6. Woolf, C. J. and Wall, P. D. The relative effectiveness of C primary afferent fibres of different origins in evoking a prolonged facilitation of the flexor reflex in the rat. *Journal of Neuroscience*, **6**, 1433–1442 (1986)
7. Armstrong, D. Bradykinin, kallidin and kallikrein. In *Handbook of Experimental Pharmacology, Vol. 25* (ed. E. G. Erdos), Springer-Verlag, Berlin, pp. 434–481 (1970)
8. Beck, P. W. and Handwerker, H. O. Bradykinin and serotonin effects on various types of cutaneous nerve fibres. *Pflügers Archiv; European Journal of Physiology*, **347**, 209–222 (1974)
9. Ferreira, S. H. Prostaglandins, aspirin-like drugs and analgesia. *Nature*, **240**, 200–203 (1972)
10. Moncada, S., Flower, R. J. and Vane, J. R. Prostaglandins, prostacyclin, thromboxane A_2 and leukotrienes. In *The Pharmacological Basis of Therapeutics*, 7th edn. Ch. 28, (ed. A. G. Gilman *et al.*), Macmillan, New York, pp. 660–673 (1985)
11. Chahl, L. A. and Ladd, R. J. Local oedema and general excitation of cutaneous sensory receptors produced by electrical stimulation of the saphenous nerve in the rat. *Pain*, **2**, 25–34 (1976)
12. Lembeck, F. Sir Thomas Lewis's nocifensor system, histamine and substance-P containing primary afferent nerves. *Trends in Neuroscience*, **6**, 106–108 (1983)
13. Fardin, V., Oliveras, J.-L. and Besson, J.-M. A reinvestigation of the analgesic effects induced by stimulation of the periaqueductal gray matter in the rat. I. The production of behavioral side effects together with analgesia. *Brain Research*, **306**, 105–123 (1984)
14. Fields, H. L. Sources of variability in the sensation of pain. *Pain*, **33**, 195–200 (1988)

15. Rexed, B. A cytoarchitectonic atlas of the spinal cord in the cat. *Journal of Comparative Neurology*, **96**, 415–495 (1952)
16. Price, D. D. and Dubner, R. Neurons that subserve the sensory-discriminative aspects of pain. *Pain*, **3**, 307–338 (1977)
17. Willis, W. D. *The Pain System*, S. Karger, Basel (1985)
18. Torebjork, H. E. and Hallin, R. G. Identification of afferent C units in intact human skin nerves. *Brain Research*, **16**, 321–332 (1973)
19. Bishop, G. H. Neural mechanisms of cutaneous sense. *Physiological Review*, **26**, 77–102 (1946)
20. Campbell, J. N. and Long, D. M. Peripheral nerve stimulation in the treatment of intractable pain. *Journal of Neurosurgery*, **45**, 692–699 (1976)
21. Cooperman, A. M., Hall, B., Mikalacki, K., Hardy, R. and Sadar, E. Use of transcutaneous electrical stimulation in the control of postoperative pain – Results of a prospective, randomized, controlled studyy. *American Journal of Surgery*, **133**, 185–197 (1977)
22. Price, D. D., Hayes, R. L., Ruda, M. A. and Dubner, R. Spatial and temporal transformations of input to spinothalamic tract neurons and their relation to somatic sensations. *Journal of Neurophysiology*, **41**, 933–947 (1978)
23. Le Bars, D., Dickenson, A. H. and Besson, J. M. Diffuse noxious inhibitory controls (DNIC). I. Effects on dorsal horn convergent neurones in the rat. *Pain*, **6**, 283–304 (1979)
24. White, J. C. and Sweet, W. H. *Pain and the Neurosurgeon*, Charles C. Thomas, Springfield, Illinois (1969)
25. Casssinari, V. and Pagni, C. A. *Central Pain, a Neurosurgical Survey*, Harvard University Press, Cambridge, Massachusetts (1969)
26. Tasker, R. R., Tsuda, T. and Hawrylyshyn, P. Clinical neurophysiological investigation of deafferentation pain. *Advances in Pain Research Therapy*, **5**, 713–738 (1983)
27. Kevetter, G. A. and Willis, W. D. Collateralization in the spinothalamic tract: new methodology to support or deny phylogenetic theories. *Brain Research Reviews*, **7**, 1–14 (1984)
28. Ma, W. and Peschanski, M. Spinal and trigeminal projections to the parabrachial nucleus in the rat: Electron-microscopic evidence of a spino-ponto-amygdalian somatosensory pathway. *Somatosensory Research*, **5**, 247–257 (1988)
29. Albe-Fessard, D., Berkley, K. J., Kruger, L., Ralston, H. J., III, and Willis, W. D., Jr. Diencephalic mechanisms of pain sensation. *Brain Research Reviews*, **9**, 217–296 (1985)
30. Craig, A. D. and Burton, H. Spinal and medullary lamina I projection to nucleus submedius in medial thalamus: a possible pain center. *Journal of Neurophysiology*, **45**, 443–466 (1981)
31. Kaufman, E. F. S. and Rosenquist, A. C. Efferent projections of the thalamic intralaminar nuclei in the cat. *Brain Research*, **335**, 257–279 (1985)
32. Melzack, R. and Casey, K. L. Sensory, motivational and central control determinants of pain. A new conceptual model. In *The Skin Senses* (ed. D. Kenshalo), Charles C. Thomas, Springfield, Illinois, pp. 423–439 (1968)
33. Barber, T. X. Toward a theory of pain: Relief of chronic pain by prefrontal leucotomy, opiates, placebos, and hypnosis. *Psychological Bulletin*, **56**, 430–460 (1959)
34. Berthier, M., Starkstein, S. and Leiguarda, R. Asymbolia for pain: a sensory-limbic disconnection syndrome. *Annals of Neurology*, **24**, 41–49 (1988)
35. Fields, H. L. and Heinricher, M. M. Anatomy and physiology of a nociceptive modulatory system. *Philosophical Transactions of the Royal Society of London, Series B*, **308**, 361–374 (1985)
36. Basbaum, A. I. and, Fields H. L. Endogenous pain control mechanisms: review and hypothesis. *Annals of Neurology*, **4**, 451–462 (1978)
37. Basbaum, A. I. and Fields, H. L. Endogenous pain control system: brainstem spinal pathways and endorphin circuitry, *Annual Review of Neuroscience*, **7**, 309–338 (1984)
38. Fields, H. L. and Basbaum, A. I. Brainstem control of spinal pain-transmission neurons. *Annual Review of Physiology*, **40**, 217–248 (1978)
39. Snyder, S. H. and Matthysse, S. Opiate receptor mechanisms. In *Neurosciences Research Program Bulletin, Vol. 13*, MIT Press, Cambridge, Massachusetts, pp. 1–166 (1977)
40. Hughes, J., Smith, T. W., Kosterlitz, H. W., Fothergill, L. A., Morgan, B. A. and Morris, H. R. Identification of two related pentapeptides from the brain with potent opiate agonist activity. *Nature*, **258**, 577–579 (1975)
41. Frederickson, R. C. A. and Geary, L. E. Endogenous opioid peptides: review of physiological, pharmacological and clinical aspects. *Progress in Neurobiology*, **19**, 19–69 (1982)
42. Dickenson, A. The inhibitory effects of thalamic stimulation on the spinal transmission of nociceptive information in the rat. *Pain*, **17**, 213–224 (1983)
43. Chipkin, R. E., Latranyi, M. Z., Iorio, L. C. and Barnett, A. Potentiation of D-Ala^2 enkephalinamide analgesia in rats by thiorphan. *European Journal of Pharmacology*, **83**, 283–288 (1982)

44. Yaksh, T. L. Direct evidence that spinal serotonin and noradrenaline terminals mediate the spinal antinociceptive effects of morphine in the periaqueductal gray. *Brain Research*, **160**, 180–185 (1979)
45. Basbaum, A. I., Moss, M. S. and Glazer, E. J. Opiate and stimulation-produced analgesia: the contribution of the monoamines. *Advances in Pain Research Therapy*, **5**, 323–339 (1983)
46. Botney, M. and Fields, H. L. Amitriptyline potentiates morphine analgesia by a direct action on the central nervous system. *Annals of Neurology*, 13, 160–164 (1983)
47. Taiwo, U., Fabian, A., Pazoles, C. and Fields, H. L. Further studies on the mechanism of the potentiation of morphine antinociception of monoamine uptake inhibitors. *Pain*, **21**, 329–338 (1986)
48. Diamond, S. and Baltes, B. J. Chronic tension headache treated with amitriptyline – a double-blind study. *Headache*, **11**, 110–116 (1971)
49. Couch, J. R., Ziegler, D. K. and Hassanein, R. Amitriptyline in the prophylaxis of migraine. *Neurology*, **26**, 121–127 (1976)
50. Watson, C. P., Evans, R. J., Reed, K., Merskey, H., Goldsmith, L. and Warsh, J. Amitriptyline versus placebo in postherpetic neuralgia. *Neurology*, **32**, 671–673 (1982)
51. Fields, H. L. and Heinricher, M. M. Anatomy and physiology of a nociceptive modulatory system. *Philosophical Transactions of the Royal Society of London, Series B*, **308**, 361–374 (1985)
52. Fields, H. L. and Levine, J. L. Placebo analgesia – a role for endorphins? *Trends in Neuroscience*, **7**, 271–273 (1984)

2
Hyperalgesia and sensitization of primary afferent fibers

Srinivasa N. Raja, Richard A. Meyer and James N. Campbell

INTRODUCTION

Pain is one of the most important warning systems that prompt the patient to consult a physician. It is the body's way of signalling that the integrity of its tissues is threatened; thus acute pain serves a protective function. However, pain sometimes persists even after the normal healing of an acute injury or recovery from a disease. This prolonged or chronic pain serves no useful purpose. An aspect of pain not always appreciated in chronic pain states relates to the development of hyperalgesia. Hyperalgesia is best known as it relates to inflammation. It refers to the leftward shift of the stimulus–response function that relates the magnitude of pain to the intensity of applied stimuli. Hyperalgesia may manifest as pain in the absence of external stimuli (spontaneous pain), as pain that results from low-intensity ordinarily innocuous stimuli (allodynia) and as increased pain to noxious (injurious or potentially injurious) stimuli.

Hyperalgesia is a common manifestation of inflammation. The enhanced pain induced by a burn or other trauma to the skin presents as cutaneous hyperalgesia. The dysuria that accompanies a urinary tract infection, the sore throat that accompanies pharyngitis, the tender abdomen that accompanies peritonitis, are all additional examples of hyperalgesia. Of special interest to the neurologist is the hyperalgesia that accompanies insults to the nervous system, be it from herpes zoster infection, trauma to the peripheral nerve, or metabolic neuropathies such as occur with diabetes mellitus.

Most studies on the peripheral neural mechanisms of hyperalgesia have centered on changes in sensation and the neural processing of noxious stimuli following cutaneous injury. Hence, this chapter focuses on studies of hyperalgesia following cutaneous injury. We review first how physiological changes in the nervous systems encode the hyperalgesia at and around the site of cutaneous injury (primary and secondary hyperalgesia, respectively). We review how the increased sensibility to pain correlates with an enhanced responsiveness (i.e. sensitization) of nociceptive afferent fibers. We then consider what is known about how insults to the peripheral nervous system induce hyperalgesia. To accomplish this we first review, in brief, how pain is signalled under normal conditions (*see* recent review by Raja *et al.* [1] for details).

CUTANEOUS NOCICEPTORS

Information about the environment is signalled to the central nervous system by highly specialized types of sensory fibers. For example, our capacity to discriminate between cutaneous stimuli that evoke sensations of cooling, warmth, or touch is due to the presence of sensory receptors that are selectively sensitive to these stimuli. Warm fibers, which are predominately unmyelinated fibers, are strikingly sensitive to gentle warming of their receptive fields. The quality and intensity of warmth sensation is signalled exclusively by these fibers [2,3]. Similarly, studies have shown that a sub-set of thinly myelinated fibers, cold fibers, encode the sense of cooling [4]. A group of mechanoreceptive afferent fibers that are exquisitely sensitive to deformations of the skin signal touch sensation. These fibers encode sensory attributes such as texture and shape.

Other primary afferent fibers have cutaneous receptors characterized by a relatively high threshold to the appropriate stimulus, whether it be heat, mechanical, chemical or cooling stimuli. Because they respond preferentially to noxious stimuli, this sub-group of primary afferent fibers are termed nociceptors [5]. Nociceptors can be classified into sub-types based on the following three criteria: (1) conduction velocity for action potential propagation in the nerve fiber; (2) modalities of stimulation that evoke a response, and (3) characteristics of their response to natural stimuli.

Cutaneous nociceptive afferent fibers may be myelinated (A fibers) or unmyelinated (C fibers). C fibers responsive to mechanical and heat stimuli applied to their respective field have been studied in most species, including man [6–12], and are perhaps the most common type of cutaneous nociceptor. Many of these respond not only to noxious mechanical and heat stimuli but also to chemical stimuli, and hence have been referred to as polymodal nociceptors [6,13,14]. A-fiber nociceptive afferents also respond to mechanical and heat stimuli [15–18]. Some myelinated afferents have receptors that respond only to intense noxious mechanical stimuli and are thus termed high-threshold mechanoreceptors [16,17,19,20]. Other less frequently observed nociceptors that respond only to intense cold [21] or intense heat [22] have also been reported. The presence in the skin of specific chemosensitive nociceptors has been suggested recently [23,24].

C-fiber mechano-heat nociceptors (CMHs)

Response to heat stimuli

The threshold for activation by heat stimuli of CMHs in primates is typically > 38°C but < 50°C (*see* Table 2.1). The response of a typical CMH that innervates hairy skin to a sequence of heat stimuli from 41 to 49°C is shown in Figure 2.1. The CMHs demonstrate a monotonic increase in response to stimuli in the noxious range. The responses to heat of CMHs that innervate hairy skin differ from those innervating glabrous skin: CMHs that innervate hairy skin are sensitized by repeated heat stimulation, whereas those innervating glabrous skin are not [7]. However, the conduction velocity and the initial thermal thresholds of the CMHs that innervate hairy and glabrous skin are similar.

Table 2.1 Properties and presumed physiologic role of nociceptive afferents sensitive to mechanical and heat stimuli

Property	C-fiber mechano-heat afferents	A-fiber mechano-heat afferents	
		Type I	*Type II*
Receptive field area (mm²)	19 ± 3[a]	37 ± 4[c]	1–4[e]
Skin type	Glabrous and hairy	Glabrous and hairy	Hairy only
Heat threshold (°C)	43.6 ± 0.6[a]	> 49[c]	43[e]
Receptor utilization time (to heat) (ms)	> 50[b]	Long (> 600)[d]	Short (< 200)[d]
Heat response characteristic	Slowly or quickly adapting[b]	Slowly adapting[c]	Quickly adapting[d]
Mechanical threshold (bars)	6.0 ± 0.6[a]	3.5 ± 0.3[c]	1.7 (0.4 g)[e]
Conduction velocity (m/s)	0.8 ± 0.1[a]	31.1 ± 1.5[c]	15.2 ± 9.9[e]
Presumed physiologic role	Burning pain (second pain); Hyperalgesia in hairy skin	Primary hyperalgesia after injury to glabrous and possibly hairy skin	Pricking pain (first pain); ?Role in hyperalgesia

[a] From [10]
[b] From [58]
[c] From [18]
[d] From [29]
[e] From [64]
(From Raja, S. N., Meyer, R. A. and Campbell, J. N. Peripheral mechanisms of somatic pain. *Anesthesiology*, **68**, 571–590 (1988), with permission)

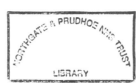

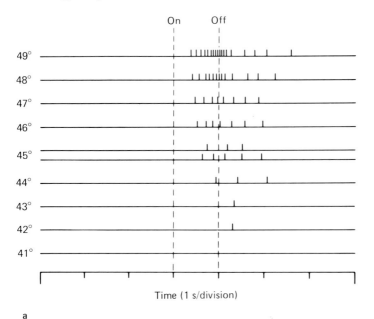

a

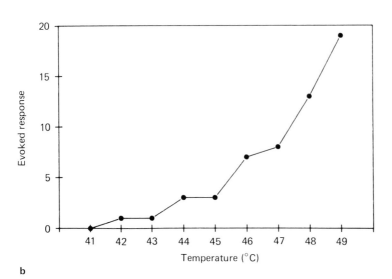

b

Figure 2.1 Response of a typical C-fiber mechano-heat nociceptor (CMH) innervating hairy skin to heat stimuli. (a) Impulse train replicas of reponses of a CMH to a thermal test sequence (TTS). The TTS consisted of a 45°C stimulus followed by a random sequence of nine 1 s stimuli ranging from 41° to 49°C presented at 29 s interstimulus intervals. Each horizontal line represents a trial where the heat stimulus shown was delivered. The lower line at 45°C corresponds to the first stimulus in the TTS while the upper line corresponds to the second 45°C stimulus within the TTS. Each vertical tick corresponds to an action potential. (b) Stimulus–response function for the same CMH

Response to mechanical stimuli

The response of CMHs to mechanical stimuli depends on skin type. On hairy skin, there are multiple punctate spots, usually confined to an area of 50 mm^2, that are responsive to mechanical stimuli. On glabrous skin, the sensitivity to mechanical stimuli is more uniform across the receptive field area. The receptive fields to mechanical stimuli and to heat are similar.

CMHs exhibit a slowly adapting response to stepped mechanical stimuli. Although the mean threshold for response (6.0 bars; 600 kPa; *see* Table 2.1) is well below the pain threshold, the response of CMHs increases monotonically as the stimulus increases into the noxious range [25, 26], unlike the response of low-threshold mechanoreceptors presented with similar stimuli. With prolonged stimuli (120 s), CMHs respond to the onset of noxious pressure stimulus with a dynamic discharge lasting 10 s followed by slowly adapting tonic discharges lasting throughout the stimulus.

A-fiber mechano-heat nociceptors (AMHs)

Response to heat stimuli

Myelinated nociceptive afferent fibers with conduction velocities in the range 5–55 m/s (A-δ and A-β range) have been observed in several species, including humans [16,18,19,27,28]. Two distinct classes of AMHs with different response characteristics to heat stimuli were noted by Dubner and Hu [15], and these have subsequently been classified as Type I and Type II AMHs (Table 2.1) [29,30]. Type I AMHs are found in both glabrous and hairy skin and have a high threshold to heat stimuli – generally greater than 49°C. Type I AMHs have a long receptor utilization time to heat stimuli (time between stimulus onset and initiation of action potential activity) and respond throughout a prolonged stimulus.

A role of type I AMHs is apparent from comparison of human pain ratings with responses of nociceptive afferent fibers during a prolonged high-intensity stimulus. A 53°C stimulus for 30 s evokes a sustained high level of pain. When exposed to the same stimulus, CMHs respond vigorously only in the first few seconds. Type I AMHs, conversely, respond vigorously, beginning several seconds after the onset of the stimulus (Figure 2.2b). Hence, it is likely that type I AMHs may signal the sustained pain during such a stimulus [31–33]. A characteristic feature of type I AMHs is the increase in responsiveness following repetitive heat stimulation or heat injury to the skin [16,18,30]. This phenomenon, termed sensitization, is discussed in the following section on hyperalgesia and sensitization (pages 28–34).

Type II AMHs were first described on the monkey face [15], but they are known to exist in other hairy skin areas. Type II AMHs are found less frequently than type I AMHs and have not been found at all on the glabrous skin of the hand. They are characterized by thresholds to heat similar to those of CMHs, short receptor-utilization time and a quickly adapting response to stepped heat stimuli (Figure 2.2a) [15,30]. Type II AMHs are thought to signal first pain (*see below*).

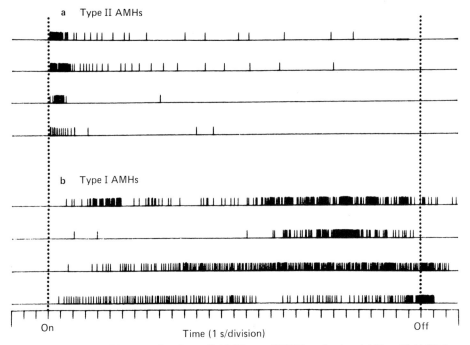

Figure 2.2 Response of four type I and type II AMHs to a 53°C 30 s stimulus. (a) Type II AMHs have a short receptor utilization time and a quickly adapting response to stepped temperature stimuli. (b) Type I AMHs have a long receptor utilization time and respond throughout the stimulus. Each horizontal line corresponds to a different fiber and each vertical tick corresponds to an action potential

Response to mechanical stimuli

The response of AMHs to mechanical stimuli of short duration (< 3 s) is proportional to stimulus intensity [18] (Figure 2.3). When exposed to prolonged stimuli (120 s), high-threshold mechanoreceptive A-δ fibers have an initial dynamic response followed by tonic discharges. The dynamic discharge rates in the first 10 s increases monotonically with increasing stimulus intensity and may encode for stimulus strength. The tonic discharges, however, adapt at a faster rate with stronger stimuli so that firing rates are similar at the end of the different stimuli. Thus, during the course of a prolonged stimulus the encoding of stimulus strength becomes progressively weaker in A-δ mechanoreceptive fibers, but not in CMHs [26]. In contrast to the response of these A-δ fibers, the response of slowly adapting low-threshold mechanoreceptors (SA-Is and SA-IIs) to prolonged noxious stimuli is inversely related to stimulus intensities in the noxious range. Thus, pain from noxious mechanical stimulation is probably signalled by activity in nociceptors and not in the SAs [25,26].

High-threshold mechanoreceptors (HTMs)

These nociceptors respond only to intense mechanical stimuli but not to heat stimuli. HTMs with myelinated afferents have large multipoint receptive fields.

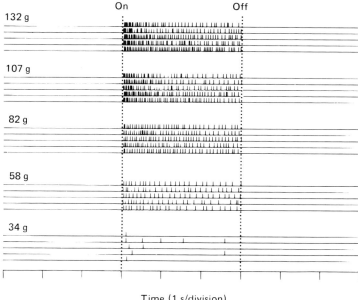

On   Off

132 g

107 g

82 g

58 g

34 g

Time (1 s/division)

a

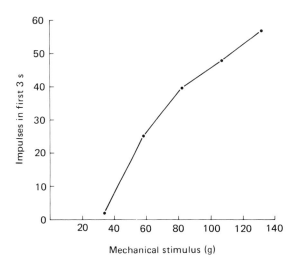

b

Figure 2.3 Response of a type I A-fiber mechano-heat nociceptor (AMH) to constant force mechanical stimuli. Each stimulus was a step indentation of the skin lasting 3 s and presented every 28 s. The force of indentation was varied randomly from 34 to 132 g. Base force was 10 g and probe size was 0.8 mm in diameter. (a) Impulse-train replicas with trials grouped by the force of the mechanical stimuli delivered. (b) Total response during the 3 s stimulus period is plotted as a function of the force of the mechanical stimulus. (From Campbell, J. N., Meyer, R. A. and LaMotte, R. H. Sensitization of myelinated nociceptive afferents that innervate monkey hand. *Journal of Neurophysiology*, **42**, 1669–1679 (1979), with permission)

Although some HTM units respond to stimuli that are not overtly noxious, their thresholds are usually much higher than those of low-threshold mechanoreceptors, and noxious pressures are required for maximal response [17,19,34]. In humans, recordings have been made from a sub-group of A-δ fibers that respond only to high-threshold mechanical stimulation and not to heat [27]. C fibers with similar properties have also been described in the cat and monkey [13,17].

Correlation of nociceptor activity and pain sensation

Heat stimuli

Several lines of evidence from psychophysical and microneurographic studies in humans and neurophysiological studies in animals indicate that CMHs code for pain from heat stimuli applied to the skin. First, as shown in Figure 2.4, there is a

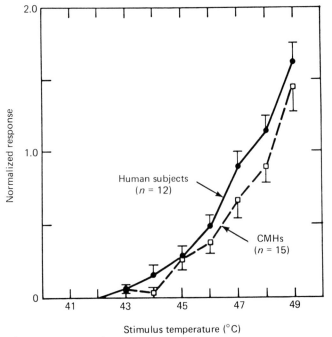

Figure 2.4 C-fiber mechano-heat nociceptors (CMHs) code for pain from heat stimuli applied to the skin. Normalized responses of human subjects and CMHs in monkey exposed to identical heat stimuli (TTS, same as in Figure 2.1) on glabrous skin. Human judgements of pain were measured by the magnitude estimation technique. Subjects assigned an arbitrary number (the modulus) to the intensity of pain evoked by the first 45°C stimulus and judged the painfulness of all subsequent stimuli relative to this modulus. The response to a given stimulus was normalized by dividing by the modulus for each human subject or by the average response to the first 45°C stimulus for the CMHs. (From Meyer, R. A. and Campbell, J. N. Peripheral neural coding of pain sensation. *Johns Hopkins APL Technical Digest*, **2**, 164–171 (1981), with permission)

close correlation between the pain ratings of human subjects and neurophysiolo-gical responses of CMHs in anesthetized monkeys exposed to identical heat stimuli [30]. In both cases, the response to suprathreshold heat stimuli increases monoto-nically with increasing stimulus intensity [31]. Second, the pain threshold in humans is similar to the threshold for activation of CMHs recorded in animals (about 43°C) [21]. Moreover, the heat threshold for activating CMHs recorded microneurogra-phically in awake humans is usually just below the pain threshold [35,36]. Third, both selective A-fiber ischemic blocks and C-fiber (local anesthetic) blocks indicate that C-fiber function is sufficient for thermal pain perception near the pain threshold [31,37,38]. Fourth, repeated stimulation with radiant heat results in temporal suppression of warmth and painful heat sensations [39]. Similar stimulus-interaction effects are observed in recordings from CMHs in monkey and humans [6,10]. Finally, intraneural microstimulation of presumed single identified CMHs in humans elicits aching or burning pain alone [40].

Noxious heat stimuli applied to the hairy skin of the hand or forearm evoke a double pain sensation, an initial stinging pain followed by burning pain. This is often referred to as *first pain* and *second pain*, respectively [41–43]. Latency measurements of the first-pain sensation in human subjects indicate that the responsible afferents must have conduction velocities in the A-fiber range [44]. The response properties (low heat threshold, short utilization time, and burst response to heat) of type II AMHs make them ideal candidates for subserving first-pain sensation (Figure 2.2a) [15,29]. Second-pain sensation is probably signalled by the slower-conducting C-fiber nociceptors [42].

Although there is a good correlation between discharge of nociceptors to heat stimuli and human pain ratings, there are some inconsistencies. For example, the lowest stimulus intensities that excite nociceptors are not always perceived as painful by human subjects [45,46]. Furthermore, transcutaneous electrical shocks at an intensity adequate to evoke a *single* spike of a CMH are usually not perceived at all by the awake human subject [47]. Thus, while there is considerable evidence that nociceptors signal pain, this does not mean that activity in CMHs always signals pain. Central nervous system mechanisms for attention appear to have an important role in determining whether (and how much) nociceptor activity leads to the perception of pain. It is also probable that receptors other than nociceptors signal pain in certain circumstances. For example, in causalgic conditions low-threshold mechanoreceptors may be responsible for signalling pain [48].

Mechanical stimuli

The inconsistencies between pain thresholds and thresholds for nociceptor activa-tion are more striking for mechanical stimuli than for heat stimuli. Mechanical stimulation at intensities that evoke up to 10 impulses per second in CMHs is not accompanied by the sensation of pain, whereas heat stimulation resulting in responses of < 3 impulses per second results in pain [49]. The mechanical threshold for activation of CMHs and type I AMHs is lower than the mechanical threshold for pain on glabrous skin in humans [10,18,26]. During long-lasting noxious mechanical stimulation in human volunteers, the intensity of pain elicited is directly proportional to the intensity of the stimulus and has a tendency to increase throughout the 120 s stimulus period [50]. In contrast, discharges of polymodal C-fiber nociceptors in man show an initial high-frequency discharge followed by adaptation. Thus, the time course of the stimulus-induced pain sensations does not correlate with the activity in C-fiber nociceptors [50]. These discrepancies have led some investigators to suggest that the threshold, intensity and modality of sensations, including pain, are dependent on central processing of information from afferent fibers [51].

It is likely that spatial and temporal summation of nociceptor impulses at central levels are needed to evoke pain under most circumstances [42]. Thus, a punctate mechanical stimulus that results in a relatively vigorous response in a few nociceptors is not perceived as painful, whereas a large heat stimulus that evokes a weak response in a large number of receptors results in pain sensation. Another possibility is that mechanical stimulation also activates low-threshold mechano-receptors that have an inhibitory influence, in the central nervous system, on the input from nociceptive afferents. This second hypothesis is supported by the observation that pain induced by intraneural electrical stimulation at C-fiber strength can be substantially reduced by vibration of the skin within the projected pain region [52]. The central nervous system, therefore, has an important modulatory role in inhibiting or summating the information it receives from the peripheral nociceptors.

HYPERALGESIA AND SENSITIZATION OF NOCICEPTORS FOLLOWING CUTANEOUS INJURY

Tissue injury results in hyperalgesia, the perceptual companion of inflammation. A remarkable lowering of the threshold for pain occurs such that the inflamed skin becomes the source of increased pain. Light touching or gentle warming of the skin induces pain. Hyperalgesia occurs not only at the site of injury, but also in the area surrounding the injury.

An important property of the function of nociceptors is their change in response properties following injury to the tissue they innervate. Sensitization of nociceptors is one neurophysiological correlate of hyperalgesia and is characterized by a decrease in threshold, an increased response to suprathreshold stimuli and, occasionally, by spontaneous activity. A relevant question is whether hyperalgesia can be explained by proportional changes in the sensitivity of cutaneous nociceptors [53].

Primary and secondary hyperalgesia: psychophysical studies

Lewis identified two distinct types of hyperalgesia: primary and secondary hyperalgesia [54–56]. *Primary hyperalgesia* refers to changes that occur within the site of injury, whereas *secondary hyperalgesia* refers to changes that occur in the area surrounding the site of injury [55–57]. The hyperalgesia that follows a cutaneous injury was more recently characterized in a study of the responses of human volunteers to mechanical and heat stimuli before and after a heat injury (localized burn) to the glabrous skin of the hand [58,59]. Within the zone of a cutaneous injury, hyperalgesia is present to both heat and mechanical stimuli. Similar results were observed following mechanical injury or injection of noxious chemicals [60,61]. In the region surrounding the injury (zone of secondary hyperalgesia),

hyperalgesia is present to mechanical but not to heat stimuli. This dissociation of mechanical and heat hyperalgesia in the area surrounding an injury suggests that the neural mechanisms for these sensations are different.

The characteristics of primary hyperalgesia following a burn to the hairy skin differs from that in glabrous skin. In hairy skin, whereas the pain threshold is markedly decreased as in the glabrous skin, the response to suprathreshold heat stimuli (e.g. ≥ 49°C) does not differ from the response before the injury (Figure 2.5 a,b) [62].

Primary hyperalgesia: neural mechanisms

Sensitization of C-fiber [7,13,22,63] and A-fiber [16,19,31] nociceptors to heat stimuli after injury has been reported and might account for the hyperalgesia to heat at the site of injury.

Hyperalgesia to heat stimuli

To determine which nociceptors code for primary hyperalgesia, Meyer and Campbell [31] performed a correlational analysis of psychophysical studies of hyperalgesia in humans with responses of AMHs and CMHs in monkeys (Figure 2.6). Identical test heat stimuli ranging from 41 to 49°C were presented to the glabrous skin of the hand in humans and monkeys before and after a localized heat injury (53°C, 30 s stimulus). In humans, the burn led to prominent primary hyperalgesia within minutes, characterized by increased pain from both mechanical and heat stimuli. Following the burn, the heat threshold for type I AMHs in monkey was greatly decreased and the response to suprathreshold stimuli was increased. Similar sensitization of AMHs by heat was reported by other investigators [16,19,64]. In contrast, following the burn the heat threshold of the CHMs increased and the response to suprathreshold stimuli was decreased. Similar lack of sensitization of CMHs innervating monkey glabrous skin was observed by others [11]. These data suggest that type I AMHs, not CMHs, code for the thermal hyperalgesia that follows a burn to the glabrous skin.

Whereas CMHs that innervate the glabrous skin of the hand do not sensitize, regardless of the intesity of the burn injury, CMHs that innervate hairy skin sensitize with both mild and strong burn injuries [7]. LaMotte and coworkers compared the responses of CMHs that innervated hairy skin of monkey with responses of human subjects (Figure 2.5) before and after a 50°C 100 s injury [53,65]. The decreased threshold in the CMHs correlated with the decreased pain threshold in human subjects. However, the increased responses at the higher temperatures (e.g. 49°C) did not correlate with the unchanged painfulness in humans at these temperatures. In these studies the response of type I AMHs was not affected, and type II AMHs were not studied. The source of this discrepancy between the sensitization of monkey CMHs on hairy skin and the hyperalgesia in humans is not clear. A decreased discharge of type II AMHs (not recorded) at the higher temperatures could explain this discrepancy. Alternatively, changes in central processing of nociceptive input could explain the incongruity.

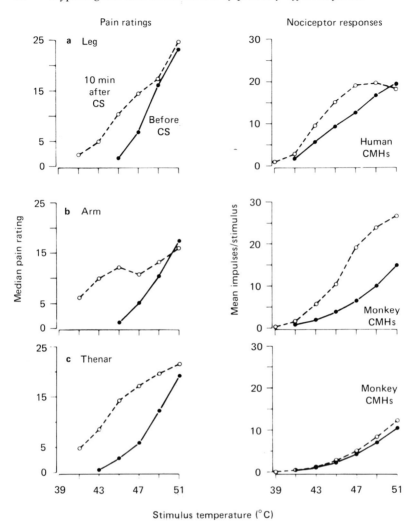

Figure 2.5 Comparison of median scaling functions for the magnitude of pain with mean intensity–response functions of CMH nociceptors for each stimulus delivered before and 10 min after a conditioning stimulus (CS, 50°C 100 s heat injury) to the skin. Left column; median maximum pain ratings of each stimulus for subjects tested on three different areas of skin before and 10 min after the CS; right column, the mean number of impulses evoked by each stimulus in CMHs in monkeys before and after the CS. In both left and right columns, the responses before and after the CS are represented by solid and dashed lines respectively. (a) Pain ratings were recorded in humans (left panel) simultaneously with evoked discharges in CMHs (right panel) during heat stimulation of the leg or dorsum of the foot. (b) Pain ratings on the volar forearm in humans are compared with the responses of CMHs with receptive fields in the hairy skin of the monkey wrist or hand. (c) Pain ratings for the thenar eminence of the glabrous skin of the hand in humans are compared with the responses of CMHs with receptive fields on the glabrous skin of the monkey hand. (From LaMotte, R. H. Can the sensitization of nociceptors account for hyperalgesia after skin injury? *Human Neurobiology*, **3**, 47–52 (1984), with permission)

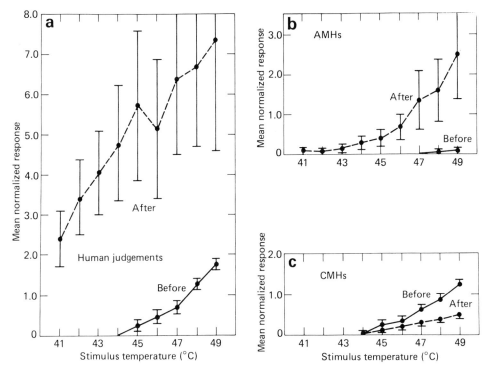

Figure 2.6 Neurophysiologic mechanisms of primary hyperalgesia to heat following a burn. Normalized response to the heat sequence 5 min before and 10 min after a 53°C 30s burn to the glabrous skin of the hand. The burn resulted in increases in the magnitude of pain (hyperalgesia) in human subjects that were matched by enhanced responses (sensitization) in the type I AMHs. In contrast, the burn resulted in decreased sensitivity of the CMHs. (a) Human judgements of pain (*n* = 8). (b) Type I AMHs in monkeys (*n* = 14). Because the AMHs did not respond to the first 45°C stimulus before the burn, the data were normalized by dividing by the response to the first 45°C stimulus after the burn. (c) CMHs in monkeys (*n* = 15). Standard error bars are shown. (From Meyer, R. A. and Campbell, J. N. Myelinated nociceptive afferents account for the hyperalgesia that follows a burn applied to the hand. *Science*, **213**, 1527–1529 (1981), with permission. Copyright 1981 by the AAAS)

Hyperalgesia to mechanical stimuli

The primary hyperalgesia that follows injury is characterized by increased pain in response not only to heat stimuli but also to mechanical stimuli. One would expect sensitization of nociceptors to mechanical stimuli to account for this phenomenon; however, the thresholds to mechanical stimulation of either CMHs or AMHs are not significantly changed following a heat injury [18,66]. Suprathreshold responses were not adequately tested.

Although earlier studies failed to demonstrate sensitization of nociceptors to mechanical stimuli after many types of cutaneous injury, in a recent study sensitization was observed following sustained mechanical stimulation. Repeated constant force stimuli, 120 s in duration, were applied on or adjacent to the receptive fields (RFs) of A-fiber and C-fiber nociceptors on the rat tail. The A-δ but not C-fiber nociceptors developed spontaneous activity, lowered von Frey thresholds (Figure 2.7) and expanded receptive fields after the mechanical injury stimulus [26].

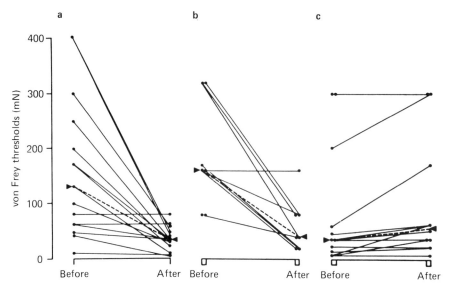

Figure 2.7 Changes in threshold to mechanical stimulation of nociceptors induced by conditioning noxious mechanical stimulation, (a) to the most sensitive spot inside the receptive fields (RFs) of A-δ high-threshold mechanoreceptive (HTM) fibers (*n* = 15 inside RF), (b) to an originally unresponsive site closely outside RFs of HTM A-δ fibers (*n* = 10 outside RF), (c) to the center of RFs of CMH fibers (*n* = 14 inside RF). Black triangles and broken lines refer to the median values. (From Reeh, P. W., Bayer, J., Kocher, L. and Handwerker, H. O. Sensitization of nociceptive cutaneous nerve fibers from the rat's tail by noxious mechanical stimulation. *Experimental Brain Research*, **65**, 505–512 (1987), with permission)

Other mechanisms could account for the hyperalgesia to mechanical stimuli that occurs at the site of injury. Recruitment of input from nociceptors with adjacent receptive fields (spatial summation) is one such possible mechanism. Following a burn injury adjacent to the receptive field of a primary afferent nociceptor, the receptive field for that primary afferent was found to spread to include part of the area of the burn injury [66]. The threshold to mechanical stimuli in this expanded receptive field area was similar to that in other regions of the receptive field of that fiber. The net result is that within the area of injury a given suprathreshold mechanical stimulus will activate more nociceptors than it would have before injury. Assuming that spatial summation contributes to pain intensity, this finding could account for hyperalgesia.

It has been argued that nociceptors that are yet to be identified may account for mechanical hyperalgesia [67]. Mechanical responsiveness may develop following injury in a receptor previously unresponsive. This idea is not without precedents. Heppelman *et al.* [68] observed that previously unresponsive C and A-δ fibers that innervate the knee joint of the cat develop responses to knee motion in the physiological range after inflammation of the joint. Recently, a new technique to search for such receptors has been described [69]. More than half of the C-fiber primary afferents found with this technique did not respond to mechanical or heat stimuli and, therefore, were not typical CMH nociceptors. Some of these receptors appeared to be specifically sensitive to chemical agents. There are other recent reports of C-fiber receptors that respond to chemical stimuli but not to mechanical or heat stimuli [24,70].

Hyperalgesia to mechanical stimuli may involve central mechanisms. A burn may induce prolonged central changes, such that there is increased synaptic efficacy between central pain-signalling neurons and low-threshold mechanoreceptive afferent fibers [71]. Another central mechanism may relate to the concept that low-threshold mechanoreceptor input normally inhibits pain elicited by nociceptor input [52,72–74]. Injury may decrease the input of low-threshold mechanoreceptors to the central nervous system, when the skin is stimulated mechanically. Thus, the input of the nociceptors is unopposed and may result in mechanical hyperalgesia.

Secondary hyperalgesia: neural mechanisms

In the past, both peripheral as well as central mechanisms have been suggested to explain secondary hyperalgesia. Lewis observed that electrical stimulation of a nerve trunk in man led to hyperalgesia in the distribution of that nerve, even if the proximal end of the nerve was blocked with a local anesthetic during the stimulation period [56]. Recently, LaMotte *et al.* [75] have also observed that intrafascicular electrical stimulation leads to tenderness in the distribution of the fascicle. Lewis proposed that secondary hyperalgesia was due to a peripheral mechanism resulting from the spread of sensitization from adjoining nociceptors that were directly injured. According to this hypothesis, activation of part of the nociceptive receptor by the injury stimulus leads to antidromically propagated action potentials in other branches of the afferent fiber, resulting in the release of sensitizing substances. The flare that surrounds an injury is thought to involve a similar axon reflex mechanism [76]. This vascular response requires intact C-fiber innervation of the skin [77], and is believed to be due to release of vasoactive substances, such as substance P, from the peripheral terminals of nociceptors.

Other observations support the idea that secondary hyperalgesia is mediated, at least in part, by a peripheral mechanism. LaMotte *et al.* [61] recently studied the characteristics of chemically induced hyperalgesia. They found that intradermal injection of capsaicin resulted in hyperalgesia to light mechanical stimulation in a large skin area surrounding the injection site. Cooling the capsaicin injection site for 1–3 min greatly reduced or eliminated the hyperalgesia around the injection site, whereas rewarming brought it back. Furthermore, injection of local anesthetic into the capsaicin injection site abolished the hyperalgesia. Thus, the hyperalgesia appeared to be maintained by neural activity at the site of chemical injury. Additional observations that intradermal injection of a strip of lidocaine restricted the spread of hyperalgesia distally, but not proximally, indicated that the neural activity probably spread by a cutaneous axon reflex mechanism. The above experiments, when repeated during selective conduction block in A or C fibers, demonstrated that the hyperalgesia induced by capsaicin was mediated by C fibers and by slowly conducting A-δ fibers [78]. Thus, the mechanism of secondary hyperalgesia is proposed to be similar to that of primary hyperalgesia in that both result from sensitization of nociceptors.

In support of Lewis' spreading-sensitization hypothesis, Fitzgerald [79] reported that adjacent injuries and antidromic electrical stimulation of the peripheral nerve in rabbits results in sensitization to heat of C-fiber nociceptors. However, in rats and monkeys, antidromic stimulation does not sensitize CMHs [80,81]. Injury adjacent to the receptive field of nociceptors also failed to alter the responses of monkey CMHs to heat [60]. Thalhammer and LaMotte [82] determined that injury of one half of the receptive field did not change the sensitivity of the other half to heat stimuli, nor did it alter the mechanical threshold. These neurophysiological observations corroborate the psychophysical observations that hyperalgesia to heat does not occur in the region of secondary hyperalgesia. However, they do not provide an explanation of the mechanical hyperalgesia.

Because psychophysical studies indicate that secondary hyperalgesia is characterized by hyperalgesia to mechanical stimuli, neurophysiologic studies should focus on the change in mechanical sensitivity following an injury. Studies in monkeys have failed to demonstrate a change in the mechanical threshold of A-fiber or C-fiber nociceptors following a heat injury adjacent to their receptive field [66,82]. However, it has been observed recently that conditioning noxious mechanical stimulation outside the receptive field of A-fiber, but not C-fiber, nociceptors in rats resulted in a lower mechanical threshold in the uninjured part of their receptive field [26]. In addition, following conditioning stimuli outside the receptive field, a proportion of the A-fiber mechanoreceptors developed prominent dynamic responses to mechanical stimulation. Whether this sensitization occurs in other species as well and is sufficient to account for secondary hyperalgesia remains to be proven.

Hardy and his colleagues [57,83] were unable to replicate Lewis's antidromic stimulation experiments. They, therefore, postulated that secondary hyperalgesia may result from central changes brought about by the sensitized nociceptors. Input from sensitized nociceptors in turn sensitizes dorsal horn 'pain' neurons that receive sensory input from the skin surrounding the region of injury.

In support of a central mechanism for secondary hyperalgesia, sensitization of dorsal horn spinothalamic neurons to mechanical stimuli has been demonstrated following cutaneous heat injury [84]. Similarly, an enhanced response to mechanical stimuli of neurons of wide dynamic range (WDR) and high threshold in the dorsal horn of the cat and monkey has recently been reported following intradermal capsaicin injection [85]. In addition, C-fiber strength-conditioning stimuli or cutaneous injury in rats has been shown to increase the receptive field size of certain dorsal horn cells [71,86,87]. Some of the dorsal horn neurons that initially responded only to noxious mechanical stimulation, responded to low-threshold (brush and touch) stimuli following the conditioning stimuli. Although these studies suggest a role of the central nervous system in secondary hyperalgesia, they do not rule out a role for peripheral mechanisms.

BIOCHEMICAL MECHANISMS OF HYPERALGESIA

We can conclude from our discussion so far that the hyperalgesia that follows tissue injury and inflammation is based, at least in part, on sensitization of nociceptors. We now consider the potential role of chemical mediators in the mechanism of hyperalgesia.

The endogenous chemicals that may play a part in hyperalgesia can be broadly subclassified into neurogenic and non-neurogenic. Neuropeptides released from peripheral endings of nociceptive afferents following noxious chemical or physical stimulation can mediate or facilitate the inflammatory process [88]. Although studies have suggested that the neurogenically released peptides have a role in the inflammatory process, a direct relationship to pain and hyperalgesia is yet to be established. Catecholamines released from sympathetic efferent fibers may modulate the activity of nociceptors [89]. A variety of substances are released from such non-neural tissues as mast cells and vasculature, following injury: these substances include amines such as histamine and serotonin, peptides such as bradykinin and substance P, metabolites of arachidonic acid, platelet-activating factor and free radicals. Some of these substances have been shown to produce acute pain upon application to a blister base preparation [90,91]. Several studies have since indicated that some of these substances, especially bradykinin and eicosanoids, promote the pain and hyperalgesia associated with inflammation [92].

Histamine

Intradermal injection of histamine results in a local wheal and flare. As cutaneous injury is usually followed by a wheal and flare reaction, many investigators have proposed an important role of histamine in hyperalgesia. Lewis [54] noted, however, that histamine in neutral pH solution elicited only itch, regardless of dose. These observations have recently been confirmed by LaMotte [67], who noted that histamine had negligible effects on heat–pain sensation. Conversely, clinical evidence suggests that antihistamine drugs have analgesic effects. However, antihistaminic drugs have other non-specific interactions with serotonin, α-adrenergic muscarinic cholinergic receptors, calcium channels and phospholipases. Thus, there is no clear evidence of a role for histamine in hyperalgesia.

Serotonin

Degranulation of mast cells leads to the release of platelet-activating factor, which in turn results in the release of serotonin (5-hydroxytryptamine) from platelets. Serotonin causes pain when applied to a human blister base [93]. It can also potentiate pain induced by bradykinin when injected intra-arterially in cats [94] or intravenously in man [95] or applied to a blister base [93]. Recently, a novel serotonin receptor has been identified on peripheral neurons [93,96]. Specific antagonists of this receptor can block both the direct painful effect of serotonin and the serotonin-potentiation of bradykinin-induced pain on human blister base [93]. Although these agents block acute pain from exogenously applied serotonin, it is not clear what effect they have on hyperalgesia. Further studies are needed to define the role of serotonin in inflammatory pain and hyperalgesia.

Bradykinin

Several lines of evidence indicate an important role of bradykinin in pain and hyperalgesia. First, bradykinin produces pain in man when administered intradermally, intra-arterially or intraperitoneally [97–99]. In addition, it is released with tissue injury and is present in inflammatory exudates [100,101]. High-affinity (3H) bradykinin-binding sites are localized to regions of the nervous system involved in the transmission of nociceptive information [102]. Psychophysical studies in man indicate that bradykinin produces acute pain as well as hyperalgesia [103]. Bradykinin is known to sensitize nociceptive afferent fibers: single-fiber recordings from peripheral nerves have shown that intra-arterial administration of BK enhances the response to heat stimuli of C-fiber nociceptors [104–106]. Furthermore, bradykinin (administered intradermally in the receptive field) causes an evoked response and sensitization of C-fiber and A-fiber nociceptors in monkeys [107]. Bradykinin, when administered close arterially into spleen and other organs, produces pseudoaffective (presumably nociceptive) reflexes in animals [108,109]. Bradykinin has also been shown to excite rat dorsal root ganglia and trigeminal ganglia cells in culture [110].

Studies of the precise role(s) of bradykinin in the mechanism of pain and hyperalgesia have, until recently, been limited by the lack of precise inhibitors of its physiologic and pharmacologic activities. Recently, two bradykinin receptors have been identified: they are classified as B_1 and B_2 on the basis of their binding affinities and the agonist or antagonist activities of sequence-related bradykinin structural analogs [111–113]. Specific antagonists have been synthesized that distinguish betwen the bradykinin receptor sub-types present in smooth muscles [113]. Studies with these antagonists on the pain response of human blister base [114] and nociceptor stimulation in rabbits [115] suggest that the B_2 bradykinin receptors have a role in pain. The B_2-receptor antagonists have recently been observed to inhibit bradykinin- and urate-induced hyperalgesia in the rat paw [102].

Bradykinin may well be one of many substances linked to the production of pain and hyperalgesia associated with inflammation. Bradykinin is capable of stimulating the synthesis and release of prostaglandins by activation of phospholipase A_2 [76]. The prostaglandins, in turn, may enhance the sensitizing actions of bradykinin on nociceptors [105,116]; indeed, several arachidonic acid metabolites produce a dose-dependent potentiation of bradykinin-induced pain reactions [117].

Eicosanoids

The prostaglandins, thromboxanes and leukotrienes are a large family of arachidonic acid derivatives collectively known as eicosanoids [118]. Arachidonic acid can be metabolized by the enzyme cyclo-oxygenase to produce prostacyclin (PGI_2), thromboxane A_2 (TXA_2) and the stable prostaglandins PGE_2, PGF_{2a} and PGD_2 [119,120]. The alternate metabolic pathway for arachidonic acid is the lipoxygenase system. Lipoxygenase enzymes convert free arachidonic acid to a variety of dihydroxyeicosatetraenoic acids (HETEs), hydroperoxy dervatives (HPETEs) and leukotrienes [121–124]. Protaglandins, leukotrienes, HPETEs and HETEs, can be generated by a wide variety of cells at the site of inflammation [125].

A role for the eicosanoids in the process of inflammation is suggested by their presence in and around inflamed tissue [126,127]. In human subjects, prostaglandins and leukotrienes in concentrations similar to that found at inflamed sites do not cause overt pain but, rather, hyperalgesia to touch [126,128,129]. Subdermal PGE_1 potentiates the pain produced by subdermal bradykinin [126]. Prostaglandins have also been observed to produce prolonged hyperalgesia when injected in the rat paw [130,131]. Electrophysiologic studies of cutaneous nociceptive afferents have provided more direct evidence for the sensitizing effects of prostaglandins on unmyelinated nociceptors, as well as on A-δ mechanoreceptors [105,116,132]. Continuous intra-arterial infusions of PGE_1 and PGE_2 sensitize C-nociceptors and intensify bradykinin-induced discharges of these afferents [133]. The prostaglandins, thus, must be considered to be different from other inflammatory mediators because their principal role appears to be to enhance the inflammatory effects of other mediators such as vasoactive amines and kinins [126].

Further proof of the involvement of the eicosanoids in inflammation stems from the observation that anti-inflammatory drugs suppress their biosynthesis. Most non-steroid anti-inflammatory drugs inhibit the formation of prostaglandins and thromboxanes by interfering with cyclo-oxygenase [134,135]. Anti-inflammatory steroids act at an earlier step by the formation of a polypeptide with an antiphospholipase effect [136]. Thus, the release of arachidonic acid is blocked, resulting in inhibition of the formation not only of prostaglandins and thromboxanes but also of the leukotrienes.

The effects of lipoxygenase products and leukotrienes on pain of inflammation are less well understood. Recent studies demonstrate that mechanical or thermal trauma in rats results in increased production of leukotrienes [137]. Behavioral studies in rat indicate that the leukotriene B_4 (LTB_4)-induced hyperalgesia is dependent on the presence of polymorphonuclear leukocytes (PMNLs). When incubated with LTB_4 *in vitro*, PMNLs release a factor that induces hyperalgesia in rats that have been depleted of circulating PMNLs [138]. A recent study indicates that (8R,15S)-diHETE, a product of the 15-lipoxygenation of arachidonic acid, may be the factor that mediates the LTB_4-induced hyperalgesia [139]. Leukotriene B_4 has been shown to produce thermal hyperalgesia in humans as well [140].

Norepinephrine

Clinical studies, and physiologic studies in animals, indicate an important role of the sympathetic nervous system in nociception. The pain and hyperalgesia in patients with sympathetically maintained pain states (e.g. reflex sympathetic dystrophy, causalgia) is relieved following blockade of sympathetic efferents. Iontophoretic administration of norepinephrine in the skin of patients whose causalgic pain was relieved by sympathetic blocks, results in transient rekindling of pain [141]. Following cutaneous heat injury in cats, sympathetic stimulation enhances background activity and response to heat stimuli in a sub-set of A-δ nociceptive afferent fibers [142]. In addition, in animal models of nerve injury, an excitatory role of adrenergic agents in C and A fibers has been demonstrated [143,144]. The role of the sympathetic nervous system in pain is discussed in further detail in Chapter 4.

Calcitonin gene-related peptide

A newly recognized peptide that may be specific to nociceptors, calcitonin gene-related peptide (CGRP), appears to have potent vasodilator properties in humans and may be one of the mediators of neurogenic vasodilatation [145,146]. CGRP produces prolonged vasodilatation around the site of injection, suggesting a possible role in long-term vascular responses to injury. So far, the algesic potential of CGRP has not been investigated.

The specific cellular mechanisms by which the chemical mediators of hyperalgesia sensitize nociceptors are not known. Bradykinin, prostaglandin, serotonin and possibly other hyperalgesic mediators probably exert their effects through multiple interacting intracellular messenger systems, leading to an alteration in neuronal electrophysiology.

HYPERALGESIA AND CHRONIC PAIN

Hyperalgesia to mechanical stimuli is a hallmark symptom of certain chronic pain syndromes such as causalgia and reflex sympathetic dystrophy, as well as postherpetic neuralgia and metabolic neuropathies (e.g. diabetes mellitus) [147,148]. Light touching of the skin causes pronounced pain in patients with these syndromes. The neural basis for this pain is not well understood. As discussed earlier, under normal conditions, pain is signalled by activity in C as well as A nociceptive afferent fibers. Large-diameter (A-β) afferent fibers that innervate the skin normally signal touch sensation. However, four lines of evidence indicate that the hyperalgesia in causalgic patients is signalled by activity in myelinated fibers and not in unmyelinated nociceptive afferent fibers [149]. The evidence is, first, that a selective ischemic blockade of A-β fibers, when C and A-δ fibers were still functional, eliminated the hyperalgesia. Wallin *et al.* [141] reported a patient whose causalgia was successfully treated by surgical sympathectomy. The hyperalgesia was rekindled in this patient by intracutaneous noradrenaline iontophoresis and eliminated by a pressure block of A-fiber function. Second, a selective local anesthetic blockade of the C and A-δ fibers did not affect the hyperalgesia. Third, the pain was detected with a short latency consistent with transmission of signals via A fibers. Reaction time measurements in patients with neuralgia point similarly to the involvement of myelinated afferent fibers [150]. Fourth, transcutaneous electrical stimulation of the nerve supply to the affected area resulted in pain at stimulus strengths sufficient to activate A but not C fibers [150a].

The existence of myelinated nociceptors with conduction velocities in the A-β range have been reported [18]. It could be that these A-fiber nociceptors are sensitized and account for the hyperalgesia in the patients with peripheral nerve injuries [48,149]. A role for unmyelinated nociceptors in other forms of painful neuropathies, however, is not precluded. For example, chronic sensitization of C-fiber nociceptors was recently shown to occur in one patient with persistent hyperalgesia [151].

Crosstalk between adjacent nerve fibers provides another possible explanation for the hyperalgesia to mechanical stimuli in patients with nerve injury. Mechanical stimuli might activate low-threshold mechanoreceptors, which might in turn crosstalk with nociceptive fibers. Evidence for crosstalk between A and C fibers has been reported in several animal models of nerve injury [152–154] and is reviewed extensively by Devor and Rappaport in Chapter 3 of this book. Several clinical observations, however, indicate that crosstalk is unlikely to account for the hyperalgesia seen in these patients. First, one would expect that substantial crosstalk would result in mislocalization of pain. Yet patients are able to localize precisely the site of painful mechanical stimulation. Second, the region of hyperalgesia often extends outside the area of cutaneous innervation of the injured nerve. Crosstalk fails to explain this observation. Finally, the latency for detection of pain from mechanical stimuli is too fast for A- to C-fiber crosstalk to account for the hyperalgesia.

Nociceptors normally signal pain, but this function may not be exclusively in the domain of nociceptors. As a result of nerve injury, changes in the central nervous system may occur such that fibers, the function of which is normally concerned only with touch sensation, may now signal pain. Thus, as a result of enhanced synaptic efficacy in the CNS, activity in low-threshold mechanoreceptors may evoke pain via activation of central pain-signalling neurons. Changes in dorsal horn circuitry following cutaneous injury and following peripheral nerve lesions have been reported [71,87]. Further psychophysical and neurophysiologic work is necessary to confirm this hypothesis.

SUMMARY

Research during the last two decades has led to considerable advances in our understanding of the mechanisms of pain. Recent neurophysiologic and psychophysical studies of pain have provided convincing evidence that in normal skin a particular class of afferent fibers, termed nociceptors, signal pain.

Nociceptive afferent fibers can be unmyelinated (C fiber) or myelinated (A fiber). C-fiber nociceptors respond to intense mechanical and thermal and certain chemical stimuli and are thought to code for the location and intensity of noxious stimuli. Type I A-fiber nociceptors in the intact skin have high heat thresholds and are thought to signal the prolonged pain associated with noxious stimuli of long duration. Type II A-fiber nociceptors resemble the C-fibers in their mechanical and heat thresholds, but have shorter receptor utilization times and faster conduction velocities. They are thought to signal first-pain sensations.

Cutaneous inflammation results in hyperalgesia. Hyperalgesia to heat at the site of an injury can be explained by sensitization of A- and C-fiber nociceptors. This sensitization is probably due to local release of chemical mediators in the inflamed area. The metabolites of arachidonic acid (eicosanoids) and bradykinin appear to have an important role in the sensitization of nociceptors. The mechanism of hyperalgesia to mechanical stimuli in the region of injury as well as the region surrounding the injury is less well understood and probably results from changes in both the peripheral and central nervous systems.

Hyperalgesia is a well-known manifestation of tissue injury and nerve injury. Future work is being directed at understanding the different contributions of both the peripheral and central nervous systems to hyperalgesia. This, together with a delineation of molecular basis of sensitization of nociceptors, will undoubtedly point the way to improved therapeutic strategies.

References

1. Raja, S. N., Meyer, R. A. and Campbell, J. N. Peripheral mechanisms of somatic pain. *Anesthesiology*, **68**, 571–590 (1988)
2. Darian-Smith, I., Johnson, K. O., LaMotte, C., Shigenaga, Y., Kenins, P. and Champness, P. Warm fibers innervating palmar and digital skin of the monkey: responses to thermal stimuli. *Journal of Neurophysiology*, **42**, 1297–1315 (1979)

3. Konietzny, F. and Hensel, H. Warm fiber activity in human skin nerves. *European Journal of Physiology*, **359**, 265–267 (1975)
4. Darian-Smith, I., Johnson, K. O. and Dykes, R. 'Cold' fiber population innervating palmar and digital skin of the monkey: responses to cooling pulses. *Journal of Neurophysiology*, **36**, 325–346 (1973)
5. Sherrington, C. S. *The Integrative Action of the Nervous System*, Scribner, New York, pp. 226–230 (1906)
6. Beitel, R. E. and Dubner, R. Fatigue and adaptation in unmyelinated (C) polymodal nociceptors to mechanical and thermal stimuli applied to the monkey's face. *Brain Research*, **112**, 402–406 (1976)
7. Campbell, J. N. and Meyer, R. A. Sensitization of unmyelinated nociceptive afferents in the monkey varies with skin type. *Journal of Neurophysiology*, **49**, 98–110 (1983)
8. Croze, S., Duclaux, R. and Kenshalo, D. R. The thermal sensitivity of the polymodal nociceptors in the monkey. *Journal of Physiology*, **263**, 539–562 (1976)
9. Iggo, A. and Ogawa, H. Primate cutaneous thermal nociceptors. *Journal of Physiology*, **216**, 77P–78P (1971)
10. LaMotte, R. H. and Campbell, J. N. Comparison of responses of warm and nociceptive C-fiber afferents in monkey with human judgements of thermal pain. *Journal of Neurophysiology*, **41**, 509–528 (1978)
11. LaMotte, R. H., Thalhammer, J. G. and Robinson, C. J. Peripheral neural correlates of magnitude of cutaneous pain and hyperalgesia: a comparison of neural events in monkey with sensory judgements in human. *Journal of Neurophysiology*, **50**, 1–26 (1983)
12. Price, D. D., Hu, J. W., Dubner, R. and Gracely, R. H. Peripheral suppression of first pain and central summation of second pain evoked by noxious heat pulses. *Pain*, **3**, 57–68 (1977)
13. Bessou, P. and Perl, E. R. Response of cutaneous sensory units with unmyelinated fibers to noxious stimuli. *Journal of Neurophysiology*, **32**, 1025–1043 (1969)
14. Collins, W. F., Nulsen, F. E. and Randt, C. T. Relation of peripheral nerve fiber size and sensation in man. *Archives of Neurology*, **3**, 381–385 (1960)
15. Dubner, R. and Hu, J. W. Myelinated (A-delta) nociceptive afferents innervating the monkey's face. *Journal of Dental Research*, **56**, A167 (1977)
16. Fitzgerald, M. and Lynn, B. The sensitization of high threshold mechanoreceptors with myelinated axons by repeated heating. *Journal of Physiology*, **365**, 549–563 (1977)
17. Georgopoulos, A. P. Functional properties of primary afferent units probably related to pain mechanisms in primate glabrous skin. *Journal of Neurophysiology*, **39**, 71–83 (1976)
18. Campbell, J. N., Meyer, R. A. and LaMotte, R. H. Sensitization of myelinated nociceptive afferents that innervate monkey hand. *Journal of Neurophysiology*, **42**, 1669–1679 (1979)
19. Burgess, P. R. and Perl, E. R. Myelinated afferent fibres responding specifically to noxious stimulation of the skin. *Journal of Physiology*, **190**, 541–562 (1967)
20. Dubner, R. and Bennett, G. J. Spinal and trigeminal mechanisms of nociception. *Annual Review of Neuroscience*, **6**, 381–418 (1983)
21. LaMotte, R. H. and Thalhammer, J. G. Response properties of high-threshold cutaneous cold receptors in the primate. *Brain Research*, **244**, 279–287 (1982)
22. Beck, P. W., Handwerker, H. O. and Zimmerman, M. Nervous outflow from the cat's foot during noxious radiant heat stimulation. *Brain Research*, **67**, 373–386 (1974)
23. Dash, M. S. and Deshpande, S. S. Human skin nociceptors and their chemical response. In *Advances in Pain Research and Therapy, Vol. 1*, (ed. J. J. Bonica *et al.*), Raven Press, New York, pp. 47–52 (1976)
24. LaMotte, R. H., Simone, D. A., Baumann, T. K., Shain, C. N. and Alreja, M. Hypothesis for novel classes of chemoreceptors mediating chemogenic pain and itch. *Pain*, Suppl. 4, S15 (1987)
25. Handwerker, H. O., Anton, F. and Reeh, P. W. Discharge patterns of afferent cutaneous nerve fibers from the rat's tail during prolonged noxious mechanical stimulation. *Experimental Brain Research*, **65**, 493–504 (1987)
26. Reeh, P. W., Bayer, J., Kocher, L. and Handwerker, H. O. Sensitization of nociceptive cutaneous nerve fibers from the rat tail by noxious mechanical stimulation. *Experimental Brain Research*, **65**, 505–512 (1987)
27. Adriaensen, H., Gybels, J., Handwerker, H. O. and Van Hees, J. Response properties of thin myelinated (A-delta) fibers in human skin nerves. *Journal of Neurophysiology*, **49**, 111–122 (1983)
28. Zotterman, Y. Touch, pain and tickling: an electrophysiological investigation on cutaneous sensory nerves. *Journal of Physiology*, **95**, 1–28 (1939)
29. Campbell, J. N. and Meyer, R. A. Primary afferents and hyperalgesia. In *Spinal Afferent Processing* (ed. T. L. Yaksh), Plenum Press, New York, pp. 59–81 (1986)
30. Meyer, R. A., Campbell, J. N. and Raja, S. N. Peripheral neural mechanisms of cutaneous

hyperalgesia. In *Advances in Pain Research and Therapy, Vol. 9*, (ed. H. L. Fields *et al.*), Raven Press, New York, pp. 53–71 (1985)

31. Meyer, R. A. and Campbell, J. N. Myelinated nociceptive afferents account for the hyperalgesia that follows a burn applied to the hand. *Science*, 213, 1527–1529 (1981)

32. Meyer, R. A. and Campbell, J. N. Peripheral neural coding of pain sensation. *Johns Hopkins APL Technical Digest*, 2, 164–171 (1981)

33. Price, D. D., Hayes, R. L., Ruda, M. and Dubner, R. Spatial and temporal transformations of input to spinothalamic tract neurons and their relation to somatic sensation. *Journal of Neurophysiology*, 41, 933–946 (1978)

34. Perl, E. R. Myelinated afferent fibres innervating the primate skin and their response to noxious stimuli. *Journal of Physiology*, 197, 593–615 (1968)

35. Gybels, J., Handwerker, H. O. and Van Hees, J. A comparison between the discharges of human nociceptive nerve fibers and the subject's ratings of his sensations. *Journal of Physiology*, 292, 193–206 (1979)

36. Van Hees, J. and Gybels, J. M. Pain related to single afferent C fibers from human skin. *Brain Research*, 48, 397–400 (1972)

37. Sinclair, D. C. and Hinshaw, J. R. A comparison of the sensory dissociation produced by procaine and by limb compression. *Brain*, 73, 480–498 (1950)

38. Torebjörk, H. E. and Hallin, R. G. Perceptual changes accompanying controlled preferential blocking of A and C fibre responses in intact human skin nerves. *Experimental Brain Research*, 16, 321–332 (1973)

39. Adriaensen, H., Gybels, J., Handwerker, H. O. and Van Hees, J. Suppression of C-fiber discharges upon repeated heat stimulation may explain characteristics of concomitant pain sensations. *Brain Research*, 302, 203–211 (1984)

40. Torebjörk, E. and Ochoa, J. Specific sensations evoked by activity in single identified sensory units in man. *Acta physiologica scandinavica*, 110, 445–447 (1980)

41. Lewis, T. and Pochin, E. E. The double pain response of the human skin to a single stimulus. *Clinical Science*, 3, 67–76 (1937)

42. Price, D. D. and Dubner, R. Mechanisms of first and second pain in the peripheral and central nervous systems. *Journal of Investigative Dermatology*, 69, 167–171 (1977)

43. Sinclair, D. C. and Stokes, B. A. R. The production and characteristics of 'second pain'. *Brain*, 87, 609–618 (1964)

44. Campbell, J. N. and LaMotte, R. H. Latency to detection of first pain. *Brain Research*, 266, 203–208 (1983)

45. Torebjörk, E. Nociceptor activation and pain. *Philosophical Transactions of the Royal Society of London [Biol]*, 308, 227–234 (1985)

46. Torebjörk, H. E., LaMotte, R. H. and Robinson, C. J. Peripheral neural correlates of magnitude of cutaneous pain and hyperalgesia: simultaneous records in humans of sensory judgments of pain and evoked responses in nociceptors with C-fibers. *Journal of Neurophysiology*, 51, 325–339 (1984)

47. Handwerker, H. O., Adriaensen, H. F. M., Gybels, J. M. and Van Hees, J. Nociceptor discharges and pain sensations: results and open question. In *Pain Management in Man: Neurophysiological Correlates of Pain* (ed. B. Bromm), Elsevier, Amsterdam, pp. 55–64 (1984)

48. Campbell, J. N., Raja, S. N. and Meyer, R. A. Painful sequelae of nerve injury. In *Pain Research and Clinical Management, Vol. 3, Proceedings of the Vth World Congress on Pain* (ed. R. Dubner *et al.*), Amsterdam, Elsevier, pp. 135–143 (1988)

49. Van Hees, J. Human C-fiber input during painful and nonpainful skin stimulation with radiant heat. In *Advances in Pain Research and Therapy, Vol. 1* (ed. J. J. Bonica *et al.*), Raven Press, New York, pp. 35–40 (1976)

50. Adriaensen, H., Gybels, J., Handwerker, H. O. and Van Hees, J. Nociceptor discharges and sensations due to prolonged noxious mechanical stimulation – a paradox. *Human Neurobiology*, 3, 53–58 (1984)

51. Wall, P. D. and McMahon, S. B. The relationship of perceived pain to afferent nerve impulses. *Trends in Neuroscience*, 9, 254–255 (1986)

52. Bini, G., Crucci, G., Hagbarth, K. E., Schady, W. and Torebjörk, E. Analgesic effect of vibration and cooling on pain induced by intraneural electrical stimulation. *Pain*, 18, 239–248 (1984)

53. LaMotte, R. H. Can the sensitization of nociceptors account for hyperalgesia after skin injury? *Human Neurobiology*, 3, 47–52 (1984)

54. Lewis, T. Clinical observations and experiments relating to burning pain in extremities, and to so-called 'erythromelagia' in particular. *Clinical Science*, 1, 175–211 (1933)

55. Lewis, T. Experiments relating to cutaneous hyperalgesia and its spread through somatic fibres. *Clinical Science*, 2, 373–423 (1935)

56. Lewis, T. *Pain*, Macmillan, New York (1942)

57. Hardy, J. D., Wolff, H. G. and Goodell, H. Experimental evidence on the nature of cutaneous hyperalgesia. *Journal of Clinical Investigation*, **29**, 115–140 (1952)
58. Meyer, R. A. and Campbell, J. N. Evidence for two distinct classes of unmyelinated nociceptive afferents in monkey. *Brain Research*, **224**, 149–152 (1981)
59. Raja, S. N., Campbell, J. N. and Meyer, R. A. Evidence for different mechanisms of primary and secondary hyperalgesia following heat injury to the glabrous skin. *Brain*, **107**, 1179–1188 (1984)
60. Campbell, J. N., Khan, A. A., Meyer, R. A. and Raja, S. N. Responses to heat of C-fiber nociceptors in monkey are altered by injury in the receptive field but not by adjacent injury. *Pain*, **32**, 327–332 (1988)
61. LaMotte, R. H., Simone, D. A., Baumann, T. K., Shain, C. N. and Alreja, M. Hypothesis for novel classes of chemoreceptors mediating chemogenic pain and itch. In *Pain Research and Clinical Management, Vol. 3* (ed. R. Dubner *et al.*), Elsevier, Amsterdam, pp. 529–535 (1988)
62. LaMotte, R. H., Thalhammer, J. G. and Robinson, C. J. Peripheral neural correlates of magnitude of cutaneous pain and hyperalgesia: A comparison of neural events in monkey with sensory judgements in human. *Journal of Neurophysiology*, **50**, 1–26 (1983)
63. Beitel, R. E. and Dubner, R. Response of unmyelinated (C) polymodal nociceptors to thermal stimuli applied to monkey's face. *Journal of Neurophysiology*, **39**, 1160–1175 (1976)
64. Dubner, R., Price, D. D., Beitel, R. E. and Hu, J. W. Peripheral neural correlates of behavior in monkey and human related to sensory-discriminative aspects of pain. In *Pain in the Trigeminal Region* (ed. D. J. Anderson *et al.*), Elsevier North Holland, Amsterdam, pp. 57–66 (1977).
65. LaMotte, R. H., Thalhammer, J. G., Torebjörk, H. E. and Robinson, C. J. Peripheral neural mechanisms of cutaneous hyperalgesia following mild injury by heat. *Journal of Neuroscience*, **2**, 765–781 (1982)
66. Thalhammer, J. G. and LaMotte, R. H. Spatial properties of nociceptor sensitization following heat injury of the skin. *Brain Research*, **231**, 257–265 (1982)
67. LaMotte, R. H. Psychophysical and neurophysiological studies of chemically induced cutaneous pain and itch: the case of the missing nociceptor. *Progress in Brain Research*, **74**, 331–335 (1988)
68. Heppelman, B., Hebert, M. K., Schaible, H. G. and Schmidt, R. F. Morphological and physiological characteristics of the innervation of cats normal and arthritic knee joint. In *Effects of Injury in Trigeminal and Spinal Somatosensory System* (ed. L. S. Pubols *et al.*), Alan R. Liss, New York, pp. 19–27 (1987)
69. Meyer, R. A., and Campbell, J. N. A novel electrophysiological technique for locating cutaneous nociceptive and chemospecific receptors. *Brain Research*, **441**, 81–86 (1988)
70. Koltzenburg, M. and McMahon, S. B. Plasma extravasation in the rat urinary bladder following mechanical, electrical and chemical stimuli: evidence for a new population of chemosensitive primary sensory afferents. *Neuroscience Letters*, **72**, 352–356 (1986)
71. Cook, A. J., Woolf, C. J., Wall, P. D. and McMahon, S. B. Dynamic receptive field plasticity in rat spinal cord dorsal horn following C-primary afferent input. *Nature*, **325**, 151–153 (1987)
72. Melzack, R. and Wall, P. D. Pain mechanisms: a new theory. *Science*, **150**, 971–979 (1965)
73. Noordenbos, W. *Pain*, Elsevier, Amsterdam, pp. 1–182 (1959)
74. Van Hees, J. and Gybels, J. C. Nociceptor activity in human nerve during painful and non-painful skin stimulation. *Journal of Neurology, Neurosurgery and Psychiatry*, **44**, 600–607 (1981)
75. LaMotte, R. H. Torebjörk, E. and Lundberg, L. Neural mechanisms of cutaneous hyperalgesia in humans: peripheral or central? *Society of Neuroscience Abstracts*, **13**, 189 (1987)
76. Lembeck, F., Popper, H. and Juan, H. Release of prostaglandins by bradykinin as an intrinsic mechanism of its algesic effect. *Naunyn-Schmiedeberg's Archives of Pharmacology*, **294**, 69–73 (1976)
77. Chapman, L. F., Ramos, A. O., Goodell, H. and Wolff, H. G. Neurohumoral features of afferent fibers in man. *AMA Archives of Neurology*, **4**, 617–650 (1961)
78. Simone, D. A., Baumann, T. K., and LaMotte, R. H. Dose-dependent pain and mechanical hyperalgesia in humans after intradermal injection of capsaicin. *Pain*, **38**, 99–107 (1989)
79. Fitzgerald, M. The spread of sensitization of polymodal nociceptors in the rabbit from nearby injury and by antidromic nerve stimulation. *Journal of Physiology*, **297**, 207–216 (1979)
80. Meyer, R. A., Campbell, J. N. and Raja, S. N. Antidromic nerve stimulation in monkey does not sensitize unmyelinated nociceptors to heat. *Brain Research*, **441**, 168–172 (1988)
81. Reeh, P. W., Kocher, L. and Jung, S. Does neurogenic inflammation alter the sensitivity of unmyelinated nociceptors in the rat? *Brain Research*, **384**, 42–50 (1986)
82. Thalhammer, J. G. and LaMotte, R. H. Heat sensitization of one-half of a cutaneous nociceptor's receptive field does not alter the sensitivity of the other half. In *Advances in Pain Research and Therapy, Vol. 5* (ed. J. J. Bonica *et al.*), Raven Press, New York, pp. 71–75 (1983)
83. Hardy, J. D., Wolff, H. G. and Goodell, H. *Pain Sensation and Reactions*, Williams and Wilkins, Baltimore, pp. 65–85 (1952)

84. Kenshalo, D. R., Leonard, R. B., Chung, J. M. and Willis, W. D. Responses of primate spinothalamic neurons to graded and to repeated noxious heat stimuli. *Journal of Neurophysiology*, **42**, 1370–1389 (1979)

85. Simone, D. A., Baumann, T. K., Collins, J. G., and LaMotte, R. H. Sensitization of cat dorsal horn neurons to innocuous mechanical stimulation after intradermal injection of capsaicin. *Brain Research*, **486**, 185–189 (1989)

86. Woolf, C. J. Long term alterations in the excitability of the flexion reflex produced by peripheral tissue injury in the chronic decerebrate rat. *Pain*, **18**, 325–343 (1984)

87. Woolf, C. J. Evidence for a central component of post-injury pain hypersensitivity. *Nature*, **306**, 686–688 (1983)

88. Payan, D. G., McGillis, J. P., Renold, F. K., Mitsuhashi, M. and Goetzl, E. J. Neuropeptide modulation of leukocyte function. *Annals of the New York Academy of Sciences*, **496**, 182–191 (1987)

89. Roberts, W. J. and Elardo, S. M. Sympathetic activation of A-delta nociceptors. *Somatosensory Research*, **3**, 33–44 (1985)

90. Armstrong, D., Jepson, J. B., Keele, C. A. and Stewart, J. W. Pain-producing substance in human inflammatory exudates and plasma. *Journal of Physiology*, **135**, 350–370 (1957)

91. Keele, C. A. and Armstrong, D. *Substances Producing Pain and Itch*, Edward Arnold, London, pp. 107–219 (1964)

92. Vane, J. R. Prostaglandins as mediators of inflammation. In *Advances in Prostaglandin and Thromboxane Research, Vol. 2* (ed. J. J. Bonica *et al.*), Raven Press, New York, pp. 597–603 (1983)

93. Richardson, B. P., Engel, G., Donatsch, P. and Stadler, P. A. Identification of serotonin M-receptor subtypes and their specific blockade by a new class of drugs. *Nature*, **316**, 126–131 (1985)

94. Fock, S. and Mense, S. Excitatory effects of 5-hydroxytryptamine, histamine and potassium ions on muscular group IV afferent units: a comparison with bradykinin. *Brain Research*, **105**, 459–469 (1976)

95. Sicuteri, F., Fanciullacci, M., Franchi, G. and Del Bianco, P. L. Serotonin-bradykinin potentiation on the pain receptors in man. *Life Sciences*, **4**, 309–316 (1965)

96. Richardson, B. P. and Engel, G. The pharmacology and function of 5-HT3 receptors. *Trends in Neuroscience*, **9**, 424 (1986)

97. Coffman, J. D. The effect of aspirin on pain and hand flow responses to intra-arterial injection of bradykinin in man. *Clinical Pharmacology and Therapeutics*, **7**, 26–37 (1966)

98. Cormia, F. E. and Dougherty, J. W. Proteolytic activity in development of pain and itching: cutaneous reactions to bradykinin and kallikrein. *Journal of Investigative Dermatology*, **35**, 21–26 (1960)

99. Lim, R. K. S., Miller, D. G., Guzman, F. *et al*. Pain and analgesia evaluated by intraperitoneal bradykinin-evoked pain method in man. *Clinical Pharmacology and Thermodynamics*, **8**, 521–542 (1967)

100. DiRosa, M., Giroud, J. P. and Willoughby, D. A. Studies of the mediators of the acute inflammatory response induced in rats in different sites by carrageenan and turpentine. *Journal of Pathology*, **104**, 15–29 (1971)

101. Melmon, K. L., Webster, M. E., Goldfinger, S. E. and Seegmiller, J. E. The presence of a kinin in inflammatory synovial effusion from arthritides of varying etiologies. *Arthritis and Rheumatism*, **10**, 13–20 (1967)

102. Steranka, L. R., Manning, D. C., DeHass, C. J. *et al*. Bradykinin as a pain mediator: receptors are localized to sensory neurons and antagonists have analgesic actions. *Proceedings of the National Academy of Sciences of the United States of America*, **85**, 3245–3249 (1988)

103. Manning, D. C., Khan, A. A., Campbell, J. N., Meyer, R. A. and Raja, S. N. Bradykinin induced cutaneous pain is independent of wheal and flare. *Pain*, Suppl. 4, s16 (1987)

104. Beck, P. W. and Handwerker, H. O. Bradykinin and serotonin effects on various types of cutaneous nerve fibers. *Pflügers Archiv; European Journal of Physiology*, **347**, 209–222 (1974)

105. Chahl, L. A. and Iggo, A. The effects of bradykinin and prostaglandin E1 on rat cutaneous afferent nerve activity. *British Journal of Pharmacology*, **59**, 343–347 (1977)

106. Szolcsanyi, J. Effect of pain-producing chemical agents on the activity of slowly conducting afferent fibres. *Acta physiologica hungarica*, **56**, 86 (1980)

107. Khan, A. A., Raja, S. N., Campbell, J. N., Hartke, T. V. and Meyer, R. A. Bradykinin sensitizes nociceptors to heat stimuli. *Society of Neuroscience Abstracts*, **12**, (1), 219 (1986)

108. Guzman, F., Braun, C. and Lim, R. K. S. Visceral pain and the pseudaffective response to intra-arterial injection of bradykinin and other algesic agents. *Archives internationales de pharmacodynamie et de therapie*, **136**, 353–384 (1962)

109. Moncada, S., Ferreira, S. H. and Vane, J. R. Inhibition of prostaglandin biosynthesis as the mechanism of analgesia of aspirin-like drugs in the dog knee joint. *European Journal of Pharmacology*, **31**, 250–260 (1975)
110. Baccaglini, P. I. and Hogan, P. G. Some rat sensory neurons in culture express characteristics of differentiated pain sensory cells. *Proceedings of the National Academy of Sciences of the United States of America*, **80**, 594–598 (1983)
111. Brass, K. M., Manning, D. C., Perry, D. C. and Snyder, S. H. Bradykinin analogues: Differential agonist and antagonist activities suggesting multiple receptors. *British Journal of Pharmacology*, **94**, 3–5 (1988)
112. Regoli, D. and Barabe, J. Pharmacology of bradykinin and related kinins. *Pharmacology Reviews*, **32**, 1–46 (1980)
113. Vavrek, R. J. and Stewart, J. M. Competitive antagonists of bradykinin. *Peptides*, **6**, 161–164 (1985)
114. Whalley, E. T. Receptors mediating the increase in vascular permeability to kinins: comparative studies in rat, guinea-pig and rabbit. *Naunyn Schmiedeberg's Archives of Pharmacology*, **336**, 99–104 (1987)
115. Griesbacher, T. and Lembeck, F. Effect of bradykinin antagonists on bradykinin-induced plasma extravasation, venoconstriction, prostaglandin E2 release, nociceptor stimulation and contraction of the iris sphincter muscle in the rabbit. *British Journal of Pharmacology*, **92**, 333–340 (1987)
116. Handwerker, H. O. Influences of algogenic substances and prostaglandins on the discharges of unmyelinated cutaneous nerve fibers identified as nociceptors. In *Advances in Pain Research and Therapy, Vol. 1* (ed. J. J. Bonica et al.), Raven Press, New York, pp. 41–45 (1976)
117. Hori, Y., Katori, M., Harada, Y., Uchida, Y. and Tanaka, K. Potentiation of bradykinin-induced nociceptive response by arachidonate metabolites in dogs. *European Journal of Pharmacology*, **132**, 47–52 (1986)
118. Corey, E. J., Niwa, H., Falck, J. R., Mioskowski, C., Arai, X. and Margat, A. Recent studies on the chemical synthesis of eicosanoids. In *Advances in Prostaglandins and Thromboxane Research, Vol. 6* (ed. B. Samuelsson et al.), Raven Press, New York, pp. 19–25 (1980)
119. Kuehl, F. A., Jr and Egan, R. W. Prostaglandins, arachidonic acid, and inflammation. *Science*, **210**, 978–984 (1980)
120. Samuelsson, B., Granstrom, E., Green, K., Hamberg, M. and Hammarstrom, S. Prostaglandins. *Annual Review of Biochemistry*, **44**, 669–695 (1975)
121. Granstrom, E. Biochemistry of the prostaglandins, thromboxanes, and leukotrienes. In *Advances in Pain Research and Therapy, Vol. 1* (ed. J. J. Bonica et al.), Raven Press, New York, pp. 605–616 (1983)
122. Piper, P. Pharmacology of leukotrienes. *British Medical Bulletin*, **39**, 255–259 (1983)
123. Samuelsson, B. and Hammarstrom, S. Nomenclature for leukotrienes. *Prostaglandins*, **19**, 645–648 (1980)
124. Wolfe, L. S. Eicosanoids: Prostaglandins, thromboxane, leukotrienes and other derivatives of carbon-20 unsaturated fatty acids. *Journal of Neurology*, **38**, 1–14 (1982)
125. Ford-Hutchinson, A. W., Bray, M. A., Doig, M. V., Shipley, M. E. and Smith, M. J. H. Leukotriene B, a potent chemokinetic and aggregating substance released from polymorphonuclear leukocytes. *Nature*, **286**, 264–265 (1980)
126. Ferreira, S. H. Peripheral and central analgesia. In *Advances in Pain Research and Therapy, Vol. 5* (ed. J. J. Bonica et al.), Raven Press, New York, pp. 627–634 (1983)
127. Greaves, M. W., Sondergaard, J. and McDonald-Gibson, W. Recovery of prostaglandins in human cutaneous inflammation. *British Medical Journal*, **2**, 258–260 (1971)
128. Collier, H. O. J. and Schneider, C. Nociceptive responses to prostaglandins. *Nature*, **236**, 141–143 (1972)
129. Beubler, E. and Juan, H. Is the effect of diphenolic laxatives mediated via release of prostaglandin E? *Experientia*, **34**, 386–387 (1978)
130. Kuhn, D. C. and Willis, A. L. Prostaglandin E2 inflammation and pain threshold in rat paws. *British Journal of Pharmacology*, **49**, 183P–184P (1973)
131. Tyers, M. B. and Haywood, H. Effects of prostaglandins on peripheral nociceptors in acute inflammation. *Agents and Actions*, (Suppl) **6**, 65–78 (1979)
132. Pateromichelakis, S. and Rood, J. P. Prostaglandin E-induced sensitization of A-delta moderate pressure mechanoreceptors. *Brain Research*, **232**, 89–96 (1982)
133. Handwerker, H. O. Pharmacological modulation of the discharge of nociceptive C fibers. In *Sensory Functions of the Skin in Primates* (ed. Y. Zotterman), Pergamon Press, Oxford, pp. 427–439 (1976)

134. Ferreira, S. H. and Vane, J. R. New aspects of the mode of action of non-steroid anti-inflammatory drugs. *Annual Review of Pharmacology*, **14**, 57–73 (1974)
135. Lundberg, J. M., Rokaeus, A., Hokfelt, T., Rosell, S., Brown, M. and Goldstein, M. Neurotensin-like immunoreactivity in the preganglionic sympathetic nerves and in the adrenal medulla of the cat. *Acta physiologica scandinavica*, **114**, 153–155 (1982)
136. Blackwell, G. J., Carnuccio, R., DiRosa, M., Flower, R. J., Parente, L. and Persico, P. Macrocortin: A polypeptide causing the anti-phospholipase effect of glucocorticoids. *Nature*, **287**, 147–149 (1980)
137. Denzlinger, C., Rapp, S., Hagmann, W. and Keppler, D. Leukotrienes as mediators in tissue trauma. *Science*, **230**, 330–332 (1985)
138. Levine, J. D., Gooding, J., Donatoni, P., Borden, L. and Goetzl, E. J. The role of polymorphonuclear leukocyte in hyperalgesia. *Journal of Neuroscience*, **5**, 3025–3029 (1985)
139. Levine, J. D., Lam, D., Taiwo, Y. O., Donatoni, P. and Goetzl, E. J. Hyperalgesic properties of 15-lipoxygenase products of arachidonic acid. *Proceedings of the National Academy of Sciences of the United States of America*, **83**, 5331–5334 (1986)
140. Bisgaard, H. and Kristensen, J. K. Leukotriene B produces hyperalgesia in humans. *Prostaglandins*, **30**, 791–797 (1985)
141. Wallin, B. G., Torebjörk, E. and Hallin, R. G. Preliminary observations on the pathophysiology of hyperalgesia in the causalgic pain syndrome. In *Sensory Functions of the Skin of Primates with Special Reference to Man* (ed. Y. Zotterman), Pergamon, Oxford, pp. 489–499 (1976)
142. Roberts, W. J. and Elardo, S. M. Sympathetic activation of A-delta nociceptors. *Somatosensory Research*, **3**, 33–44 (1985)
143. Korenman, E. M. D. and Devor, M. Ectopic adrenergic sensitivity in damaged peripheral nerve axons in the rat. *Experimental Neurology*, **72**, 63–81 (1981)
144. Wall, P. D. and Gutnick, M. Properties of afferent nerve impulses originating from a neuroma. *Nature*, **248**, 740–743 (1974)
145. Brain, S. D., Tippins, J. R., Morris, H. R., MacIntyre, I. and Williams, T. Potent vasodilator activity of calcitonin gene-related peptide in human skin. *Journal of Investigative Dermatology*, **87**, 533–536 (1986)
146. Piotrowski, W. and Foreman, J. C. Some effects of calcitonin gene-related peptide in human skin and on histamine release. *British Journal of Dermatology*, **114**, 37–46 (1986)
147. Bonica, J. J. Causalgia and other reflex sympathetic dystrophies. In *Advances in Pain Research and Therapy, Vol. 13* (ed. J. J. Bonica), Raven Press, New York, pp. 141–166 (1979)
148. Sunderland, S. *Nerves and Nerve Injuries*, Churchill Livingstone, New York, pp. 348–350 (1978)
149. Campbell, J. N., Raja, S. N., Meyer, R. A. and Mackinnon, S. E. Myelinated afferents signal the hyperalgesia associated with nerve injury. *Pain*, **32**, 89–94 (1988)
150. Lindblom, U. and Verrillo, R. T. Sensory functions in chronic neuralgia. *Journal of Neurology, Neurosurgery and Psychiatry*, **42**, 422–435 (1979)
150a.Price, D.D., Bennett, G. J. and Rafii, A. Psychophysical observations on patients with neuropathic pain relieved by a sympathetic block. *Pain*, **36**, 273–288 (1989)
151. Cline, M. and Ochoa, J. Chronically sensitized C nociceptors in skin. Patient with hyperalgesia, hyperpathia and spontaneous pain. *Society of Neuroscience Abstracts*, **12**, 331–331 (1986)
152. Seltzer, Z. and Devor, M. Ephaptic transmission in chronically damaged peripheral nerves. *Neurology*, **29**, 1061–1064 (1979)
153. Blumberg, H. and Janig, W. Activation of fibers via experimentally produced stump neuromas of skin nerves: ephaptic transmission or retrograde sprouting. *Experimental Neurology*, **76**, 468–482 (1982)
154. Meyer, R. A., Raja, S. N., Campbell, J. N., Mackinnon, S. E. and Dellon, A. L. Neural activity originating from a neuroma in the baboon. *Brain Research*, **325**, 255–260 (1985)

3
Pain and the pathophysiology of damaged nerve

Marshall Devor and Z. Harry Rappaport

INTRODUCTION

The relative importance of peripheral and central factors in the aetiology of neuropathic and radiculopathic pain has been debated extensively over the years. There can be little doubt that both are important. Without wishing to minimize the part played by changes in information processing within the central nervous system (CNS) following nerve injury, we focus in this chapter exclusively on peripheral processes. Specifically, we show how recent advances in the study of nerve pathophysiology in experimental models of nerve injury indicate a striking congruence between the abnormal electrical behavior of sensory axons, and symptomatology seen in various clinical pain syndromes. This match encourages the hypothesis that pathophysiologic changes in the peripheral nervous system (PNS) are a principal cause of neuropathic and radiculopathic pain. For each pathophysiologic process discussed we first set out the experimental evidence, and then briefly point out some of the clinical syndromes that display similar features. More in-depth discussions of clinical aspects of many of these syndromes appear in other chapters of this book.

Peripheral neuropathic and radiculopathic pain: definition

Peripheral neuropathic pain is pain associated with a disturbance of function, or a pathologic change in a peripheral nerve (derived from Merskey [1]). Radiculopathic, or cranial root pain is similar, but relates to sensory (dorsal) spinal or cranial roots. Functional disturbances in dorsal root ganglia (DRGs) are generally included in the category of radiculopathy on the basis of the spatial distribution of symptoms. As discussed later, however, functional properties of DRGs differ from those of nerves and roots.

Irritation or damage to peripheral nerves or sensory roots triggers the development of distinctive clinical syndromes which include both negative and positive symptoms. The immediate effect is partial or total conduction block in the injured nerve with corresponding sensory (and motor) loss. Because of overlap of the sensory components of adjacent nerves and spinal roots, the loss of sensation observed on clinical examination is often minor compared with the actual distribution of the nerve/root involved, even if transection is total. Accompanying positive complaints, which generally evolve after some delay, include spontaneous paresthesias and pain, and peculiar sensations including pain upon light tactile or other stimulation of the skin or deep tissue. These sensations tend to have a more widespread distribution than the negative symptoms, and generally follow the classic nerve or dermatomal pattern. There may, however, be spread beyond these boundaries.

It is important to note that the association of positive symptoms, including pain, with injury or disease in a particular nerve or root does not necessarily mean that the neural process responsible for the pain resides in that nerve/root. Nerve injury can trigger changes in the CNS by virtue of the absence of afferent input (so-called 'deafferentation pain'), excess input ('centralization' of pain), or as a result of altered trophic relationships between center and periphery. The central changes then become the primary culprits [2] (*see* Chapter 7). Indeed, the view that nerve injury evokes chronic pain by deafferentation is so widely held that it may come as a surprise to some readers that a particular syndrome is even discussed here in terms of pathophysiology in the PNS. The fact is, however, that for the majority of clinical entities there are insufficient data to know with any certainty the relative importance of peripheral and central processes. One should therefore try to keep an open mind.

'Normal' versus neuropathic pain

In the absence of unusual central gating, pain is felt when impulses reach a conscious brain along specialized fine myelinated (A-δ) and/or unmyelinated (C) nociceptive afferents. It is the match between the high threshold of these afferents in the periphery and the interpretation (pain) assigned by the brain to impulses arriving along them that makes this an effective signalling system. Pain may be considered 'normal' as long as it results from activity in nociceptive afferents elicited by intense stimuli. Even chronic pain is 'normal' by this standard if it is evoked by a maintained or recurrent noxious stimulus.

Neuropathic pain, in contrast, results from a change in the normal functioning of peripheral nerves or central processing channels, and it may occur in the absence of any noxious stimulus. How can a change in neural physiology cause pain? There are at least four ways. First, the sensitivity of nociceptor endings in skin or other peripheral tissues may increase ('sensitization'). Second, neuropathic pain might arise if otherwise normal nociceptive afferents for some reason began to produce impulses at abnormal (ectopic) locations along their course, for example at sites of injury. Third, neuropathic pain could result from a breakdown in the normal isolation between adjacent axons in a nerve trunk, permitting low-threshold fibers to activate nociceptors. Finally, neurons in the CNS, the activity of which evokes a conscious appreciation of pain, could begin firing spontaneously, or could come to be activated by peripheral stimuli normally inadequate to activate them. All four types of change have been seen in experimental nerve-injury preparations.

Nerve injury: the injured axon and its intact neighbors

When an axon is disconnected from its cell body it undergoes irreversible (Wallerian) degeneration. The part still connected to the cell body seals off and forms a terminal end-bulb. It may also die back for up to a few millimeters, and the myelin sheath adjacent to the end-bulb is invariably disrupted. Dying back is a self-limiting process, however, and within a short time fine axon sprouts emerge from near the cut end and begin to elongate. Under favorable conditions these regenerating sprouts reach peripheral target tissue where growth stops. Peripheral receptor function is then restored and excess sprouts are culled. If the forward progress of regenerating sprouts is blocked, sprouting from end-bulbs is retarded or, alternatively, outgrowing sprouts grow back on themselves in a swollen, tangled mass, a 'neuroma' [3–5].

If an entire nerve trunk has been divided with regeneration prevented, as in limb amputation, a 'nerve-end neuroma' is created. Partial division, or total division with partial regeneration, as after surgical nerve repair, yields a 'neuroma-in-continuity' at the site of anastomosis. Trauma may also cause small axon fascicles, or even individual axons, to be compromised at multiple and scattered levels forming 'disseminated microneuromas'. Microneuromas can also form when regeneration is arrested downstream of the injury. Finally, any incision, or even minor abrasion of skin, injures axons near their sensory terminals. In all of these situations of axonal growth or arrest, the axonal end-structure may become a source of positive as well as negative symptoms, by virtue of the development of ectopic impulse generation (electrogenesis).

Curiously, neighboring axons that have not themselves been injured, also shift into a growth mode at their endings in skin or deep tissue ('collateral sprouting'). This type of growth, probably triggered by reduced interfiber competition, favors nociceptive afferents. The result is selective proliferation of nociceptor terminals in partially denervated skin near the borders of total denervation [6,7]. Abnormalities in cutaneous sensibility in partial nerve injury may therefore derive both from innervated skin adjacent to the denervated region, and from ectopic sites proximally along the trunk of the injured nerve.

ECTOPIC ELECTROGENESIS IN SEVERED AXONS

Spontaneous impulse discharge in experimental nerve-end neuromas

The first experimental evidence that positive sensory symptoms can originate in the region of injured axons came from electrophysiologic recordings from dorsal rootlets in rats in which an experimental neuroma was made by cutting the sciatic nerve and capping its end against regeneration. Despite the cut, the roots carried massive spontaneous afferent discharge. It was clear that many of the impulses originated in the neuroma because pressing on it augmented the discharge and anaesthetizing it reduced the discharge [8,9]. However, not all of the fibers in the dorsal rootlets studied run in the sciatic nerve, and some of the spontaneous discharge may have derived from such intact axons. To confirm the neuroma as the source of ectopic discharge, Govrin-Lippmann and Devor [10], and subsequently several other groups (*see*, for example, [11–15]) made similar recordings but from the injured nerve itself just central to the neuroma (Figure 3.1b). This experimental approach confirmed the neuroma as an important site of ectopic electrogenesis in both myelinated (A) and unmyelinated (C) axons in a variety of different species, and also permitted quantitative evaluation of the discharge.

The function of somatosensory axons in mid-nerve is to propagate the neural message generated at sensory end-structures rapidly and accurately without missing impulses, or adding extra ones. For this reason the design properties of conducting axons, acquired during the course of evolution, make them inherently incapable of generating repetitive discharge. In experimental preparations, for example, direct depolarization produced by injecting current into mid-nerve axons via a microelectrode evokes an action potential at the onset of the stimulus, and perhaps also on offset, but there is no sustained firing during the course of the depolarization [16]. Similarly, steady pressure on a healthy nerve does not evoke repetitive discharge, and does not produce paresthesias referred to the peripheral distribution of the nerve. A sharp rap may do so, particularly at locations where the nerve passes over a bony prominence, but the discharge and the sensation die down quickly. Even complete transection yields only a brief 'injury discharge' which generally lasts only seconds [17,18]. The common notion that pain results from nerve entrapment, or from 'something pressing on a nerve' misses a key element of the neuropathic process.

Acute entrapment or pressure is at most momentarily painful. For these stimuli to evoke ongoing paresthesias and pain requires that axons fundamentally alter their electrical properties and change from impulse conductors to impulse generators (neural pacemakers). Whereas normal axons in mid-nerve are incapable of repetitive impulse generation (electrogenesis) but capable only of impulse propagation, end-bulbs and sprouts of injured axons acquire an impulse-generating capability. As a result, they become capable of producing prolonged impulse trains in response to a broad range of depolarizing stimuli, even stimuli with a very gradual onset. In fact many discharge spontaneously without any (intentional) stimulus at all. They became spontaneous ectopic pacemaker sites. The acquisition by injured nerve fibers of ectopic pacemaker capability is among the fundamental pathophysiologic changes that underly the emergence of neuropathic pain [19].

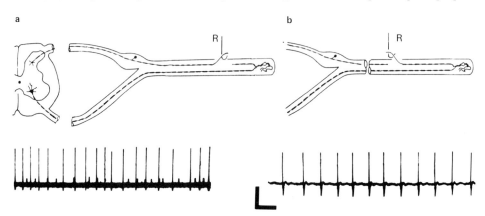

Figure 3.1 Spontaneous discharge originating in the DRG (a) and the nerve-end neuroma (b) in a chronic cut rat sciatic nerve. The top panel shows the experimental set-up, including the position of the recording electrodes (R). Actual impulse trains from these ectopic sources are shown below. Note that in the trace on the left there are two fibers, with distinct action potential amplitudes. The discharge originating in the DRG has a low frequency ($\approx$ 0.5 Hz) with irregular intervals between consecutive spikes; the discharge originating in the neuroma has a high frequency (22 Hz) and regular interspike intervals (rhythmic discharge). Calibration: 1 s/500 μV for a; 50 ms/700 μV for b. (From Wall, P. D. and Devor, M. Sensory afferent impulses originate from dorsal root ganglia as well as from the periphery in normal and nerve-injured rats. *Pain*, **17**, 321–339 (1983), [20] with permission)

Neuromas and pain

The obvious relationship between pain and swollen palpable neuromas rich, on histological examination, in tangled axon sprouts, has led to the notion that swelling and sprouts are an essential feature of neuroma pain (e.g. Kugelberg [21]). Correspondingly, when such obvious neuromas are absent, or pain returns after their removal, a peripheral explanation of the sensory abnormality is often abandoned. New histological data from functionally hyperexcitable neuromas in experimental preparations, however, refute both of these conclusions. Abnormal electrical activity matures well before a swollen neuroma is palpable, and before the classic morphological picture of massively tangled axonal sprouts is evident in histology [22] (Figure 3.2). A functional neuroma need not be swollen or rich in sprouts. Indeed, in the early stages of neuroma formation, in small nerves, and in the case of disseminated microneuromas, it probably never is. Thus it is a mistake to conclude that the absence of a classic neuroma rules out a peripheral neuropathic process.

Is it correct even to use the term 'neuroma' when the classic indicators are absent? In light of our interest in the functional aspects of injured nerves, we have chosen to adopt a broad definition of neuroma that does not place undue emphasis on structural characteristics which have never been linked mechanistically to function. Thus, we adopt the definition of the eminent anatomist Santiago Ramon y Cajal [23] who uses the term 'neuroma' to refer to the 'portion of nervous tissue which is included in a system of neuroglial trabeculae or tracts' at the proximal stump of a cut nerve, and places it in contrast to the 'glioma' of the distal stump.

Mechanosensitivity in experimental neuromas

Spontaneous discharge is only one measure of the global hyperexcitability that develops in injured nerve with the development of pacemaker capability. Hyperexcitability is also reflected in sensitivity to a broad range of depolarizing stimuli (*see below*). An important example is mechanosensitivity. When recordings are made from individual regenerating axons in an experimentally injured nerve, or from axons trapped in a neuroma, it is often possible to find a highly localized spot where minimal force produces (or facilitates) repetitive discharge [8,9,12–14,18,24,25]. The discharge may be limited to a short burst at the moment of stimulus onset and/or release, or it may be sustained for the duration of force application. In some fibers the discharge continues for an extended period of time after the end of the stimulus ('mechanical afterdischarge', *see* Figure 3.7).

Painful neuroma: clinical perspective

In the clinical setting, painful neuromas are usually located at sites that are subjected to mechanical stimulation, such as in the oral cavity, superficially along the side of a finger, or in an amputation stump. There is often no pain when mechanical disturbance or weight bearing is absent. Nerve block relieves mechanically evoked pain, but ongoing sensations, although reduced, usually persist. A good example of this is the phantom limb. Activation of neuromas by palpation, for example, often does produce a sensation referred into the phantom. There may even be a clear topography where an ulnar nerve neuroma, for example, projects to

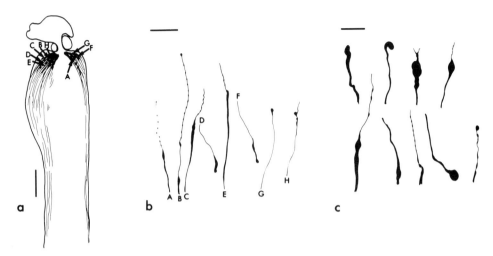

Figure 3.2 Structure of an electrically active rat nerve-end neuroma (15 days post injury). The end-structure of individual sensory axons (A–H in a and b, and at higher magnification in c is visualized with intracellular WGA-HRP reaction product. Such end-bulbs are the probable source of spontaneous and evoked ectopic neuroma discharge. Calibration bars: a, 1 mm; b, 100 μm; c, 50 μm (From Fried, K. and Devor, M. End-structure of afferent axons injured in the peripheral and central nervous system. *Somatosensory and Motor Research*, **6**, 79–99 (1988) with permission)

the ulnar surface of the phantom [26]. On the other hand, anesthetic nerve block or even proximal plexus block, often does not eliminate phantoms totally even for the duration of the block. It is widely concluded that phantoms must be generated in the CNS. However, elimination of neuromas as a primary source does not exhaust the possible contribution of PNS pathophysiology to neuropathic pain. As discussed below, there are alternative ectopic pacemaker sites in the PNS, for example the dorsal root ganglia (DRGs).

In contrast to ongoing sensation, there is an obvious association between mechanosensitivity and sites of injury along nerves. Pressure or light percussion of neuromas usually elicits symptoms such as paresthesias and sharp lancinating pain felt in the distribution of the nerve (Tinel's sign). The sensation long outlasts the stimulus, recalling 'mechanical afterdischarge' in experimental neuromas. Anesthetic block of the proximal nerve always abolishes these responses, but only for the duration of action of the anesthetic.

The idea of providing relief by surgically removing neuromas is futile as another neuroma, palpable or not, will soon re-form. There is no basis for expecting the new neuroma to be less hyperexcitable than the old. On the other hand, there is an obvious rationale, where possible, for dissecting neuromas free of surrounding cicatrix and embedding them deeply into adjacent well-vascularized soft tissue [27]. Distancing the neuroma in this way from compression by mechanical stimuli can abolish the exacerbation of symptoms due to mechanosensitivity. A similar approach is the use of appliances such as braces and prostheses designed to minimize mechanical stimulation of sensitive neuromas.

Neuromas-in-continuity with the nerve, such as form after partial nerve section or nerve section with surgical repair, are more problematic than nerve-end neuromas as any manipulation risks further damage to functional fibers continuing through the neuroma. In contrast to nerve-end-neuromas, ongoing paresthesias and pain *are* often ascribed to such sites. The reasons for the difference in spontaneous sensations between nerve-end and in-continuity neuromas are not clear. There is no reason, a priori, to expect ectopic pacemaker sites in in-continuity neuromas to differ much from those in nerve-end neuromas in their underlying excitability. However, the distal nerve trunk holds in-continuity neuromas under traction and, as a result, mechanical stimulation, including that generated by limb movements, may well be more intense [28]. Recalling that elevated discharge can long outlast the mechanical stimulus itself, even intermittent changes in the traction force on the nerve may sum to yield elevated baseline activity. This situation may be exaggerated still further when tiny microneuromas are disseminated along a stretch of nerve, as after partial trauma or a range of other peripheral neuropathies [29]. Here, of course, the presence of what is fundamentally neuroma pathophysiology would probably not be suspected, as there would not necessarily be any swelling or even discrete tender spots on examination.

Neurolysis, aimed at relieving traction forces, can relieve pain and improve neurologic function, but there is a real risk of injuring previously through-conducting fibers and adding them to the pool trapped in the in-continuity neuroma. Excision of the neuroma and re-anastomosis of the nerve ends may be performed in the hope that more fibers will regenerate successfully the second time. However, unless the original anastomosis was spontaneous, or was performed under extremely unfavorable surgical conditions, this hope may not justify the risk of adding additional injury. Although statistics are sparse, excision of in-continuity neuromas and re-anastomosis for the treatment of pain alone is best avoided [30].

Ectopic neuroma pacemakers in man

The recently developed method of percutaneous microneurographic recording from single nerve fibers in conscious man [31] has created the possibility of observing abnormal discharge in nerve injury patients, and directly comparing it with abnormal sensation. So far, practitioners have been justifiably reluctant to insert electrodes into problematic nerves in humans for essentially experimental purposes. This is so particularly in light of the experimental evidence that individuals may carry a genetic predisposition for developing abnormal neural discharges (*see below*). Patients with neuropathic pain, after all, are probably pre-selected for this trait, their a priori risk being particularly great. None the less, a few reports have been published in which microneurographic recordings were made during episodes of spontaneous and evoked paresthesias and pain in man. In each instance spontaneous and evoked discharges were observed, particularly in fibers that were thought to be unmyelinated and therefore probably nociceptors [32–37].

An example of this approach is the study of Nystrom and Hagbarth [34] in which abnormal paroxysmal activity was observed in the peroneal and median nerve fibers of two amputees with ongoing pain in their phantom foot and hand respectively. This discharge was augmented by percussion of the neuroma, a maneuver which in both cases produced a Tinel sign and accentuated the phantom pain. Local anesthetic infiltration of the nerve-end neuroma abolished the mechanosensitivity of the axons and the mechanically evoked sensation. Much of the ongoing discharge and pain persisted, however, suggesting the involvement of additional, more proximal ectopic sources (*see below*).

QUALITY OF NEUROPATHIC SENSATION

Experimental nerve injury: types of fibers/patterns of discharge

From experiments on dorsal versus ventral roots, on nerves that are purely cutaneous, and on mixed nerves following de-efferentation, it is clear that the great bulk of spontaneous neuroma activity is generated in sensory, rather than in motor or autonomic, fibers. Measurements of axon conduction velocity in early rat neuromas show that A-αβ and A-δ afferents are represented according to their numbers in the nerve. Spontaneously active C afferents are under-represented at short postoperative times and over-represented at long postoperative times [38,39]. Thus, in rat neuromas of long standing, the spontaneous ectopic barrage is dominated by C fibers.

Most spontaneously active neuroma A afferents (about 90% in rats) discharge rhythmically, with highly regular intervals between adjacent impulses within a train (Figure 3.1b). This is the firing pattern that is expected of intrinsic electrogenesis at a single active pacemaker site ('autorhythmicity'). Spontaneous firing rates usually range from 15 to 30 Hz, but can rise to > 200 Hz on mechanical stimulation. To generate such rates in normal afferents requires a substantial sensory stimulus. In just over one-third of the rhythmic firing fibers, the discharge is interrupted by silent pauses, resulting in a 'bursty' pattern (*see* Figure 3.6). Bursty firing has also been noted in microneurographic studies in humans (references in the previous section). Occasionally, fibers with complex cycling rhythms are encountered. Finally, some A fibers fire in a slow irregular pattern. Curiously, nearly all spontaneously active C fibers, in rat neuromas at least, have a slow, irregular discharge pattern [39]. This suggests that there may be some interesting differences in the mechanism of electrogenesis in A versus C fibers that might be exploitable therapeutically.

It is reasonable to assume that the quality of sensation generated at ectopic sources in injured nerve bears a close relationship to the types of sensory fibers that contribute to the afferent barrage. Unfortunately, it has not been ascertained in experimental neuroma preparations whether all of the different sensory receptor types contribute equally or whether certain types predominate. The experimental problem, of course, is that the identity of the peripheral receptor is lost when the nerve is cut. Animals with chronic neuromas frequently exhibit self-attack ('autotomy'), a probable behavioral indicator of anesthesia dolorosa [40], and acute palpation of neuromas elicits vocalization and escape behavior.

Sensory quality of neuropathic symptoms: clinical perspective

In patients, the intense sensation experienced upon firm percussion of a neuroma is often likened to an electric shock 'shooting' along the course of the nerve. Electric shocks differ from natural somatic stimuli in that they activate all types of sensory axons in near synchroneity and at a uniform frequency determined by the power source (usually 50 or 60 Hz). Natural stimuli (burn, touch, prick) produce a symphony of afferent activity. The 'unnatural' electric shock-like sensation evoked by a sharp rap on a neuroma is therefore understandable in terms of brief, synchronous activation of perhaps all fiber types.

In a mixed nerve, the quality of ongoing sensation, or sensation following moderate neuroma stimulation, ranges widely among individuals and over time. When a particular, recognizable, sensation is experienced, we presume that the afferent fiber types that dominate are those activated during the corresponding natural stimulus – thermal and polymodal nociceptors in the case of burning pain, muscular or periosteal nociceptors for cramping, stabbing pain, type II slowly adapting mechanoreceptors for dull pressure, etc. [41,42]. Sometimes, of course, the sensation does not mimic everyday experience and is simply called paresthesia or dysesthesia. Here, some atypical mix of afferent types and firing patterns is presumably present. Abnormal central processing of abnormal afferent signals probably has a further distorting role.

For more specialized types of nerves the quality of the sensation evoked by ectopic electrogenesis is, of course, expected to correspond to the type of nerve involved. A deep, cramping-type sensation might be expected of ectopic pacemakers along a muscle nerve (e.g. neurogenic myalgia, fibrositis, temporomandibular joint (TMJ) syndrome, myofascial pain), whereas a more superficial sensation such as 'pins-and-needles' would be typical of injured cutaneous nerves. Certain recognizable disease entities may be characterized by the quality of sensation felt and these, in turn, presumably reflect the particular afferent fiber types most involved (e.g. burning pain in causalgia). Injury to visceral nerves such as may occur in intra-abdominal operative procedures, or during cardiac ischemia, may result in deep, poorly localized pains, often with distant reference [43].

Indeed, the hypothesis of ectopic pacemakers as a prime mover in nerve pathophysiology can be extended to a number of diseases that go beyond the range of somatovisceral sensation. Thus, one may speculate that ectopic discharge in an injured auditory nerve could be a cause of tinnitus, in the vestibular nerve vertigo, and in the glossopharyngeal and vagus nerves nausea, and cardiovascular and enteric disturbances.

Experimental neuromas: variability in the amount of spontaneous neuroma discharge

The amount of ectopic discharge observed in experimentally damaged nerves is often very different from preparation to preparation and an analysis of the sources of this variability holds out hope of understanding the reasons for the tremendous variability in sensory symptoms among human nerve-injury patients. A number of controlling variables have already been identified.

Time since the injury

From the earliest quantitative measurements of neuroma electrogenesis it was clear that the amount of discharge depends heavily on the time since nerve injury [10]. In rat sciatic nerve, for example, there is virtually no spontaneous activity from the time that the acute 'injury discharge' dies down (seconds to a few minutes) until the third postoperative day. Activity in A fibers then rises to high levels for about two weeks, with nearly 25% active. Subsequently, the A-fiber discharge falls back to a lower, but sustained level.

Afferent fiber type

In the rat neuroma model, spontaneous activity in afferent C fibers emerges only as activity in A fibers begins to decline. Thus, during the first few postoperative weeks the neuroma is dominated by A-fiber activity, which is later superseded by C-fiber activity.

Nerve studied

We have found that peak spontaneous activity levels in neuromas of the saphenous nerve in rats were consistently lower than in the sciatic nerve (M. Devor, unpublished data).

Species of animal

The natural history of spontaneous discharge of A afferents in CBA-strain mouse sciatic nerve resembles that of (Sabra-strain) rats except that two early peaks can be distinguished [12]. Nerves of random-bred cats, however, yield a substantially different natural history [13]. Rabbits, apparently, produce little or no ectopic neuroma discharge (S. J. W. Lisney and J. Diamond, personal communication). The natural history of ectopic neuroma activity in baboon and in man has not yet been determined.

Individual differences and genetic predisposition

Even when figures are taken from A fibers in a single nerve, in male rats of uniform age there is still substantial animal-to-animal variability in the percentage incidence of spontaneous activity. One of the most striking quantitative differences between the various experimental preparations is the variability between different strains of rats. Following behavioral clues (autotomy), Devor *et al.* [44] examined neuromas of Lewis-strain rats and found them to be much less active, on average, than neuromas of Sabra-strain rats. First-generation offspring of Sabra × Lewis parents had low levels of activity resembling the Lewis parent (Figure 3.3). Together, these observations indicate substantial genetic variability in the propensity of injured sensory fibers to develop ectopic hyperexcitability.

Variability of pain symptoms: clinical perspective

In the clinic, the tremendous variability of chronic pain symptoms among individuals with apparently similar injuries has been a constant source of mystery. Indeed, this observation routinely raises the suspicion of 'hidden agendas' with respect to patients whose suffering appears to be excessive. Without minimizing the role of social variables such as attention seeking, pending litigation, or outright hypochondria, the possibility of substantial individual variability in the underlying nerve pathophysiology should not be neglected.

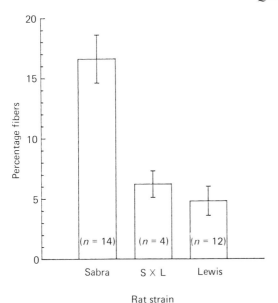

Figure 3.3 Genetic variability of ectopic hyperexcitability in experimental nerve-end neuromas. Comparison of the percentage of neuroma A fibers with spontaneous discharge (mean ± s.e.m.) in neuromas of Sabra-strain rats, Lewis-strain rats, and F1 hybrids 3–16 days after operation. (From Devor, M., Inbal, R. and Govrin-Lippmann, R. Genetic factors in the development of chronic pain. In *Genetics of the Brain* (ed. I. Lieblich), Elsevier, Amsterdam, pp. 273–296 (1982), with permission)

It is obviously difficult, perhaps impossible using the usual epidemiologic approaches, to determine whether a tendency to develop neuropathic pain has an important heritable component. Family and cross-cultural studies do show correlated differences in pain response [45,46] but these are generally interpreted as reflecting effects of socialization. Nor can one expect to find matched nerve lesions in many individuals in a family lineage, or among homozygous twins (but *see* [47]).

The one clinical fact that does suggest an inherent individual predisposition for developing pathophysiologic nerve responses is the outcome of repeat injuries in the same individual. The logic is simple. If a particular type of injury, say below-the-knee amputation, yields chronic pain of a certain intensity in, say 10% of cases, then after re-operation only 10% of these, or 1% of the original amputees, ought to be left in pain. Clinical experience shows, however, that if pain developed once it often does so again – so often, in fact, that re-operation should, in practice, usually be avoided [43]. We are not aware of statistical data on whether the occurrence of neuropathic pain in one nerve is associated with an elevated likelihood of pain if a second nerve is subsequently injured. Certainly, it is common for one site to be painful and the second benign. The sural nerve, for example, is commonly sacrificed to provide material for cable grafting in painful nerve injuries in the arm, without giving rise to obvious neuropathic pain in the calf. This is to be expected, however, from the experimental finding of different levels of ectopic electrogenesis in different nerves.

The question of heritability of neuropathic pain in man is not resolved. This factor, more than any other, could account for the gross variability of sensory symptoms in the human patient population.

Experimental nerve injury: chemo- and thermosensitivity

Once ectopic pacemaker *capability* has developed in damaged nerve fibers, a broad range of chemical, physical and metabolic factors that influence nerve membrane potential can excite repetitive discharge. Mechanosensitivity, and the Tinel sign, were mentioned above. Other examples include ischemia, anoxia (Figure 3.4) increased extracellular K^+, pharmacologic blockade of K^+ conductances, various peptides and related neuroactive substances [9,12,13,48–55].

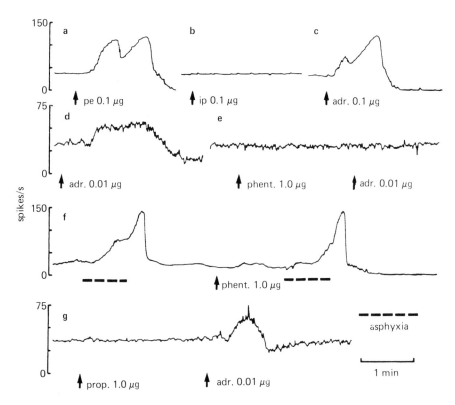

Figure 3.4 Effect of α- and β-adrenergic agonists and antagonists on the discharge of single neuroma axons in the rat. a–c, excitation by close-arterially injected phenylephrine (pe, an α-agonist) and adrenaline (adr.), but not isoprenalin (ip, a β-agonist); d–g, excitation by adrenaline is blocked by phentolamine (phent., an α-antagonist), but not propanolol (prop., a β-antagonist); f, phentolamine did not block excitation caused by asphyxia. (From Korenman, E. M. D. and Devor, M. Ectopic adrenergic sensitivity in damaged peripheral nerve axons in the rat. *Experimental Neurology*, **72**, 63–81 (1981), with permission)

A particularly interesting example, and one not easily predictable a priori, is the fact that many afferents in experimental neuromas are excited by systemic or close arterially injected sympathomimetics, and by electrical stimulation of sympathetic efferent nerves. Use of selective pharmacologic agonists and antagonists indicates mediation by α-adrenergic receptors (Figure 3.3). Sympathetic excitation is not due simply to vasoconstriction-induced asphyxia, but rather appears to reflect a direct action of α-agonists on injured afferents [9,48,56].

Another type of sensitivity in neuroma afferents that could shed light on neuralgia symptomatology is the response to warming and cooling. In myelinated neuroma fibers, the rate of spontaneous discharge increases with warming and additional, previously silent, fibers are recruited. Cooling suppresses firing. Unmyelinated axons, in contrast, tend to be suppressed by warming and excited by cooling [55] (Figure 3.5).

It is important to emphasize that these various sensitivities are not a characteristic of normal or acutely injured sensory nerve fibers in mid-nerve, but develop ectopically as a consequence of injury. The primary change is the development of ectopic pacemaker capability; aggravating stimuli merely activate the pacemaker.

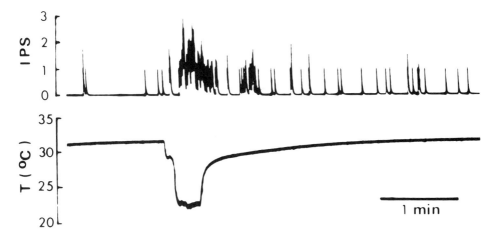

Figure 3.5 This neuroma C fiber was excited by cooling the neuroma. IPS, impulses/s. (From Matzner, O. and Devor, M. Contrasting thermal sensitivity of spontaneously active A- and C-fibers in experimental nerve-end neuromas. *Pain*, **30**, 373–384 (1987) with permission)

Aggravating factors in neuropathic pain: clinical perspective

Reflex sympathetic dystrophy (RSD)

A range of painful neuropathic conditions with sympathetic involvement are grouped under the heading RSD. These include causalgia (burning pain), Sudek's atrophy, the shoulder–hand syndrome and others ([57] and *see*, for example, Chapter 5). The main indications of sympathetic involvement are vasomotor and sudomotor symptoms (cold sweaty limb, or hot dry limb), 'trophic' changes in skin texture and in the growth of nails, and the impressive relief provided by surgical sympathetic ganglionectomy or regional intravenous administration of the peripheral sympatholytic drug guanethidine [58].

The unique interaction of efferent (sympathetic) and afferent (sensory) indicators in RSD has provoked a great deal of theoretical discussion, to which the new data on adrenergic chemosensitivity in experimentally injured nerve adds a new dimension. Specificaly, it has been suggested that sympathetic outflow releases noradrenalin from endings of sympathetic efferents trapped at the site of injury and at disseminated microneuromas further distally, and that this activates ectopic pacemaker activity in afferents that have developed ectopic adrenergic chemosensitivity. [50].

This theory neatly accounts for ongoing pain referred to the limb, and for its relief by sympathectomy. It does not, however, account for the extreme sensitivity of the skin to weak stimuli (allodynia). This symptom requires additional factors, such as surviving afferent endings in skin becoming hyperexcitable under the influence of injury and/or sympathetic efferent activity, or sympathetically mediated crosstalk among low- and high-threshold afferents. Case reports of RSD following CNS damage [59], assuming that they do not involve peripheral trauma as well, remain unexplained.

Vascular insufficiency and cold intolerance

In recordings from the ulnar nerve in healthy subjects, Ochoa and Torebjork [33] observed spontaneous high-frequency firing from nerve fibers following production of ischemia by a 20 min suprasystolic inflation of a blood-pressure cuff. This remained after ulnar nerve block central to the recording site, indicating a peripheral source, presumably intact sensory receptors in the skin. The spontaneous discharges correlated with paresthesias reported by the subject.

Cold weather is often listed among the aggravating factors in both phantom and stump pain, even in well-perfused amputation stumps [60]. Similarly, vascular insufficiency combined with nerve trauma, such as stump pain in diabetic amputees, is often notoriously painful. In the clinical setting it is often impossible to unravel these two effects. Poor circulation in an extremity usually lowers temperature, and exposure to cold often triggers peripheral vasoconstriction with corresponding vascular insufficiency. The ectopic neural pacemaker hypothesis predicts that both ought to be painful, on the grounds that ischemia and anoxia globally activate ectopic discharge in experimental neuromas, and that cold selectively activates damaged C fibers [48,55].

ECTOPIC ELECTROGENESIS IN DEMYELINATED AXONS

Experimental demyelination

Demyelination *per se* is expected to reduce fiber excitability to the extent of causing conduction block. However, molecular reorganization of the demyelinated axolemma can lead to renewal of conduction [61–63] and even to elevated local excitability. Axons that have been experimentally demyelinated, but are otherwise in continuity, may develop bursting spontaneous discharge, mechanosensitivity and afterdischarge that closely resembles ectopic neuroma activity [64–67]. Indeed, as neuroma formation does not occur in the absence of myelin disorganization, some of the pathophysiologic properties of neuromas could, in fact, be associated with demyelination.

Positive sensory symptoms in demyelinating disease

Demyelinating neuropathies and nerve entrapment

A number of peripheral demyelinating neuropathies present positive sensory symptoms together with the characteristic sensory and motor loss. An example is neuropathic and/or radiculopathic pain in the sensory variety of the Guillain–Barré syndrome (acute inflammatory demyelinating polyradiculopathy). Approximately 12 weeks after a non-specific viral illness, patients develop severe lancinating girdle pains [68,69]. The pain may be constant with phasic accentuations. However, paroxysms of pain do occur either spontaneously or in response to mechanical stimulation. Postinfectious and post-vaccination brachial plexopathy are additional painful conditions associated with peripheral demyelination.

Local demyelination is often produced by chronic pressure from mechanical nerve entrapment. In the carpal tunnel syndrome, for example, percussion of the entrapped and partly demyelinated median nerve gives rise to tingling paresthesias radiating into the median fingers, much as is encountered when pressing over a divided nerve early in regeneration. Ischemia produced by inflating a pressure cuff around the upper arm to above systolic pressures often increases the pain. In entrapment neuropathies or radiculopathies, sensitivity may also be present at a distance from the actual site of injury. Thus, in radicular pain secondary to a herniated low lumbar disk, there is often tenderness to palpation at the sciatic notch or along the sciatic nerve in the thigh [70]. We interpret this symptom as reflecting mechanosensitivity of regenerating sprouts freely growing, or arrested in disseminated microneuromas.

In microneurographic recordings from a patient with entrapment of the ulnar nerve at the elbow, Nordin *et al.* [36] observed ectopic multi-unit nerve activity correlating in intensity and time course to the sensations (Tinel's sign) evoked by tapping the nerve. Similar abnormal nerve discharges were recorded in a patient with thoracic outlet syndrome when paresthesias were evoked by elevating the arm.

Tumors (neurofibromas) along the course of nerves are generally painless, but they may be associated with pain if they form in an enclosed space and apply chronic pressure to a nerve or root. The same is true for non-neural space-occupying tumors that impinge on nerve or roots. Once again, it is not the pressure *per se*, but the pathophysiologic increase in nerve excitability that is the primary change.

Diabetic neuropathy, and several of the toxic neuropathies (e.g. arsenic and thallium neuropathy) produce disseminated demyelination and positive sensory symptoms including paresthesias and pain [69]. To the best of our knowledge, microneurographic recordings have not yet been performed in such cases. Burchiel *et al.* [71] have observed abnormal electrogenesis in an animal model of diabetic neuropathy. Finally, bacterial infection of nerve can cause a polyneuritis with disseminated myelin damage and pain.

Demyelination in the CNS may also be a source of positive sensory symptoms. Spinal cord white matter lesions in multiple sclerosis (MS), for example, are often accompanied by paresthesias, or burning or tingling pain quite similar to that seen in the demyelinating peripheral neuropathies [72,73]. If a plaque in the dorsal column were the origin of such activity, abnormal impulse discharges generated there would propagate centrally causing sensory symptoms, and also antidromically, out along corresponding peripheral nerves. Nordin *et al.* [36] took advantage of this bidirectional conduction and made microneurographic recordings from the median nerve in an MS patient with Lhermitte's sign. Abnormal, presumably antidromic, discharges were observed in close correlation with paresthesias felt in the hand upon neck flexion [36].

Cranial neuralgias and tic douloureux

One of the current concepts of the pathophysiology of trigeminal and related cranial neuralgias stresses vascular compression of the nerve root [74] and, indeed, decompression and mechanical separation of the root from the vessel can be an effective treatment [75]. As noted, root compression *per se* is not expected to provoke action potentials. However, sustained compression does produce local demyelination [76]. The resulting ectopic pacemaker region would then be capable of spontaneous firing, of afterdischarge following activity evoked at peripheral 'trigger points' and of discharge evoked by mechanical pounding of the vessel on the ectopic pacemaker site itself. Note again the dual effects of the compressing blood vessel. Removal of the mechanical component of excitation by separation of the root from the vessel yields immediate relief of symptoms due to mechanosensitivity. Sensory consequences of ectopic spontaneous electrogenesis in the root, and of neuralgia attacks triggered from the skin (afterdischarge), subside over the next few days as remyelination proceeds. The question of how, according to this hypothesis, ectopic activity in large-diameter myelinated axons can evoke pain is discussed below.

Symptomatically typical trigeminal neuralgia may also occur in patients with MS. Demyelinating plaques in these cases are located in the pontine tegmentum, among other locations, suggesting involvement of ascending second-order trigeminal fibers [77].

ECTOPIC ELECTROGENESIS IN DORSAL ROOT GANGLIA (DRGs)

Discharge originating in DRGs in experimental preparations

In contrast to sensory axons in nerve trunks, sensory cell somata in DRGs normally possess pacemaker capability and will fire in response to mechanical distortion even without any conditioning injury. Indeed, a small number discharge spontaneously [64,78]. The incidence of spontaneous and evoked DRG discharge, however, is significantly augmented by chronic peripheral nerve injury. Thus, after nerve injury, the DRG makes a significant contribution to the ectopic afferent barrage over and above that generated by ectopic neuroma pacemaker sites [14,78–80] (Figures 3.1a, 3.7c and d).

The endogenous pacemaker capability of DRG neurons may be particularly problematic when the cell has been infected with certain strains of herpes simplex virus. Mayer and collaborators [81] have recently shown that such infections can cause DRG cells to become electrically coupled in a syncytium. This, of course, would tend to amplify both ectopically and naturally generated impulse activity, and cause it to spread beyond the population of neurons in which it was initially evoked.

DRG as a source of neuropathic and radiculopathic pain: clinical perspective

Spinal trauma

Except in the case of sharp percussion, acute pressure on peripheral nerves or sensory roots does not produce impulses or sensation. Chronic pressure, of course, induces ectopic pacemaker development and mechanosensitivity as discussed above. In contrast, acute pressure or traction on sensory ganglia, such as may result from intervertebral disk herniation or frank displacement of a vertebra, does produce impulses and typically causes acute pain which persists. If the spinal nerve or root is involved, an additional axonally derived component of abnormal afferent discharge may be recruited subsequently.

Specific clinical evidence of this comes from microneurographic recordings made by Nordin *et al.* [36] in a man with L5–S1 herniated disk and radiculopathic pain in the foot. Mechanical stretch applied to the root/DRG/spinal nerve by flexing the neck, putting the chin on the chest, evoked intense paresthesias in the leg. Correlated with this sensation were bursts of (antidromic) impulses recorded in the sural nerve. Note that all three ectopic impulse generators (root, DRG and spinal nerve) produce dermatomal reference; it is, therefore, not trivial to identify the principal source. Similarly, treatment aimed at one source, say decompression of the DRG, may not totally relieve symptoms.

Nerve injury

The fact that peripheral nerve block central to the site of injury sometimes does not relieve sensory symptoms even for the duration of the block is frequently taken as evidence of a CNS process. A prominent example is the amputation phantom. This conclusion, however, ignores the effect of nerve injury on ectopic DRG activity. In contrast to DRG involvement following spinal trauma, in which all elements of the ganglion are equally likely to fire abnormally, nerve injury will lead to excess discharge only in those DRG neurons that have actually been axotomized. Therefore, reference is expected to follow the peripheral distribution of the nerve, and not the dermatomal distribution of the DRGs that are the heart of the problem. For this reason the attention of the physician is naturally drawn to the injured nerve, and after failing to obtain relief with nerve block, to the CNS!

Diagnostic distinction between DRG and CNS processes could, in principle, be accomplished by local anesthetic block of the relevant DRGs or dorsal roots (note the plurals) although, in practise, care would have to be taken to avoid spread to the spinal cord. Another possible approach is the use of peripheral microneurographic recording combined with appropriate nerve blocks. For example, Nystrom and Hagbarth [34] recorded ongoing neural activity in the median nerve of a hand amputee with phantom limb pain. Local anesthetic block of the nerve end neuroma eliminated mechanically evoked discharges and Tinel's sign, as mentioned above, but did not eliminate the ongoing activity or the phantom. DRG activity is a prime suspect in this patient. Spinal root or DRG block was not performed.

Dorsal rhizotomy is said not always to be effective in relieving phantom limb and other neuropathic pains [82], an observation that, if correct, would tend to exclude peripheral sources, whether in the nerve, DRG or spinal root. Before a general conclusion can be reached from such clinical observations, however, it is essential to document that all of the relevant roots have been cut. This criterion has rarely been met. Furthermore, it is necessary to ascertain that rhizotomy has not actually eliminated the original neuropathic pain, and at the same time replaced it with a new, true deafferentation phantom of the sort that occurs in paraplegics and during spinal anesthesia [83,84]. The difference between the original and the new pain may not necessarily be volunteered by the patient, who may not be aware of, or interested in, the significance of the distinction. Information of this sort can only be obtained by detailed clinical documentation of symptoms both before and after the rhizotomy.

Postherpetic neuralgia

After herpes zoster infection of DRGs, postherpetic neuralgia may develop in a dermatomal distribution in the partially anesthetic skin some 4–6 weeks following the herpetic eruption [85]. There are two components to the pain: a deep burning or aching sensation which serves as a constant background, and a superficial one which is characterized by dysesthesias and sharp lancinating spontaneous bursts, and bursts triggered by touch. The congruity of dermatomal symptoms and the location of virus-infected DRGs, suggests the possible involvement of the DRG as an impulse source (*see* Chapter 9).

AMPLIFICATION MECHANISMS ASSOCIATED WITH ECTOPIC NEURAL PACEMAKERS

Afterdischarge, and the significance of 'threshold for repetitive firing'

The concept of a 'threshold' for neural excitation is well known. As the strength of a stimulus pulse is gradually increased there comes a level where the fiber suddenly fires an all-or-none action potential on each pulse; this is its threshold. Less well known is the concept of 'threshold for repetitive firing' at pacemaker sites. Most neural pacemakers are incapable of firing at very low frequencies. With weak stimulation (tonic depolarization), the pacemaker is silent. As the depolarization is gradually increased there comes a level where repetitive firing begins. At this 'threshold', firing rate jumps suddenly from zero to a substantial rate (say, about 20 impulses per second for a neuroma fiber). Beyond this point, additional increases in stimulation strength produce gradually increasing firing rates (Figure 3.6). The important point is the non-linearity at rhythmic threshold [86,87]. Starting at a

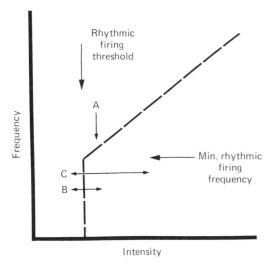

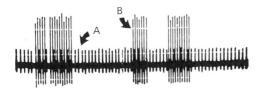

Figure 3.6 Sketch of the normal relationship between generator potential (steady-state stimulus intensity) and discharge frequency in neural pacemakers. Note the sharp non-linearity where firing rate jumps from zero to the minimum rhythmic firing frequency. An ectopic pacemaker site with a stable suprathreshold membrane potential is expected to produce tonic rhythmic discharge like the axon marked A. A pacemaker with membrane potential straddling the rhythmic firing threshold is expected to produce on-off, or bursty discharge like fiber B. Membrane potential trajectories like C yield discharge patterns such as in Figure 3.7b

point just below threshold, a very slight increase in stimulus strength produces a very large increase in response. Correspondingly, starting from a point just above rhythmic threshold, a very slight decrease in stimulus strength may yield a very large decrease in response. Ectopic neural pacemakers in injured and demyelinated nerves, dorsal roots and DRGs tend to be placed very near rhythmic threshold; they are, therefore, often subject to this amplification effect [14,54,67].

Neuroma fibers with bursting discharge are good examples. They appear to be straddling rhythmic firing threshold, sometimes above threshold and sometimes below (Figure 3.6). Some fibers rest just below rhythmic threshold, such as the one illustrated in Figure 3.7b. A brief stimulus, mechanical or electrical, sent this fiber into rhythmic firing which continued long after the stimulus had ceased ('afterdischarge'). The stimulus had not so much evoked the prolonged response as it had engaged the built-in rhythmic firing tendency of the ectopic pacemaker. Curiously, for about a minute at the end of each barrage the repetitive firing mechanism of the fiber became refractory, and single-stimulus pulses during this period evoked only single-impulse responses. The resemblance of this behavior to the refractoriness of trigger points in trigeminal neuralgia following a paroxysmal attack may be more than just coincidental.

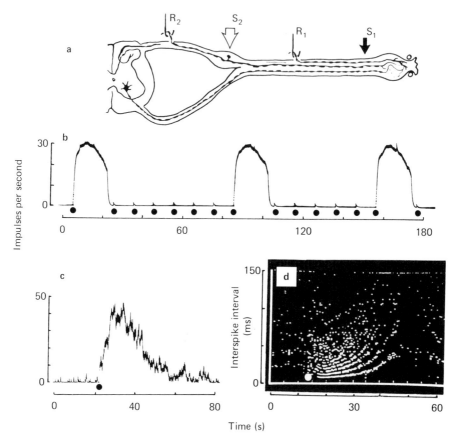

Figure 3.7 Afterdischarge at ectopic neuroma and DRG pacemaker sites. The fiber in b (recorded from position R1 in panel a) did not fire spontaneously, but produced about 20 s of rhythmic discharge when stimulated (S1, black dots) by a single 0.1 ms electrical pulse (or a brief mechanical stimulus – not shown). The pacemaker was refractory for about 1 min after each such paroxysmal burst. The fiber in c and d (recorded from position R2 in panel a) had slow, irregular spontaneous discharge generated at a DRG pacemaker site. A single 0.5 s mechanical probe of the DRG (150 mg von Frey hair) triggered elevated discharge for > 1 min. Discharge pattern during the burst is shown in d where each white dot indicates a single action potential, height above the abscissa indicating the interval since the previous action potential. Dots close to the abscissa indicate short interspike intervals and therefore high firing rate. (From Devor, M. The pathophysiology of damaged peripheral nerves. In: *Textbook of Pain* (eds. P. D. Wall and R. Melzack), Churchill Livingstone, Edinburgh, pp 63–81 (1989), with permission)

Amplification by 'extra spikes'

Calvin *et al.* [88], proposed an additional mode of impulse multiplication in damaged nerves. Their argument begins with the fact that the duration of the absolute refractory period in mammalian myelinated axons is only slightly longer than that of the action potential itself [89]. Therefore, if the duration of a propagating impulse were to increase in a pathologic condition, the broadened action potential might re-excite the membrane it had just passed over. This re-excitation would send an 'extra spike' in the reverse direction down the axon. Many such sites along the length of an axon – patches of myelin disruption, for example – could create reverberation, and a shower of 'extra spikes' every time a normal one propagated up the axon. Specific evidence for 'extra spike' production has been obtained experimentally at sites of focal demyelination and at the T junction of DRGs [66,88,90,91].

'Hyperpathia': clinical perspective

The quality of sensation is peculiar in a broad range of neuropathic conditions. In addition to sensory modality (e.g. light touch evoking pain) there may be peculiarities in time and space. For example, sensation may appear after a delay and then rapidly build up to an explosive crescendo, aftersensation may be present, response to repeated stimuli may wind up, and it may radiate beyond the immediate site of stimulation. Symptoms of this sort identify 'hyperpathia' [92]. Although generally ascribed to changes in CNS processing of sensory signals, many of the hyperpathic phenomena, particularly explosiveness, wind up and aftersensation, bear a striking resemblance to threshold behavior and afterdischarge in ectopic neural pacemakers. The same is true for other neuropathic and radiculopathic conditions involving paroxysmal pain and aftersensation, such as tic douloureux, or glossopharyngeal neuralgia.

Functional crosstalk between nerve fibers in experimental preparations

One of the most problematic features of neuropathic pain is the frequent occurrence of pain upon weak stimulation of the skin or other peripheral tissues ('allodynia') [1] where the stimulus is applied away from ectopic pacemaker sites associated with the injured nerve. The classic interpretation of such cutaneous hypersensibility is sensitization of peripheral cutaneous nociceptor endings [93] and this explanation is probably correct in some conditions [37]. However, recent data based on the timing of abnormal sensation, selective nerve block and microneurographic recording ([94,95] and *see* Chapter 2) suggest that sensitization is frequently not the correct explanation. Another possibility, short of abnormal CNS processing, is intermodal crosstalk in the periphery.

'Crossed afterdischarge'

As discussed above, 'afterdischarge' at ectopic pacemaker sites reflects the prolonged engagement of a fiber's endogenous rhythmic firing capability by a momentary mechanical, electrical or other stimulus applied directly to the pace-maker. The brief stimulus kicks the pacemaker from just below rhythmic firing threshold to just above (Figure 3.6). Recent experimental data show that the same endogenous rhythmic firing mechanisms can also be engaged by impulse activity in neighboring fibers. An example is illustrated in Figure 3.8. Here, the spontaneous rate of discharge of a neuroma fiber was increased for nearly 30 s as a result of a 5 s burst of activity in its neighbors. The fiber itself was not stimulated. This phenomenon, which we call 'crossed afterdischarge' [54,96], reflects an effective breakdown in the normal insulation of nerve fibers one from another at sites of injury. Note the potential for excitation of one fiber type by activity in others. Such intermodal crosstalk surely distorts sensory quality.

Note, too, that after the end of the intense period of firing in the fiber in Figure 3.8, the discharge rate temporarily fell below baseline. The most likely explanation is that intense firing hyperpolarizes the pacemaker, presumably due to sodium pumping or activation of a prolonged, activity-related potassium current (e.g. $g^{K^+}_{Ca^{2+}}$. This suppression may contribute to the temporary relief of neuropathic pain symptoms following high-frequency transcutaneous electrical nerve stimula-tion (TENS), and may explain the refractoriness of trigger points in trigeminal neuralgia in the aftermath of a paroxysmal attack.

Crossed afterdischarge always involves repetitive firing and a gradual build up of activity with time; it is distinctly different from 'ephaptic crosstalk' discussed next. The mechanism underlying crossed afterdischarge appears to be activation of the fiber in question by depolarizing substances released locally as a result of impulse activity in the neighbors. Many substances are potentially involved, including potassium ions, neuroactive peptides and catecholamines (as discussed above with

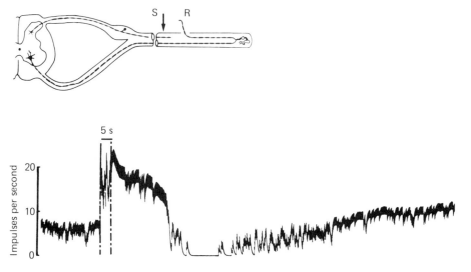

Figure 3.8 Crossed afterdischarge in a neuroma afferent. This fiber, recorded at position R, fired spontaneously at about 7 Hz. Five seconds of stimulation (S, 100 Hz) to neighboring axons in the nerve, but not the recorded fiber itself, increased the firing rate for 25–30 s followed by aftersuppression. (From Lisney, S. J. W. and Devor, M. Afterdischarge and interactions among fibers in damaged peripheral nerve in the rat. *Brain Research*, **415**, 122–136 (1987), with permission)

respect to sympathetic coupling and reflex sympathetic dystrophy). Interestingly, some fibers show depression upon repetitive activity of neighbors, suggesting that some endogenous substance(s) released from nerves can hyperpolarize and suppress ectopic neural pacemakers [96]. The identity of the substance(s) is obviously of interest.

Electrical ('ephaptic') crosstalk

An additional form of fiber-to-fiber interaction characteristic of neuromas and demyelination plaques in nerves and spinal roots is 'ephaptic (electrical) crosstalk'. In the mid-1940s Granit and Skoglund [97] discovered that acute transection can short-circuit neighboring axons in a nerve so that current from the cut end of one fiber can excite others. This acute ephaptic coupling is unlikely to be of much functional significance, however, because it decays and vanishes within minutes. However, it has recently been discovered that, several weeks after injury, ephaptic crosstalk once again develops but now in an enduring form [98].

An example of 'ephaptic' crosstalk is given in Figure 3.9. Here electrical stimulation of dorsal root fibers ending in a sciatic nerve neuroma evoked a time-locked impulse in a single axon contained in a fine ventral root filament (Figure 3.9a). Stimulation of the ventral root filament, in turn, drove the coupled axon in the dorsal root (Figure 3.9b). Such high safety-factor, bidirectional ephaptic crosstalk occurs in nerve-end neuromas [15,98–102] in regenerating nerve far distal to the site of injury [98] and in patches of demyelination [65,101]. It appears to be a consequence of close membrane appositions [18,101,102] with consequent passage of current directly from one member of a coupled axon pair into the other. As the coupled fibers are frequently of different types, this is another mechanism whereby nociceptors might become activated following stimulation of low-threshold sensory afferents. Electrical coupling in virus-infected DRG cell syncytia [81] was mentioned above.

Augmented dorsal root reflex

Impulses that propagate into the spinal terminals of afferent fibers partially depolarize the terminals of their neighbors [103]. A small minority of afferent terminals are so intensely depolarized that they reach threshold and generate propagated action potentials (the dorsal root reflex). This, then, is an additional form of fiber-to-fiber crosstalk. Calvin *et al.* [88] suggested that augmentation of the dorsal root reflex could account for pain elicited by stimulation of low-threshold trigeminal afferents in tic douloureux. Unfortunately, recent data indicating that primary afferent depolarization and the dorsal root reflex are substantially *reduced* by peripheral nerve trauma do not favor this hypothesis [104,105].

Fiber-to-fiber crosstalk: clinical perspective

The surprising link between sensation and sympathetic efferent activity was discussed above in the context of noradrenalin-related crossed afterdischarge and reflex sympathetic dystrophy. Functional crosstalk based on crossed afterdischarge

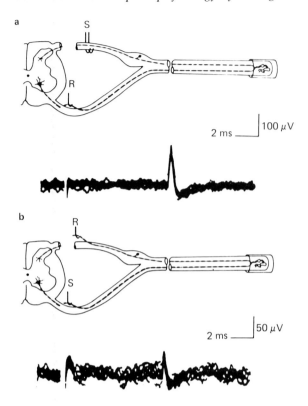

Figure 3.9 Bidirectional ephaptic (electrical) crosstalk be-tween two axons in a nerve-end neuroma. R,S, as in Figure 3.8. a, Stimulation of dorsal root fibers; b, stimulation of ventral root filament (*see text*). (Modified from Seltzer, Z. and Devor, M. Ephaptic transmission in chronically damaged peripheral nerves. *Neurology*, **29**, 1061–1064 (1979), with permission)

involving other mediators (particularly potassium and peptides) may well prove to play an important part in allodynia and hyperalgesia. Specifically, activity evoked in low-threshold afferents by gentle stroking of the skin could activate nociceptive fibers upstream along the nerve by crossed afterdischarge. The same holds for ephaptic interactions in injured and demyelinated nerves and roots.

Regional spread, as in hyperpathia, is an additional peculiarity of sensation which, in principle, could be accounted for in terms of fiber-to-fiber crosstalk. The clinical observation is that sensation evoked by stimulating a particular patch of skin radiates beyond it. Here, the explanation would be spread of activity from axons activated by the stimulus to passive neighbors, either by crossed afterdischar-ge or by ephaptic interactions. If the pathophysiologic process were limited to a nerve, then the maximal boundaries of sensory spread would be the peripheral distribution of the nerve. However, most peripheral nerve trunks send primary afferents in several adjacent dorsal roots, and crosstalk in the roots could therefore spread sensation across several dermatomes.

Putting it all together: tic douloureux

Trigeminal neuralgia (tic douloureux) provides a specific clinical example of what might be expected when various of the pathophysiologic features of ectopic neural pacemakers – including spontaneous electrogenesis, afterdischarge and cros-stalk – operate in tandem. In this condition, touching a specific localized trigger point in the face provokes paroxysmal 'lightning-like' pain in the distribution of one or more trigeminal divisions. The clinical history often suggests loss or block of some afferent fibers in the corresponding nerve, DRG or trigeminal root, and hints at a pathology in which ectopic pacemaker activity of the type discussed here might be expected.

Momentary light touch, or movement as during chewing, initiates attacks which outlast the stimulus by tens of seconds. This behavior recalls the amplification mechanisms of afterdischarge and 'extra spike' cascade, which, indeed, are most prominent among myelinated axons of the type that would be activated by weak stimuli. The fact that sensation spreads beyond the local trigger site recalls crosstalk in one of its various forms. When the spread is into a second trigeminal division, the crosstalk presumably occurs in the trigeminal ganglion or root. Crossed activation of neighboring nociceptive afferents would be expected to yield pain. Finally, after the end of a lightning attack, there is usually a refractory period during which the characteristic trigger stimulus is no longer effective, although there is no anesthesia and cutaneous stimuli continue to be felt. This behavior recalls the refractoriness of ectopic neural pacemakers after an intense discharge (Figure 3.7b).

In this brief exercise a few of the experimentally defined properties of ectopic pacemakers have been arranged into a constellation that efficiently accounts for most, if not all, of the clinical features of trigeminal neuralgia. Of course, many other neuropathic pain entities could be handled similarly (Table 3.1). The fact that

Table 3.1 Possible basis of some neuropathic pain states derived from experimental studies of peripheral nerve pathophysiology

Disease state	Possible pathophysiologic mechanisms (excluding CNS changes)
Trigeminal neuralgia	Ectopic electrogenesis (demyelination); afterdischarge; crosstalk (including crossed afterdischarge).
Postherpetic neuralgia	Ectopic DRG[*] discharge; DRG crosstalk; receptor sensitization (?)
Phantom limb	Ectopic neuroma discharge; ectopic DRG discharge
RSD (reflex sympathetic dystrophy)	Ectopic neuroma discharge; crosstalk; α-adrenergic chemosensitivity; receptor sensitization (?)
Compression radiculopathy	DRG mechanosensitivity; root mechanosensitivity (demyelination); afterdischarge
Tinel's sign	Mechanosensitivity of ectopic pacemaker sites (neuromas, regenerating sprouts, demyelination)

[*] DRG, dorsal root ganglion

such explanations can be generated, however, does not mean that they describe what is actually going on in the clinical entity. In particular, any reference to central changes that could also account for some or all of the symptomatology have been specifically avoided [2,106]. Such models are useful for guiding clinical investigation; they should not be misconstrued as proven fact.

MECHANISM OF CREATION OF ECTOPIC PACEMAKERS IN INJURED NERVE

The primary pathophysiologic change in injured nerve that leads to ectopic hyperexcitability, and related amplification and crosstalk phenomena, is the creation of ectopic pacemaker capability. How are ectopic pacemakers created? Although still speculative, an answer is beginning to emerge which views the process as a subtle disruption of the cellular processes that control excitability in normal nerves [38,50,107].

Repetitive firing mechanisms

The basic requirements for pacemaker capability derive from fundamental biophysical principles, and from knowledge of membrane properties at normal pacemaker sites such as the axon hillock and sensory receptors [87]. Although a number of conditions must be met, the principal one is the presence of a patch of membrane with a sufficiently large number of voltage-dependent inward current channels. In the case of peripheral nerve fibers, these are voltage-sensitive sodium channels, large glycoproteins synthesized in the cell soma and transported distally along the axon. At sensory endings, action potentials are triggered when the depolarizing generator current produced by stimulation evokes near-simultaneous opening of large numbers of sodium channels. After the end of an action potential, assuming that the generator current is sustained, the membrane depolarizes again, triggering a second and then a third action potential. A number of factors control the trajectory of the membrane potential between spikes, and hence the discharge rate and pattern.

In general, the higher the sodium-channel content, the more excitable the membrane, and the more likely is it to fire repetitive action potentials on weak and gradual depolarization. Sensory receptor endings have large numbers of sodium channels and are specialized for impulse generation. The axon membrane in mid-nerve contains only enough to fire upon sudden, intense depolarization. Therefore, it reliably propagates action potentials generated at sensory endings, but originates none.

Neuromas

Evidence concerning the mechanism of hyperexcitability in neuroma end-structures is still fragmentary, but the picture emerging is as follows. During normal metabolic housekeeping in sensory neurons, sodium channels, and other membrane-bound proteins responsible for sensory transduction and propagation, are transported down the length of the axon. Once they arrive, they are implanted in the axolemma at locations and in numbers appropriate for normal function by membrane fusion during the process of exocytosis [108]. In normal axolemma and sensory endings, the steady-state channel content is determined by the equilibrium between channel delivery and channel re-uptake. Indeed, this equilibrium is probably an important factor determining whether a normal sensory ending will be a nociceptor or a low-threshold mechanoreceptor.

After nerve injury, the equilibrium is upset. The reason proposed is that all (or most) of the channel protein originally intended to serve the entire distal axon, including the terminal sensory arbor, is now delivered to the neuroma end-bulb and sprouts. The original source now serves a much smaller sink. As a result, channels dam up in the axolemma of the neuroma, causing hyperexcitability [107,109]. This cellular model of neuroma pathophysiology is illustrated in Figure 3.10. Note that the degree of neuroma hyperexcitability, according to the model, is a function of the amount of channel protein inserted into the membrane, and the kinetics (sensitivity) of the individual channel molecules. It is at this level that genetic differences between individuals might be expressed, yielding less or more ectopic activity, and less or more pathophysiologic paresthesias and pain.

Demyelination

In mid-nerve in normal myelinated axons, sodium channels are concentrated at nodes of Ranvier; the channel density of the axolemma under the internodal myelin is much lower [110]. Following demyelination, however, sodium channel density in the internode is believed to increase, and there is a concomitant increase in electrical excitability [61–63]. As in neuromas, it is likely that internodal sodium channels represent new and additional channel protein transported from the cell body, rather than redistributed nodal channels. In any event, the increased internodal excitability is believed to be responsible for the renewal of impulse propagation and for ectopic firing.

Dorsal root ganglion cells

Just as at the cut nerve end, sodium-channel protein otherwise destined for export down the axon is expected to back up in the cell body, yielding hyperexcitability. Indeed, increased excitability based on sodium electrogenesis has been documented in a number of different cell types, including primary afferents in sensory ganglia, following axotomy or block of axoplasmic transport along the nerve [111–117].

DRUG THERAPY

The ultimate test of the ectopic pacemaker hypothesis is whether it can provide a rationale for known clinically effective treatment modalities, and predict new ones.

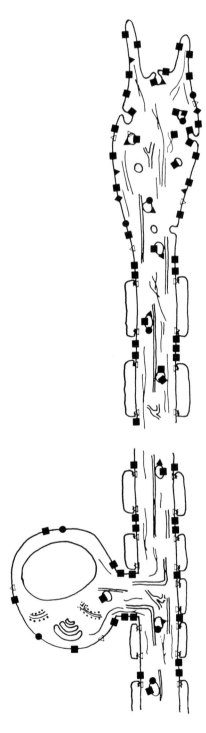

Figure 3.10 Proposed mechanism for the creation of ectopic neuroma and dorsal root ganglion (DRG) pacemaker sites in damaged nerve. Sodium channels (■) and other membrane proteins associated with electrical excitability of sensory nerve cells (▽, potassium channels; ●, calcium channels; ▲, α-adrenergic receptors; ◆, stretch-activated channels) are inserted in excess in the axolemma within the neuroma, and also in neurolemma in the DRG, because the membrane they were originally targeted for has been lost due to the injury. In other words, the source of transported proteins is too large for the residual membrane sink, resulting in channel accumulation (modified from Devor, 1983 [50])

Control of abnormal discharge in experimental neuromas

A number of approaches have proved effective at modulating ectopic electro-genesis in experimental nerve-injury models, including some with known clinical efficacy.

Corticosteroids

Depot-form corticosteroids are frequently injected into painful mechanosensitive 'trigger points' with the idea of reducing inflammation [118]. Devor *et al.* [119] showed that several commonly used steroids (triamcinolone hexacetonide, triamci-nolone diacetate, and dexamethasone) applied locally to experimental neuromas produce a profound and long-lasting suppression of spontaneous and evoked neuroma hyperexcitability. Although an anti-inflammatory action was not ruled out, the onset time was rapid, suggesting a more direct action on the axon membrane (Figure 3.11).

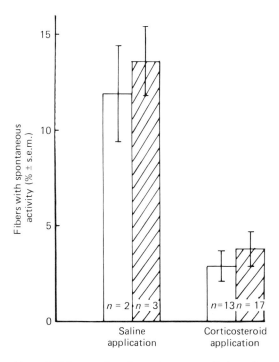

Figure 3.11 Suppression of ectopic neuroma discharge by corticosteroids applied locally at the time of the nerve injury, or several days later. ▨, Drug applied to acutely cut nerve; □, drug applied to 3–10-day neuroma. (Data from Devor, M., Govrin-Lippmann, R. and Raber, P. Corticosteroids suppress ectopic neuronal discharge ori-ginating in experimental neuromas. *Pain*, **22**, 127–137 (1985) with permission)

Sympathetic block and sympathectomy

As discussed above, afferent nerve fibers ending in experimental neuromas are sensitive to α-adrenergic agonists. Sympathetic activation is blocked by α-adrenergic antagonists, but spontaneous discharge and mechanosensitivity are not. These observations have a direct bearing on the clinical efficacy of sympathectomy in reflex sympathetic dystrophy where sympathetic activation of afferents appears to be a major contributor to pain. As sympathetic innervation is ubiquitous, sympathetic activity might be a minor contributor to pain in a wider range of neuropathic conditions. To the best of our knowledge the clinical usefulness of regional α-block in this context has never been explored.

Glycerol

Burchiel and Russell [120] found that topical glycerol suppresses experimental neuroma activity, and Rappaport *et al.* [121] showed that it suppresses autotomy, a putative behavioral indicator of anesthesia dolorosa. The injection of glycerol into the trigeminal cistern has found use in recent years in the treatment of pain in trigeminal neuralgia [122]. The mechanism of action might be reduced excitability at ectopic trigeminal pacemaker sites.

Sodium-channel blockers and anticonvulsants

Lidocaine, tetrodotoxin and other sodium-channel blockers eliminate spontaneous neuroma discharge and, at higher concentrations, nerve propagation [123]. Yaari and Devor [124] applied the anticonvulsant phenytoin (diphenylhydantoin) to experimental neuromas and reported a dose-dependent and rapidly reversible block of spontaneous discharge *without* blocking propagation (Figure 3.12). This compound is known to block sodium channels in a use-dependent (i.e. activity-dependent) manner, which should make it particularly effective against high-frequency bursty discharge.

Clinically, phenytoin, carbamazepine, and related anticonvulsants have a place in the treatment of trigeminal and other neuralgias [125]. The site of action is generally presumed to be in the CNS, but this belief needs re-evaluation. If it were possible to construct a phenytoin-like drug that did not pass the blood–brain barrier, it might prove possible to increase the dose safely and to obtain even better results.

Axoplasmic transport blockers (antimitotics)

Reasoning that the ectopic impulse generator in injured nerve fibers develops as a result of axoplasmic transport of excess channel protein, Devor and Govrin-Lippmann [38] applied the transport blockers colchicine and vinblastine to the nerve just central to the site of injury. A single application produced prolonged suppression of neuroma hyperexcitability, without blocking nerve conduction (Figure 3.13). Cutaneous and systemic application of antimitotic drugs has been used clinically in the treatment of several forms of neuropathic pain, although the proposed mechanism of action is entirely different [126,127].

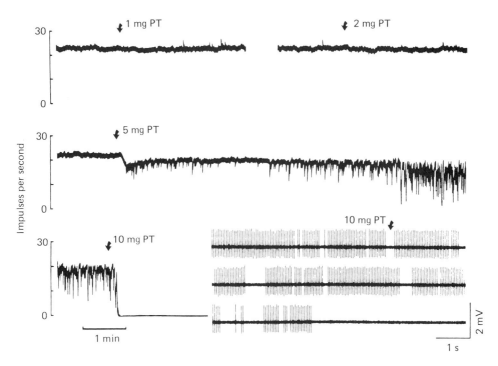

Figure 3.12 Suppression of ectopic neuroma discharge with bath-applied phenytoin (PT, diphenylhydantoin). (From Yaari, Y. and Devor, M. Phenytoin suppresses spontaneous ectopic discharge in rat sciatic nerve neuromas. *Neuroscience Letters*, **58**, 117–122 (1985), with permission)

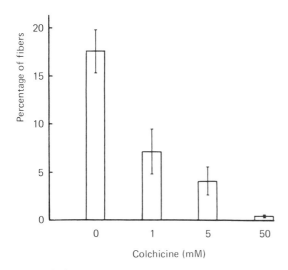

Figure 3.13 Reduction of spontaneous discharge generated in experimental nerve-end neuromas by perineural application of the axoplasmic transport blocker colchicine (data from Devor, M. and Govrin-Lippmann, R. Axoplasmic transport block reduces ectopic impulse generation in injured peripheral nerves. *Pain*, **16**, 73–85 (1983))

'CENTRALIZATION' OF NEUROPATHIC PAIN

At the beginning of this chapter it was pointed out that peripheral nerve damage, in addition to inducing pathophysiologic changes in the PNS, can alter sensory signal processing in the CNS. Even when the source is plainly peripheral, such as in the Tinel sign, the abnormal afferent barrage is always filtered through central processing networks before conscious appreciation. Correspondingly, the effectiveness of a centrally directed treatment is no proof that the pain pathophysiology is central.

Nor do CNS and PNS changes necessarily develop independent of one another. There has long been a suspicion that the very existence of abnormal discharge in the periphery might alter CNS processing in such a way that, in time, pain might be sustained even in the absence of the peripheral source. Fear of such 'centralization' of pain reasonably motivates prompt treatment of peripheral sources.

SUMMARY

Basic science and clinical research findings over the last 20 years have brought about a general appreciation of the complexity and subtlety of spinal and brain-stem mechanisms of pain – so much so, that positive symptoms associated with peripheral nerve injury are usually discussed under the heading 'deafferentation pain'. By contrast, there has been little change in the common conception of peripheral nerves as elements that either propagate or, if injured, fail to propagate, action potentials. This chapter has reviewed pathophysiologic processes through which damaged nerves can come to contribute actively to chronic pain both by injecting abnormal discharge into the nervous system, and by amplifying and distorting naturally generated signals. Far from producing deafferentation, nerve injury may present the CNS with an exaggerated afferent input!

Data reviewed suggest that the primary pathophysiologic change in injured nerves, spinal roots and DRGs, is an increase in electrical excitability. The probable cause is abnormal differentiation of the axonal membrane at the cut nerve end, at sites of demyelination and in axotomized sensory neurons. Normal nerves are capable of generating rhythmic discharge only at specialized terminal structures; damaged nerves acquire this capability at ectopic pacemaker sites. Once an ectopic pacemaker capability has been established, there may be spontaneous discharge, and sensitivity to a broad range of depolarizing stimuli – mechanical, chemical, physical and metabolic.

Associated with abnormal impulse generation in damaged nerves are several processes that can amplify normal or pathophysiologic impulse discharge. The most striking of these results from the fact that rhythmic impulse generators have threshold properties. In fibers and DRG cells that are silent but near their threshold for rhythmic firing, small stimuli that bring the rhythmic generator to threshold have disproportionately large effects. Other impulse amplification and distortion mechanisms include 'extra-spike' production and receptor sensitization. Several different types of fiber-to-fiber interaction in injured nerve could, in principle, produce nociceptor activity when only low-threshold fibers were originally activated.

There is a fundamental difference between the mechanisms of 'normal' and neuropathic pain: 'normal' pain is pain that arises from acute or chronic stimulation of normal afferent nociceptor endings by intense stimuli; neuropathic pain is pain that occurs spontaneously, or in response to weak stimuli due to abnormalities of neural excitability. Finally, it must be re-emphasized that peripheral nerve injury induces changes in the central processing of afferent signals at the same time that it triggers pathophysiologic changes in the peripheral nerve itself [2]. In no sense is it necessary to choose between PNS and CNS in the etiology of chronic neuropathic pain, but only to understand the separate role of each.

ACKNOWLEDGEMENT

The support of the United States–Israel Binational Science Foundation, the Israel Academy of Arts and Sciences and the Leonard Wolinsky Memorial Fund is gratefully acknowledged. We wish to thank W. H. Calvin and P. D. Wall for their contribution to many of the ideas developed in this chapter.

References

1. Merskey, H. (ed). Pain terms: a current list with definitions and notes on usage. *Pain*, Suppl. 3, S215–S221 (1986)
2. Devor, M. Central changes mediating neuropathic pain. In *Pain Research and Clinical Management, Vol. 3 Proceedings of the Vth World Congress on Pain* (ed. R. Dubner, G. F. Gebhart and M. R. Bond), Elsevier, Amsterdam, pp. 114–128 (1988)
3. Cajal, S. Ramon y. *Degeneration and Regeneration of the Nervous System*, (transl. R. M. May), Hafner, New York (1968)
4. Spencer, P. S. The traumatic neuroma and proximal stump. *Bulletin of the Hospital for Joint Diseases (Johns Hopkins)*, **35**, 85–102 (1974)
5. Duce, I. R. and Keen, P. The formation of axonal sprouts in organ culture and their relationship to sprouting in vivo. *International Review of Cytology*, **66**, 211–256 (1982)
6. Devor, M., Schonfeld, D., Seltzer, Z. and Wall, P. D. Two modes of cutaneous reinnervation following peripheral nerve injury. *Journal of Comparative Neurology*, **185**, 211–220 (1979)
7. Inbal, R., Rousso, M., Ashur, H., Wall, P. D. and Devor, M. Collateral sprouting in skin and sensory recovery after nerve injury in man. *Pain*, **28**, 141–154 (1987)
8. Wall, P. and Gutnick, M. Properties of afferent nerve impulses originating from a neuroma. *Nature*, **248**, 740–743 (1974)
9. Wall, P. and Gutnick, M. Ongoing activity in peripheral nerves: the physiology and pharmacology of impulses originating from a neuroma. *Experimental Neurology*, **43**, 580–593 (1974)
10. Govrin-Lippmann, R. and Devor, M. Ongoing activity in severed nerves: source and variation with time. *Brain Research*, **159**, 406–410 (1978)
11. Wiesenfeld, Z. and Lindblom, U. Behavioural and electrophysiological effects of various types of peripheral nerve lesions in the rat: a comparison of possible models for chronic pain. *Pain*, **8**, 285–298 (1980)
12. Scadding, J. W. Development of ongoing activity, mechanosensitivity, and adrenalin sensitivity in severed peripheral nerve axons. *Experimental Neurology*, **73**, 345–364 (1981)
13. Blumberg, H. and Janig, W. Discharge pattern of afferent fibers from a neuroma. *Pain*, **20**, 335–353 (1984)
14. Burchiel, K. J. Effects of electrical and mechanical stimulation on two foci of spontaneous activity which develop in primary afferent neurons after peripheral axotomy. *Pain*, **18**, 249–265 (1984)
15. Meyer, R. A., Raja, S. N., Campbell, J. N., Mackinnon, S. E. and Dellon, A. L. Neural activity originating from a neuroma in the baboon. *Brain Research*, **325**, 255–260 (1985)
16. Ruiz, J. A., Kocsis, J. D. and Preson, R. J. Repetitive firing characteristics of mammalian myelinated axons: an intra-axonal analysis. *Society for Neuroscience Abstracts*, **7**, 904–935 (1981)
17. Wall, P. D., Waxman, S. and Basbaum, A. I. Ongoing activity in peripheral nerve: injury discharge. *Experimental Neurology*, **45**, 576–589 (1974)

18. Devor, M. and Bernstein, J. J. Abnormal impulse generation in neuromas: electrophysiology and ultrastructure. In *Abnormal Nerves and Muscles and Impulse Generators* (ed. J. Ochoa and W. Culp), Oxford University Press, Oxford, pp. 363–380 (1982)

19. Calvin, W. Some design features of axons and how neuralgias may defeat them. In *Advances in Pain Research and Therapy, Vol. 3* (ed. J. J. Bonica, D. Albe-Fessard and J. C. Liebeskind), Raven Press, New York, pp. 297–309 (1980)

20. Wall, P. D. and Devor, M. Sensory afferent impulses originate from dorsal root ganglia as well as from the periphery in normal and nerve-injured rats. *Pain*, **17**, 321–339 (1983)

21. Kugelberg, E. 'Injury activity' and 'trigger zones' in human nerves. *Brain*, **69**, 310–324 (1946)

22. Fried, K. and Devor, M. End-structure of afferent axons injured in the peripheral and central nervous system. *Somatosensory and Motor Research*, **6**, 79–99 (1988)

23. Cajal, S. Ramon y. *Degeneration and Regeneration of the Nervous System* (1968, translated by R. M. May), Hafner, New York, p. 251 (1928)

24. Konorski, J. and Lubinska, L. Mechanical excitability of regenerating nerve-fibres. *Lancet*, **250**, 609–610 (1946)

25. Arndt, J. O., Krossa, M. and Samodelov, L. F. Regeneration of barosensitivity in the aortic nerve of cats when severed and transposed on various vessels in the neck. *Journal of Physiology*, **311**, 453–461 (1981)

26. Chronholm, B. Phantom limbs in amputees. *Acta psychiatrica neurologica scandinavica*, Suppl. 72, 1–310 (1951)

27. Herndon, J. H., Eaton, R. G. and Little, J. W. Management of painful neuromas in the hand. *Journal of Bone and Joint Surgery*, **58A**, 369–373 (1976)

28. Kline, D. G. and Hackett, E. R. Management of neuroma in continuity. In *Neurosurgery* (ed. R. H. Wilkins and S. S. Rengachary), McGraw-Hill, New York, pp. 1864–1871 (1985)

29. Dyck, P. J., Thomas. P. K. and Lambert, E. H. (eds). *Peripheral Neuropathy*. Saunders, Philadelphia (1974)

30. Noordenbos, W. and Wall, P. D. Implications of the failure of nerve resection and graft to cure chronic pain produced by nerve lesions. *Journal of Neurology, Neurosurgery and Psychiatry*, **44**, 1068–1073 (1981)

31. Vallbo, A. B., Hagbarth, K. E., Torebjork, H. E. and Wallin, B. G. Somatosensory, proprioceptive, and sympathetic activity in human peripheral nerves. *Physiological Review*, **59**, 919–957 (1979)

32. Torebjork, H. E., Ochoa, J. L. and McCann, F. V. Paraesthesiae: abnormal impulse generation in sensory nerve fibers in man. *Acta physiologica scandinavica*, **105**, 518–520 (1979)

33. Ochoa, J. and Torebjork, H. E. Paraesthesiae from ectopic impulse generation in human sensory nerves. *Brain*, **103**, 835–854 (1980)

34. Nystrom, B. and Hagbarth, K. E. Microelectrode recordings from transected nerves in amputees with phantom limb pain. *Neuroscience Letters*, **27**, 211–216 (1981)

35. Ochoa, J., Torebjork, H. E., Culp, W. L. and Schady, W. Abnormal spontaneous activity in single sensory nerve fibers in humans. *Muscle and Nerve*, **5**, 574–577 (1982)

36. Nordin, M., Nystrom, B., Wallin, U. and Hagbarth, K-E. Ectopic sensory discharges and paresthesiae in patients with disorders of peripheral nerves, dorsal roots and dorsal columns. *Pain*, **20**, 231–245 (1984)

37. Cline, M. and Ochoa, J. Chronically sensitized C nociceptors in skin. Patient with hyperalgesia, hyperpathia and spontaneous pain. *Society for Neuroscience Abstracts*, **12**, 331 (1986)

38. Devor, M. and Govrin-Lippmann, R. Axoplasmic transport block reduces ectopic impulse generation in injured peripheral nerves. *Pain*, **16**, 73–85 (1983)

39. Devor, M. and Govrin-Lippmann, R. Spontaneous neural discharge in neuroma C-fibers in rat sciatic nerve. *Neuroscience Letters*, Suppl. 22, S32 (1985)

40. Wall, P., Devor, M., Inbal, F. R., Scadding, J. W., Schonfeld, D., Seltzer, Z. and Tomkiewicz, M. M. Autotomy following peripheral nerve lesions: experimental anaesthesia dolorosa. *Pain*, **7**, 103–113 (1980)

41. Vallbo, A. B., Olsson, K. A., Westberg, K-G and Clark, F. J. Microstimulation of single tactile afferents from the human hand: sensory attributes related to unit type and properties of receptive fields. *Brain*, **107**, 727–749 (1984)

42. Torebjork, E. Nociceptor activation and pain. *Philosophical Transactions of the Royal Society of London, Series B*, **308**, 227–234 (1985)

43. White, J. C. and Sweet, W. H. *Pain and the Neurosurgeon*. Thomas, Springfield, Illinois, pp. 525–589 (1969)

44. Devor, M., Inbal, R. and Govrin-Lippmann, R. Genetic factors in the development of chronic pain. In *Genetics of the Brain* (ed. I. Lieblich), Elsevier, Amsterdam, pp. 273–296 (1982)

45. Wolff, B. B. and Langley, S. Cultural factors and the response to pain: a review. In *Pain: Clinical and Experimental Perspectives* (ed. M. Weisenberg), Mosby, St. Louis, pp. 144–151 (1975)

46. Violon, A. and Giugea, D. Familial models for chronic pain. *Pain*, **18**, 199–203 (1984)
47. Schott, G. D. Pain and its absence in an unfortunate family of amputees. *Pain*, **25**, 229–231 (1986)
48. Korenman, E. M. D. and Devor, M. Ectopic adrenergic sensitivity in damaged peripheral nerve axons in the rat. *Experimental Neurology*, **72**, 63–81 (1981)
49. Devor, M. Potassium channels moderate ectopic excitability of nerve-end neuromas in rats. *Neuroscience Letters*, **40**, 181–186 (1983)
50. Devor, M. Nerve pathophysiology and mechanisms of pain in causalgia. *Journal of the Autonomic Nervous System*, **7**, 371–384 (1983)
51. Low, P. A. Endoneurial potassium is increased and enhances spontaneous activity in regenerating mammalian nerve fibers – implications for neuropathic positive symptoms. *Muscle and Nerve*, **8**, 27–33 (1985)
52. Burchiel, K. J. and Russell, L. C. Effect of potassium channel blocking agents on spontaneous discharges from neuromas in rats. *Journal of Neurosurgery*, **63**, 246–249 (1985)
53. Koschorke, G. M., Helme, R. D. and Zimmerman, M. Substance P suppresses the response to bradykinin and to heat of non-myelinated fibers in experimental neuroma of the cat's sural nerve. *Society for Neuroscience Abstracts*, **11**, 118 (1985)
54. Lisney, S. J. W. and Devor, M. Afterdischarge and interactions among fibers in damaged peripheral nerve in the rat. *Brain Research*, **415**, 122–136 (1987)
55. Matzner, O. and Devor, M. Contrasting thermal sensitivity of spontaneously active A- and C-fibers in experimental nerve-end neuromas. *Pain*, **30**, 373–384 (1987)
56. Devor, M. and Janig, W. Activation of myelinated afferents ending in a neuroma by stimulation of the sympathetic supply in the rat. *Neuroscience Letters*, **24**, 43–47 (1981)
57. Schwartzman, R. J. and McLellan, T. L. Reflex sympathetic dystrophy: a review. *Archives of Neurology*, **44**, 555–561 (1987)
58. Hannington-Kiff, J. G. *Pain Relief*. Lippincott, Philadelphia (1974)
59. Loh, L., Nathan, P. W. and Schott, G. D. Pain due to lesions of central nervous system removed by sympathetic block. *British Medical Journal*, **282**, 1026–1028 (1981)
60. Sherman, R. A., Sherman, C. J. and Parker, L. Chronic phantom and stump pain among American veterans: results of a survey. *Pain*, **18**, 83–95 (1984)
61. Bostock, H. and Sears, T. A. The internodal axon membrane: electrical excitability and continuous conduction in segmental demyelination. *Journal of Physiology*, **280**, 273–301 (1978)
62. Rasminsky, M., Kearney, R. E., Aguayo, A. J. and Bray, G. M. Conduction of nervous impulses in spinal roots and peripheral nerves of dystrophic mice. *Brain Research*, **143**, 71–85 (1978)
63. Foster, R. E., Whalen, C. C. and Waxman, S. G. Reorganisation of the axon membrane in demyelinated peripheral nerve fibres: morphological evidence. *Science*, **210**, 661–663 (1980)
64. Howe, J. F., Loeser, J. D. and Calvin, W. H. Mechanosensitivity of dorsal root ganglia and chronically injured axons: a physiological basis for radicular pain of nerve root compression. *Pain*, **3**, 25–41 (1977)
65. Rasminsky, M. Ectopic generation of impulses and cross-talk in spinal nerve roots of 'dystrophic' mice. *Annals of Neurology*, **3**, 351–357 (1978)
66. Burchiel, K. J. Ectopic impulse generation in focally demyelinated trigeminal nerve. *Experimental Neurology*, **69**, 423–429 (1980)
67. Calvin, W. H., Devor, M. and Howe, J. Can neuralgias arise from minor demyelination? Spontaneous firing, mechanosensitivity and afterdischarge from conducting axons. *Experimental Neurology*, **75**, 755–763 (1982)
68. Ropper, A. H. and Shahani, B. T. Pain in Guillain–Barré syndrome. *Archives of Neurology*, **41**, 511–514 (1984)
69. Dyck, P. J., Low, P. A. and Stevens, J. C. Diseases of peripheral nerves. In *Clinical Neurology*, *Vol. 4*. (ed. A. B. Baker and R. J. Joynt), Harper & Row, Philadelphia, pp. 60–73 (1986)
70. Kein, H. A. and Kirkaldy-Willis, W. H. Low back pain. *CIBA Clinical Symposia*, **32**, 27 (1980)
71. Burchiel, K. J., Russell, L. C., Lee, R. P. and Sima, A. A. F. Spontaneous activity of primary afferent neurons in diabetic BB/Wistar rats: a possible mechanism of chronic diabetic neuropathic pain. *Diabetes*, **43**, 1210–1213 (1985)
72. Waxman, S. G. and Ritchie, J. M. (eds) *Demyelinating Disease: Basic and Clinical Electrophysiology*, Raven Press, New York (1981)
73. Clifford, D. B. and Trotter, J. L. Pain in multiple sclerosis. *Archives of Neurology*, **41**, 1270–1272 (1984)
74. Kerr, F. W. L. Pathology of trigeminal neuralgia: light and electron microscopic observations. *Journal of Neurosurgery*, **26**, 151–156 (1967)
75. Jannetta, P. J. Treatment of trigeminal neuralgia by suboccipital and transtentorial cranial operations. *Clinical Neurosurgery*, **24**, 538–549 (1977)
76. Gardner, W. J. The mechanism of tic douloureux. *Transactions of the American Neurological*

Association, **78**, 158–173 (1953)

77. Jensen, T. J., Rasmussen, P. and Reske-Nelson, E. Association of trigeminal neuralgia with multiple sclerosis: Clinical and pathological features. *Acta neurologica scandinavica*, **65**, 182–189 (1982)

78. Wall, P. D. and Devor, M. Sensory afferent impulses originate from dorsal root ganglia as well as from the periphery in normal and nerve-injured rats. *Pain*, **17**, 321–339 (1984)

79. Kirk, E. J. Impulses in dorsal spinal nerve rootlets in cats and rabbits arising from dorsal root ganglia isolated from the periphery. *Journal of Comparative Neurology*, **2**, 165–176 (1974)

80. De Santis, M. and Duckworth, J. W. Properties of primary afferent neurons from muscles which are spontaneously active after a lesion of their peripheral process. *Experimental Neurology*, **75**, 261–274 (1982)

81. Mayer, M. L., James, M. H., Russell, R. J., Kelly, J. S. and Pasternak, C. A. Changes in excitability induced by herpes simplex viruses in rat dorsal root ganglion neurons. *Journal of Neuroscience*, **6**, 391–402 (1986)

82. Iacono, R. P., Linford, J. and Sandyk, R. Pain management after lower extremity amputation. *Neurosurgery*, **20**, 496–500 (1987)

83. Bors, E. Phantom limb patients with spinal cord injury. *Archives of Neurology and Psychiatry*, **66**, 610–631 (1951)

84. Mackenzie, N. Phantom limb pain during spinal anaesthesia. *Anesthesia*, **38**, 886–887 (1983)

85. Loeser, J. D. Herpes zoster and postherpetic neuralgia. *Pain*, **25**, 149–164 (1986)

86. Calvin, W. H. Generation of spike trains in CNS neurons. *Brain Research*, **84**, 1–22 (1975)

87. Jack, J. J. B., Noble, D. and Tiens, R. W. *Electrical Current Flow in Excitable Cells*. Clarendon Press, Oxford (1975)

88. Calvin, W. H., Howe, J. F. and Loeser, J. D. Ectopic repetitive firing in focally demyelinated axons and some implications for trigeminal neuralgia. In *Pain in the Trigeminal Region*, (ed. D. Anderson and B. Matthews), Elsevier/North Holland, Amsterdam, pp. 125–136 (1977)

89. Paintal, A. S. Conduction properties of normal peripheral mammalian axons. In *Physiology and Pathobiology of Axons* (ed. S. G. Waxman), Raven Press, New York, pp. 131–144 (1978)

90. Tagini, G. and Camino, E. T-shaped cells of dorsal root ganglia can influence the pattern of afferent discharge. *Pflüger's Archiv*, **344**, 339–347 (1973)

91. Howe, J. F., Calvin, W. H. and Loeser, J. D. Impulses reflected from dorsal root ganglia and from focal nerve injuries. *Brain Research*, **116**, 139–144 (1976)

92. Noordenbos, W. *Pain*, Elsevier/North Holland, Amsterdam (1959)

93. Lewis, T. *Pain*, Macmillan, New York (1942)

94. Lindblom, U. and Verrillo, R. T. Sensory functions in chronic neuralgia. *Journal of Neurology, Neurosurgery and Psychiatry*, **42**, 422–435 (1979)

95. Campbell, J. N., Raja, S. N. and Meyer, R. A. Painful sequelae of nerve injury. In *Proceedings of Vth World Congress on Pain* (ed. R. Dubner, G. F. Gebhart and M. R. Bond), Elsevier, Amsterdam, pp. 135–143 (1988)

96. Devor, M. and Dubner, R. Centrifugal activity in afferent C-fibers influences the spontaneous afferent barrage generated in nerve-end neuromas. *Brain Research*, **446**, 396–400 (1987)

97. Granit, R. and Skoglund, C. R. Facilitation, inhibition and depression at the 'artificial synapse' formed by the cut end of a mammalian nerve. *Journal of Physiology*, **103**, 435–448 (1945)

98. Seltzer, Z. and Devor, M. Ephaptic transmission in chronically damaged peripheral nerves. *Neurology*, **29**, 1061–1064 (1979)

99. Blumberg, H. and Janig, W. Activation of fibres via experimentally produced stump neuromas of skin nerves – Ephaptic transmission or retrograde sprouting? *Experimental Neurology*, **76**, 468–482 (1982)

100. Lisney, S. J. W. and Pover, C. M. Coupling between fibres involved in sensory nerve neuromata in cats. *Journal of the Neurological Sciences*, 59, 255–264 (1983)

101. Rasminsky, M. Ephaptic transmission between single nerve fibers in the spinal nerve roots of dystrophic mice. *Journal of Physiology*, **305**, 151–169 (1980)

102. Bernstein, J. J. and Pagnanelli, D. Long-term axonal apposition in rat sciatic nerve neuroma. *Journal of Neurosurgery*, **57**, 632–684 (1982)

103. Lloyd, D. P. C. Electrotonus in dorsal roots. *Cold Spring Harbor Symposia on Quantitative Biology*, **17**, 203–219 (1952)

104. Wall, P. D. and Devor, M. The effect of peripheral nerve injury on dorsal root potentials and on transmission of afferent signals into the spinal cord. *Brain Research*, **209**, 95–111 (1981)

105. Horch, K. W. and Lisney, S. J. W. Changes in primary afferent depolarization of sensory neurones during peripheral nerve regeneration in the cat. *Journal of Physiology*, **313**, 287–299 (1981)

106. Dubner, R., Sharav, Y., Gracely, R. H. and Price, D. D. Idiopathic trigeminal neuralgia: sensory features and pain mechanisms. *Pain*, **31**, 23–33 (1987)

107. Devor, M., Keller, C. H., Deerinck, T. J., Levinson, S. R. and Ellisman, M. H. Na$^+$ channel accumulation on axolemma of afferent endings in nerve-end neuromas in *Apteronotus*. *Neuroscience Letters*, in press

108. Hammerschlag, R. and Stone, G. C. Membrane delivery by fast axonal transport. *Trends in Neuroscience*, **5**, 12–15 (1982)

109. Lombet, A., Laduron, P., Mourre, C., Jacomet, Y. and Lazdunski, M. Axonal transport of the voltage-dependent Na$^+$ channel protein identified by its tetrodotoxin-binding site in rat sciatic nerves. *Brain Research*, **345**, 153–158 (1985)

110. Waxman, S. G. and Foster, R. E. Ionic channel distribution and heterogeneity of the axon membrane in myelinated fibres. *Brain Research Review*, **2**, 205–234 (1980)

111. Pitman, R. M. The ionic dependence of action potentials induced by colchicine in an insect motoneurone cell body. *Journal of Physiology*, **247**, 511–520 (1975)

112. Goodman, C. S. and Heitler, W. J. Electrical properties of insect neurones with spiking and non-spiking somata: normal, axotomised and colchicine-treated neuron. *Journal of Experimental Biology*, **83**, 95–121 (1979)

113. Kuwada, J. Y. and Wine, J. J. Transient, axotomy-induced changes in the membrane properties of crayfish central neurons. *Journal of Physiology*, **317**, 435–461 (1981)

114. Pellegrino, M., Nencioni, B. and Matteoli, M. Response to axotomy of an identified leech neuron, in vivo and in culture. *Brain Research*, **298**, 347–352 (1984)

115. Sernagor, E., Yarom, Y. and Werman, R. Sodium-dependent regenerative responses in dendrites of axotomized motoneurons in the cat. *Proceedings of the National Academy of Sciences of the United States of America*, **83**, 7966–7970 (1986)

116. Titmus, M. J. and Faber, D. S. Altered excitability of the goldfish Mauthner cell following axotomy. II. Localization and ionic basis. *Journal of Neurophysiology*, **55**, 1440–1454 (1986)

117. Gallego, R., Ivorra, I. and Morales, A. Effects of central or peripheral axotomy on membrane properties of sensory neurones in the petrosal ganglion of the cat. *Journal of Physiology*, **391**, 39–56 (1987)

118. Travell, J. G. and Simons, D. G. *Myofascial Pain and Dysfunction: the Trigger Point Manual*. Williams and Wilkins, Baltimore (1984)

119. Devor, M., Govrin-Lippmann, R. and Raber, P. Corticosteroids suppress ectopic neuronal discharge originating in experimental neuromas. *Pain*, **22**, 127–137 (1985)

120. Burchiel, K. J. and Russell, L. C. Glycerol neurolysis: neurophysiological effects of topical glycerol application on rat saphenous nerve. *Journal of Neurosurgery*, **63**, 784–788 (1985)

121. Rappaport, Z. H., Seltzer, Z. and Zagzag, D. The effect of glycerol on autotomy. An experimental model of neuralgia pain. *Pain*, **26**, 85–91 (1986)

122. Lunsford, L. D. and Bennett, M. H. Percutaneous retrogasserian glycerol rhizotomy for tic douloureux. *Neurosurgery*, **14**, 424–430 (1984)

123. Matzner, O. and Devor, M. Sodium ion electrogenesis in nerve end neuromas. *European Journal of Neuroscience*, Suppl. 1, 173 (1988)

124. Yaari, Y. and Devor, M. Phenytoin suppresses spontaneous ectopic discharge in rat sciatic nerve neuromas. *Neuroscience Letters*, **58**, 117–122 (1985)

125. Swerdlow, M. Review: anticonvulsant drugs and chronic pain. *Clinical Neuropharmacology*, **7**, 51–82 (1984)

126. Knyihar-Csillik, E., Szucs, A. and Csillik, B. Ionophoretically applied microtubule inhibitors induce transganglionic degenerative atrophy of primary central nociceptive terminals and abolish chronic autochthonous pain. *Acta neurologica scandinavica*, **66**, 401–412 (1982)

127. Meek, J. B., Guidice, V. W., McFadden, J. W., Key, J. D., Jr and Enrick, N. L. Colchicine highly effective in disk disorders: final results of a double-blind study. *Journal of Neurological and Orthopaedic Medicine and Surgery*, **6**, 211–218 (1985)

4
Sympathetic nervous system influence on acute and chronic pain
William J. Roberts and Ronald C. Kramis

INTRODUCTION

Severe pain can be markedly reduced or eliminated in some neurological syndromes by suppressing activity in the peripheral sympathetic nervous system. In most of these syndromes, pain occurs both spontaneously and in response to gentle mechanical stimulation such as light touch or movement of individual hairs. With time, the spontaneous pain may become more severe and the painful area may increase in size. Without prompt diagnosis and appropriate treatment, the condition often becomes chronic.

The physiologic mechanisms by which sympathetic activity can contribute to pain in these syndromes have not been fully determined, in spite of extensive experimental and theoretical work. This incomplete understanding of physiologic processes hinders diagnosis and treatment of these painful disorders – and makes it especially difficult to differentiate them from disorders producing similar symptoms but lacking sympathetic involvement.

In this chapter mechanisms are discussed by which sympathetic efferent fibers can affect activity in both nociceptive and *non-nociceptive* sensory afferents. It is argued that sympathetic activation or sensitization of *either* type of afferent may, given appropriate conditions, contribute to the occurrence of pain. Specific painful syndromes are examined in the light of the mechanisms discussed. Evidence clearly indicates that sympathetic activity is a source of pain in some syndromes; for other syndromes, sympathetic involvement is less apparent.

A major portion of the chapter is devoted to the inter-related topics of reflex sympathetic dystrophy syndrome (RSDS), sensitization of spinal neurons, and sympathetic activation of low-threshold mechanoreceptors. The latter two processes appear to be causally related to the pain of RSDS, and they are probably related to the pain of other syndromes as well. The diagnosis and treatment of RSDS is not considered here as this topic is discussed by Payne in Chapter 5.

Recent evidence indicates that sympathetic activity may contribute to pain in both acute herpes zoster and inflammatory arthritis, although this is not widely recognized. Some of the evidence is described and possible mechanisms are considered by which sympathetic involvement might occur.

A final section considers post-sympathectomy neuralgia and the possible involvement of sympathetic activity in post-sympathectomy pain. Evidence is cited which suggests that post-sympathectomy pain depends upon development of hyperactivity in spinal neurons – a hyperactivity due to transection, during sympathectomy, of visceral afferents projecting through the sympathetic trunk.

TRADITIONAL VS NON-TRADITIONAL CONCEPTS OF SYMPATHETIC FUNCTION

Participation of the sympathetic nervous system in functions such as temperature regulation and metabolic preparation for 'fight or flight' is well known. The neuronal system responsible for these actions, illustrated schematically in Figure 4.1, consists of supraspinal centers that send commands to preganglionic neurons located in the intermediolateral cell column of the spinal cord. These preganglionic neurons also receive input (either direct or indirect) from primary afferent fibers. The combined input from both sources and from local interneurons determines the level of firing of these neurons. Axons of the preganglionic neurons leave the central nervous system through the ventral roots and form synapses on postganglionic neurons in the paravertebral or prevertebral ganglia. The classic transmitter released by the preganglionic neurons is acetylcholine, although enkephalins may also be released [1].

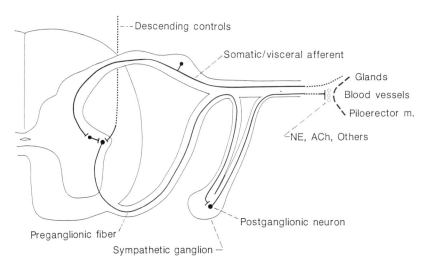

Figure 4.1 Schematic diagram of the paravertebral sympathetic nervous system showing the anatomic relationship of sympathetic pre- and post-ganglionic neurons to the spinal roots and spinal nerve. NE, norepinephrine, ACh, acetylcholine

Axons of the post-ganglionic neurons are unmyelinated in mammals, and they project through somatic or visceral nerves to target organs such as sweat glands, piloerector or vasomotor muscles and viscera. The classic neurotransmitters for these neurons are either norepinephrine or acetylcholine, although additional transmitters are now known to coexist with them. The functions of the latter relative to pain are considered later.

In contrast to the traditional functions described above, involvement of the sympathetic nervous system in the genesis of pain is not widely recognized and has received relatively little attention. A sympathetic role in pain was first demonstrated by Leriche [2], who showed that resection of sympathetic nerve fibers could alleviate the pain of causalgia. Many studies have since shown that sympathetic blocks and peripheral infusion of adrenergic blocking agents provide effective relief from certain types of pain [3–6]. These studies demonstrated that the sympathetic nervous system is causally involved in pain, but did not identify the underlying physiologic mechanisms.

Evaluation of potential sympathetic mechanisms and discussion of how they might relate to specific painful syndromes is a major purpose of this chapter.

TRADITIONAL VS NON-TRADITIONAL CONCEPTS OF NOCICEPTION AND PAIN

Nociception as used in this chapter refers to the activation of afferent neurons by stimuli that are tissue damaging (noxious) or are nearly so. Nociception is not the same as pain perception *per se*, as many factors are interposed between afferent input and perception [7]. Several types of primary afferent nociceptors exist, all of which normally respond maximally only to noxious stimuli (*see* Chapter 1). These primary afferents (hereafter called 'nociceptors') respond minimally or not at all to non-noxious stimulation unless sensitized by previous noxious stimulation (*see* Chapter 2).

Traditionally, it has been accepted that pain is elicited by peripheral stimulation only if nociceptors are activated. It has also been accepted that pain is not produced by activation of non-nociceptive primary afferents in neurologically normal individuals.

Evidence reviewed in this chapter supports a less traditional concept – that pain can occur as the result of activity in *non-nociceptive* primary afferents. These afferents have, in fact, been proposed to play a major part in the pain of reflex sympathetic dystrophy syndrome [4,8,9]. They may also contribute to pain in other syndromes, as is discussed below.

The pain that results from activation of non-nociceptive primary afferents (e.g. 'touch' afferents) in certain abnormal neurological states is proposed to depend upon sensitization of a particular type of spinal neuron, the wide-dynamic-range (WDR) or multireceptive neuron. This type of neuron, described in Chapter 1, responds to input from both nociceptive and non-nociceptive primary afferents and is thought to participate in the encoding of responses to painful stimuli [10,11]. The importance of the WDR neuron and its sensitization in relation to pain are discussed in detail in the section dealing specifically with the reflex sympathetic dystrophy syndrome (pages 93–95).

Another non-traditional idea reviewed here is the concept that sympathetic efferent fibers participate in the sensitization of primary afferent fibers [12–15]. Through this action, the sympathetic nervous system appears to contribute to the pain associated with inflammatory disorders.

SYMPATHETICALLY RELATED PAIN: NEURAL MECHANISMS

Mechanisms by which the sympathetic nervous system might contribute to the occurrence of pain include the following:

1. Sympathetic activation of primary afferent *nociceptors*; either directly, or indirectly by induction of tissue pathology.
2. Sympathetic activation of damaged or regenerating primary afferent *nociceptor axons*.
3. Sympathetic activation of *low-threshold* (non-nociceptive) primary afferents, assuming prior sensitization of WDR neurons.
4. Sympathetic activation or sensitization of nociceptor afferents by release of non-adrenergic, non-cholinergic *co-transmitters* or by release of neurally active substances, e.g. prostaglandins

These physiologic mechanisms are not mutually exclusive, and sympathetically related pain may be mediated by more than one mechanism in a single syndrome. Coexistence of multiple transmitters in sympathetic neurons and sympathetic release of neurally active substances from post-synaptic tissue are phenomena potentially relevant to each of the first three processes. They are listed separately as a fourth mechanism primarily for purposes of emphasis and discussion. Each of these four neural mechanisms is discussed in more detail below, before consideration of specific painful syndromes.

SYMPATHETIC ACTIVATION OF *NORMAL* PRIMARY AFFERENT NOCICEPTORS

Direct stimulation of nociceptors by sympathetic efferents, illustrated schematically in Figure 4.2, is an obvious mechanism that potentially explains sympathetically related pain. However, most attempts to demonstrate sympathetic activation of *unmyelinated* nociceptors, which are thought to mediate the burning and aching pain typical of most chronic pains, have been unsuccessful [16–18]. On the contrary, these studies provided evidence that sympathetic efferents do *not* excite unmyelinated nociceptors. Only one study of unmyelinated cutaneous nociceptors revealed any response to sympathetic stimulation, this being enhancement of spontaneous activity and reduction of stimulus-evoked activity [18a]. Another study reported sympathetic modulation of activity in unmyelinated afferents from tooth pulp [19]. These afferents were presumed to be nociceptors, and the modulation was thought to be secondary to changes in blood flow.

Sympathetic actions on small *myelinated* nociceptors innervating skin were tested in two studies. In one, a small sub-set of A-δ nociceptors in cats were activated by sympathetic stimulation, but only briefly and only after repeated noxious heating of the receptive field [20]. Sympathetic activation of this type of afferent was not confirmed in a study by Barasi and Lynn in rabbits [18].

Although the physiologic studies cited above provide little evidence for *direct* sympathetic activation of nociceptors, it is probable that sympathetic activity contributes *indirectly* to pain by causing release of substances such as prostaglandins, which sensitize nociceptors [13,14]. This mechanism is discussed in more

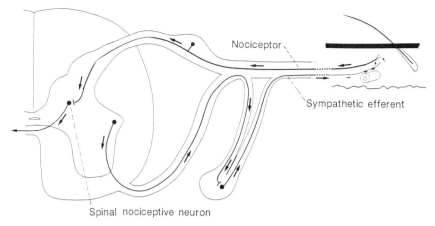

Figure 4.2 Schematic diagram showing a system hypothetically involved in sympathetic efferent activation of primary afferent nociceptors and spinal projection neurons

detail in the section on co-transmitters and sympathetically released post-synaptic substances.

Sympathetic activity may also contribute indirectly to the activation of nociceptors by causing tissue damage, like that associated with excessive sympathetically induced ischemia.

SYMPATHETIC ACTIVATION OF *DAMAGED/REGENERATING* NOCICEPTOR AXONS

Surgical resection commonly abolishes neuroma pain for several weeks; therefore it is reasonable to think that some process within the neuroma contributes to pain. This concept, illustrated schematically in Figure 4.3, has been supported by physiologic studies of sympathetic effects on primary afferents ending in stump neuromata. These studies have shown that some myelinated regenerating afferents are spontaneously active and that they can be activated by either sympathetic stimulation or application of norephinephrine on to the neuroma [21–24]. Some of the sympathetically activated afferents recorded in these studies had conduction velocities in the A-δ range, and some A-δ afferents are nociceptors; others serve as cold receptors. It could not be established in these studies that any of the activated fibers were functional nociceptors because all had been severed distal to the recording site. The possibility that sympathetically activated non-nociceptive afferents contribute to pain after nerve injury is discussed later in the chapter.

The extent of the nerve injury appears to affect the response of unmyelinated afferents to sympathetic efferent activity. More specifically, some unmyelinated primary afferents associated with *neuromata-in-continuity* are responsive to sympathetic efferent activity [25] whereas unmyelinated afferents ending in *stump neuromata* are not activated by sympathetic stimulation at physiologic rates [26]. Furthermore, those ending in stump neuromata are not ephaptically connected to sympathetic efferent fibers [27]. The unmyelinated afferents responsive to sympathetic stimulation in neuromata-in-continuity were not identified as functional nociceptors (a technically difficult feat in neuroma studies), and it is possible that

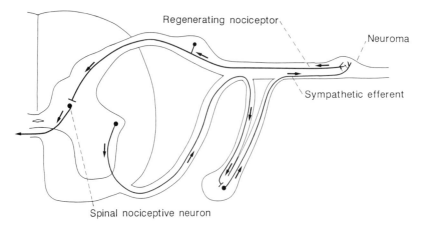

Figure 4.3 Schematic diagram showing anatomic relationships that subserve sympathetic efferent activation of regenerating nociceptors

they were low-threshold mechanoreceptors. In fact, low-threshold mechanoreceptors with unmyelinated axons are known to be sympathetically activated [18,20]

Sympathetic activation of myelinated afferents ending in stump neuromata was found not to occur in the first 24 hours after nerve transection [22]; therefore, sympathetically related pain beginning very soon after nerve injury (within hours) is not likely to result from activation of myelinated primary afferents. In some individuals, sympathetically related pain begins later, and coupling between sympathetic efferents and primary afferents in a neuroma could contribute to pain at that time.

Although the studies cited above indicate that some regenerating afferent fibers are sympathetically excitable, extrapolation of these results to clinical conditions has been questioned by Burchiel and Russell [28]. They reported that the paralytic drug gallamine, used in most animal neuroma studies, blocks potassium channels and increases spontaneous activity in regenerating primary afferent fibers. This finding suggests that gallamine may also exaggerate sympathetic actions on regenerating afferent fibers.

By recording from transected afferent fibers in two amputees with phantom limb pain, Nystrom and Hagbarth [29] studied the possible role of regenerating afferents in damaged nerves. Spontaneous afferent activity recorded proximal to the neuroma was found to persist even during anesthetic block of the neuroma. Their results showed that spontaneous afferent activity can occur after nerve injury in humans without gallamine and, in addition, that much or most of this activity originates proximal to the neuroma, perhaps from spontaneously firing dorsal root ganglion cells. They did not address the issue of sympathetic efferent modulation of afferent activity.

In summary, evidence from animal studies shows that sympathetic efferent activity can excite damaged and/or regenerating primary afferents. If the responding afferents are either nociceptors or non-nociceptive afferents projecting on to hyperexcitable WDR neurons (*see below*), then sympathetically induced activity could contribute to the pain originating from damaged nerves. The relative contribution of regenerating afferents and other uninjured afferents to pain after nerve injury is likely to vary between individuals.

SYMPATHETIC ACTIVATION OF LOW-THRESHOLD AFFERENTS

On the basis of clinical and experimental evidence, several investigators have suggested that, in certain syndromes, spontaneous and touch-evoked pain are mediated by low-threshold mechanoreceptors rather than by nociceptors [4,8,9]. They have emphasized that hyperexcitability of central neurons must exist in order for activity in low-threshold afferents to elicit pain. This idea was expanded by Roberts [9] into a formal hypothesis concerning the physiologic basis of 'sympathetically maintained pain', meaning the spontaneous pain that is abolished by sympathetic block.

This hypothesis attributes sympathetically maintained pain to the following: (1) the existence of spinal WDR neurons which receive afferent input from both nociceptive and non-nociceptive primary afferents and which send axons through traditional 'pain pathways' to brain structures involved in the experience of pain; (2) sensitization of these WDR neurons so that they respond at abnormally high rates to *non-nociceptive* afferent input; (3) activation of *non-nociceptive* afferents in the painful region by local sympathetic efferents; and (4) maintenance of spinal neuron sensitization by tonic sympathetic activation of non-nociceptive afferent fibers. The anatomic pathways involved in this process are illustrated schematically in Figure 4.4.

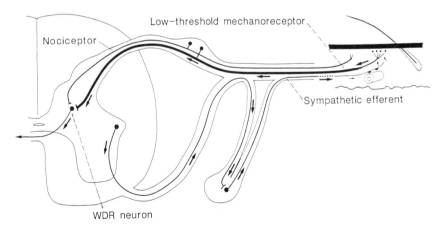

Figure 4.4 Schematic diagram showing anatomic relationships that subserve sympathetic efferent activation of low-threshold primary afferents and activation of wide-dynamic-range (WDR) neurons by convergent input from primary afferent nociceptors and low-threshold mechanoreceptors

Evidence substantiating this hypothesis is cited later in the section on reflex sympathetic dystrophy syndrome.

EFFECTS OF SYMPATHETIC CO-TRANSMITTERS AND
SYMPATHETICALLY RELEASED POST-SYNAPTIC SUBSTANCES

Sympathetic post-ganglionic neurons are not exclusively adrenergic or cholinergic – they also contain peptides and purines, which are released from their terminals [30–33]. Neuropeptide Y (NPY), for example, coexists with noradrenalin in the terminals of some sympathetic post-ganglionic neurons. Adenosine triphosphate (ATP) and norepinephrine (NE) coexist in others, and it seems likely that in still others, all three coexist [34]. For a comprehensive review *see* Hokfelt *et al.* [35].

The release of coexisting transmitters from sympathetic terminals appears to be differentially dependent on the rate of impulse activity in post-ganglionic neurons. Because the coexisting transmitters may have different physiologic functions, the level of sympathetic activity can partly determine the nature of the physiologic responses [36–38]. One transmitter may produce rapid post-synaptic potential changes, whereas a co-transmitter may operate through slower second-messenger systems, perhaps ultimately altering DNA transcription [39]. Differential rate-dependent release of NE and NPY is illustrated schematically in Figure 4.5.

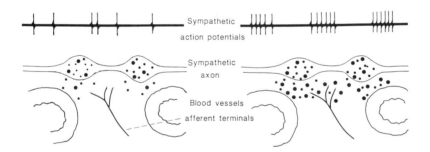

Figure 4.5 Schematic illustration showing differential release of co-transmitters from sympathetic efferent axons as a function of efferent firing rate. Note that a higher firing rate increases release of both transmitters, but that a relatively greater increase in release of neuropeptide Y (NPY) occurs. ● NE (norepinephrine); ● NE + NPY

Prostaglandins are other compounds related to both sympathetic function and pain. Although prostaglandins may serve as sympathetic co-transmitters, as proposed by Stjarne [40] and Levine *et al.* [13], stronger evidence exists that sympathetic activity causes the release of prostaglandins from cells in the vicinity of the sympathetic neuro-effector junction [41,42]. In either case, sympathetically released prostaglandins might contribute to pain, tenderness or hyperalgesia under certain abnormal conditions, as prostaglandins are known to sensitize nociceptors strongly [14,43]. Release of prostaglandins by sympathetic actions has, in fact, been proposed to contribute to inflammation and pain in rheumatoid arthritis [44]. This role for sympathetically released prostaglandins in arthritis is supported by recent demonstrations that both skin and joint nociceptors are sensitized by prostaglandin PGE_2 [12,14]. Sympathetic involvement in rheumatoid arthritis is discussed in more detail in a later section.

The possibility that non-adrenergic, non-cholinergic sympathetic transmitters are involved in mediating sympathetically related pain has received little attention and almost no experimental effort; therefore a more detailed discussion here is inappropriate. However, it is worth noting that investigations or treatments affecting only the classic sympathetic transmitters may not block sympathetic effects mediated by other substances.

REFLEX SYMPATHETIC DYSTROPHY SYNDROME AND CAUSALGIA

Description

Reflex sympathetic dystrophy syndrome (RSDS), described in detail in Chapter 5, is characterized by both spontaneous pain and stimulus-evoked pain. In most cases, allodynia, i.e. pain in response to light tactile stimulation, is present with the spontaneous pain. One subtype of RSDS, causalgia, occurs in association with traumatic injury to a major nerve [45]. As some syndromes lacking sympathetic involvement also exhibit spontaneous pain and allodynia in the absence of active tissue injury [46–48], an essential diagnostic criterion for RSDS is that sympathetic block alleviates (transiently or permanently) the spontaneous pain [49]. Overt signs of sympathetic dysfunction may or may not be present in the early stages of RSDS.

Clinical indications of sympathetic involvement

Abundant evidence indicates that sympathetic efferent activity is causally related to pain in RSDS and causalgia [8,45,50,51]. For example, spontaneous pain and allodynia are abolished in most cases by local anesthetic block of the sympathetic chain or by depletion of neurotransmitter from sympathetic terminals, as occurs following regional infusion of guanethidine.

Mechanisms

Sympathetic activation of low-threshold mechanoreceptors

Low-threshold mechanoreceptors, rather than nociceptors, are implicated in the genesis of spontaneous pain and allodynia in RSDS by several lines of evidence:

1. Selective block of only large myelinated afferents abolishes spontaneous pain and allodynia in patients with RSDS [48,52] (J. Ochoa, M. A. Cline, R. M. Dotson and W. J. Roberts, unpublished observations). Therefore, the pain and allodynia that exist prior to the block require input from large-diameter myelinated afferents. In such studies a pressure cuff is used to block conduction progressively in nerve fibers, beginning with the largest and progressing over time to the smallest. In the studies cited above, spontaneous pain and allodynia were abolished at a time when pain was still experienced in response to pinprick and noxious heat (i.e. when small myelinated and unmyelinated afferents were still conducting).

2. The threshold intensity for mechanically evoked pain in RSDS is very low and is similar to the threshold for touch perception in many patients. Thus low-threshold mechanoreceptors, which commonly signal 'touch', might be responsible for mechanically evoked pain. The possibility of mediation by low-threshold mechanoreceptors is strengthened by results from studies of sensitized nociceptors, which indicate that sensitization of most nociceptors produces little increase in mechanical sensitivity [53].
3. Sympathetic efferents can activate low-threshold mechanoreceptors in both experimental animals and humans [8,54–56]. In contrast, unmyelinated afferents that normally mediate burning and aching pain are, in most studies, not sympathetically activated [17,18].
4. Sympathetic stimulation activates only the spinal nociceptive neurons that receive input from *both* low-threshold mechanoreceptors and nociceptors (WDR neurons); spinal neurons that receive input *only from nociceptors* are *not* sympathetically activated [56,57]. This evidence further supports the proposal that low-threshold mechanoreceptors mediate sympathetically maintained pain.

Activation of nociceptors by sympathetic induction of tissue pathology

One physiologic explanation for the pain of RSDS that has achieved a degree of acceptance is the 'vicious circle' hypothesis of Livingston [58]. He proposed that trauma-induced activation of nociceptors reflexly elicits sympathetic activity which ultimately has a pathologic effect. Through mechanisms such as excessive vasoconstriction, sympathetic activity is presumed to create conditions in the injured area which produce more nociceptor activity. This in turn reflexly elicits more sympathetic activity, etc., in a vicious circle. Recently, the vicious circle hypothesis has been re-examined favorably, though with qualifications, by Janig and Kollmann [51].

Certain difficulties in using this hypothesis to explain RSDS pain become apparent when clinical findings are considered. One difficulty is that spontaneous pain and allodynia in RSDS are abruptly abolished by sympathetic block. Relief occurs too rapidly to be accounted for by reversal of the morphological and functional changes proposed by Janig and Kollman [51] to be the source of pain in RSDS. A second difficulty is that patients with RSDS do not show consistent signs of sympathetic dysfunction in the painful area [4,49,59,60].

Sympathetic activation of regenerating nociceptors

Several investigators have suggested that electrical or chemical coupling between sympathetic efferents and regenerating nociceptor afferents in damaged nerve is responsible for the spontaneous pain in causalgia [21,23,61,62].

Physiologic evidence concerning this mechanism was reviewed earlier in the section on neural mechanisms of sympathetically related pain. There is evidence for sympathetic activation of *myelinated* afferents in stump neuromata, but *not* for excitation of *unmyelinated* afferents, except in neuromata-in-continuity. The evidence regarding regenerating nociceptors remains inconclusive, but suggests that some may be sympathetically activated. Such activation could explain ongoing, sympathetically maintained pain. It would not explain *spontaneous pain* that is abolished by either nerve block or regional infusion of the adrenergic depleter, guanethidine, *distal* to a site of nerve injury [4,63]. These procedures would not affect coupling in the neuroma; thus, pain eliminated by these procedures must have been mediated by activity originating distal to the neuroma.

Sympathetic activation of regenerating afferents ending in a neuroma also fails to explain the existence of *allodynia distal* to the site of nerve injury in causalgia. This symptom probably results from mechanical activation of low-threshold mechano-receptors that project on to sensitized WDR neurons, as described earlier. Mechanical activation of *regenerating nociceptors* might contribute to allodynia that develops long after injury (i.e. long enough for regenerating fibers to reach the area of allodynia).

Summary

The evidence reviewed above strongly suggests that sympathetic activation of low-threshold mechanoreceptors and WDR neurons contributes to the pain in RSDS. Previous sensitization of WDRs is required in order that low-threshold mechanoreceptors can produce a level of WDR firing similar to that normally evoked by nociceptor input.

Pain in RSDS may also be due to nociceptor activation caused by sympathetically induced prostaglandin release or tissue pathology. This might occur, for example, in cases involving abnormal circulation and dystrophy. However, in individuals who experience rapid pain reduction at the onset of sympathetic block, tissue pathology cannot be the major source of pain.

Sympathetic activation of sensitized or regenerating nociceptors may produce pain in RSDS. However, recent demonstrations have shown that pain in patients can be abolished by selective cuff block of A fibers. This strongly supports a major role for low-threshold mechanoreceptors and argues against an exclusive role for nociceptors.

INFLAMMATORY ARTHRITIS

Description

Inflammatory rheumatoid arthritis is characterized in the early active stage by synovial inflammation, swelling, stiffness and both spontaneous and mechanically evoked pain [64].

Indications of sympathetic involvement

Herfort [65] reported positive results from sympathectomy in treating the pain of advanced rheumatoid arthritis. Similarly, Levine and colleagues [66] reported that regional guanethedine infusion in patients with active rheumatoid arthritis de-creased their pain. As guanethedine block appears to be selective for sympathetic efferents, sympathetic activity must contribute either directly or indirectly to arthritic pain. Additional evidence of sympathetic involvement was obtained in animal experiments, which showed that neonatal sympathectomy impedes the development of joint injury in adjuvant-induced arthritis [44]. These experiments also showed that hypertensive rats, which have elevated sympathetic tone, develop more joint injury than do similarly treated normotensive rats.

Mechanisms

Sympathetic activation of nociceptors

Sympathetic activity has been shown to release prostaglandins including PGE_2 from non-neural cells near the sympathetic terminals [41,67]. Levine *et al.* [13] have also suggested that PGE_2 may be released directly from sympathetic terminals in skin. Prostaglandin PGE_2 is known to sensitize nociceptors that innervate joints [12,68] and skin [14]. Thus, if sympathetic efferents cause the release of PGE_2 in joints as they do elsewhere, their activity is likely to sensitize nociceptors, augmenting their activation by arthritic inflammation.

If arthritic tissue deformation were sufficient to produce damage to terminal portions of axons innervating a joint, sensitivity of regenerating axons to sympathetically released norepinephrine might occur, as in neuromas [22].

Sympathetic activation of low-threshold afferents

Sympathetic activation of low-threshold afferents may contribute to arthritic pain because some spinal neurons activated by nociceptive joint afferents also receive convergent input from low-threshold afferents innervating joints or other tissues [69]. If the spinal neurons are hyperexcitable as a result of nociceptor input from an arthritic joint, their responses to low-threshold afferents would be enhanced (*see* earlier section on RSDS). The spinal neurons are likely to be hyperexcitable in arthritis because inflammation has been shown to activate joint C-polymodal nociceptors [68,70,71] and polymodal nociceptor activity is known to sensitize WDR neurons.

Finally, any contribution of low-threshold afferents to arthritic pain would probably be increased by movement, as movement of inflamed joints will activate such afferents directly, and it also produces vigorous reflex responses in some sympathetic efferents [72]. The increased efferent activity is likely to increase activity in low-threshold afferents through mechanisms described earlier.

Summary

Inflammation that occurs with rheumatoid arthritis activates and sensitizes nociceptors. Sympathetically induced release of prostaglandins is likely to contribute to this sensitization. It is also likely that sympathetic efferent activity is reflexly increased by the nociceptor input. The increased sympathetic efferent activity could activate low-threshold mechanoreceptors, which provide additional excitatory input on to spinal WDR neurons sensitized by nociceptor input. Both of these sympathetic actions would probably exacerbate the pain associated with the disease.

ACUTE HERPES ZOSTER

Description

Herpes zoster infection of peripheral tissues, apparently due to 're-activation' and migration of varicella-zoster viruses, can cause severe pain even before herpetic vesicles form in the infected tissue. In untreated zoster, pain occurs throughout the period of vesicle information and eruption, and it often continues after healing. The infected region is spontaneously painful, painful to touch, and typically hyperalgesic [73,74]. Postherpetic pain is discussed in detail by Watson in Chapter 9.

Clinical indications of sympathetic involvement

Involvement of the sympathetic nervous system in acute herpetic pain is indicated by the rapid and marked relief provided by sympathetic block [75–78]. In contrast, sympathetic involvement in postherpetic pain appears to be less clear [74,79]. Specifically, sympathetic blockade is usually ineffective in relieving longstanding postherpetic pain, but if applied during the acute stage, or within a few months thereafter, it appears to reduce the probability that postherpetic neuralgia will develop.

Acute herpetic pain seems to be qualitatively similar to the pain associated with RSDS and, as with RSDS pain, is relieved by sympathetic block for a period of time greater than that during which the blocking agent is active. These similarities suggest that sympathetic mechanisms involved in RSDS pain might also be operative in herpetic pain.

Recent reviews of herpes zoster and postherpetic neuralgia indicate that few studies have been well controlled in terms of sympathetic involvement [74,79]. However, the rapid alleviation of acute herpetic pain by sympathetic block seems clearly attributable to the suppression of sympathetic nervous system activity.

Mechanisms

Activation of low-threshold mechanoreceptors after sensitization of spinal neurons

The tissue damage that occurs during the formation and eruption of herpetic vesicles would undoubtedly stimulate polymodal C nociceptors by release of inflammatory mediators such as bradykinin and histamine. Research cited in the discussion of RSDS has shown that activation of these nociceptors sensitizes pain-related spinal WDR neurons.

Sensitization of WDR neurons would make excitatory input from nociceptors unusually effective in activating spinal projection neurons. It would also make input from low-threshold mechanoreceptors more effective, and possibly painful, as in RSDS. During the active phase of the disease, during which skin lesions are present, excitatory input from both nociceptors and low-threshold primary afferents would summate in spinal WDR neurons. Summation from both types of afferents would produce more activity and pain of greater intensity than that produced by inputs from nociceptors alone. Sympathetic block would reduce pain by reducing activity in sympathetically activated low-threshold afferents and by reducing sensitization of nociceptors, but it would not entirely eliminate the pain, as nociceptor activity related to vesicle eruption would remain.

Sympathetic activation of nociceptors: potential involvement of non-noradrenergic mechanisms

Evidence cited earlier in the chapter indicates that sympathetic efferents do not directly excite nociceptors. However, sympathetic activity could augment activation of nociceptors in herpetic skin lesions by releasing prostaglandins. Sympathetic activity is reported to release prostaglandin PGE_2 in many tissues ([67], and *see* Hedqvist [41] for review), and PGE_2 strongly sensitizes many types of nociceptors [14,80,81].

By enhancing the responsiveness of nociceptors to skin lesions, sympathetic release of prostaglandins would also increase sensitization of spinal WDRs. This increase might contribute to postherpetic pain because sensitization of WDRs may persist after healing [9]. Reducing the sensitization of spinal neurons during the acute phase of the disease may be the most important result of early intervention to block sympathetic activity.

POST-SYMPATHECTOMY NEURALGIA

Description

Post-sympathectomy neuralgia is reported to occur in more than one-third of all patients who undergo surgical sympathectomy [82,83]. The disorder is characterized by spontaneous pain that begins abruptly, usually about two weeks after surgery. The pain, which worsens at night, is commonly described as deep, aching or boring. It is associated with muscle tenderness and hyperesthesia in the painful area, and these are proportional to the degree of pain [82,84]. Spontaneous remission of the pain occurs in most people within 1–3 months of onset. Surprisingly, the pain and tenderness are *not* referred to the sympathectomized area, but are referred instead to *adjacent* regions which remain sympathetically innervated, as indicated by the presence of sweating. In fact, the painful area, e.g. the anteromedial and anterolateral thigh after L2, L3 ganglionectomy, is sometimes reported to show excessive sweating attributable, presumably, to sympathetic hyperactivity [84].

Clinical indications of sympathetic involvement

The fact that sympathectomy precipitates a subsequent 'neuralgia' provides an obvious link between the sympathetic nervous system and the occurrence of pain. However, sympathetic activity in the sympathectomized region is abolished, so it cannot be responsible for the pain. Instead, post-sympathectomy pain must be attributable to activity in remaining sympathetic and/or somatic neurons that in some way have been affected by the sympathectomy. A mechanism proposed below attributes post-sympathectomy pain to processes that involve visceral afferents, partially 'deafferented' spinal neurons, and sympathetic efferents that innervate tissues adjacent to the sympathectomized region.

A strong indication of the involvement of surviving sympathetic efferents in post-sympathectomy neuralgia is the finding that the pain is topographically and temporally coincident with sympathetically mediated excessive sweating [84].

Mechanisms

Spinal neuron hyperactivity due to transection of visceral afferents

Lumbar sympathectomy transects not only sympathetic efferents, as intended, but also some afferents from lower abdominal and pelvic viscera (Figure 4.6) and perhaps some afferents from the vasculature of the lower limbs [51,85–87]

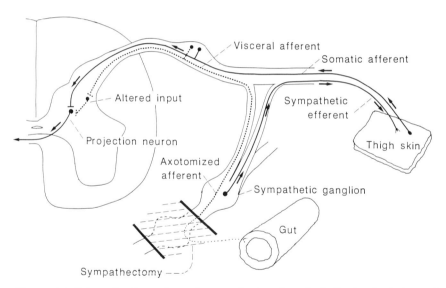

Figure 4.6 Schematic illustration of a mechanism hypothetically involved in post-sympathectomy neuralgia. Transaction of visceral afferents is proposed to cause hyperactivity in spinal projection neurons

It is proposed that transection of these visceral/vascular afferents would result in hyperactivity of certain pain-related spinal neurons normally innervated by them. The hyperactivity could result from any of several central processes which occur following peripheral axotomy of afferent neurons (for review *see* [88,89] and Chapter 3). These processes may include only alterations of synaptic effectiveness, as described by Devor and Wall [90,91]. However, as some primary afferents (up to 15%) degenerate following peripheral axotomy, processes such as collateral or terminal sprouting and denervation supersensitivity may be relevant. The importance of the latter process in the pain of another 'deafferentation' syndrome (brachial plexus avulsion) has been discussed by Fields [92]. Brachial plexus avulsion is also discussed by Burchiel in Chapter 8.

Many spinal neurons that receive afferent projections from skin, muscle and/or joints also receive projections from visceral afferents, i.e. they are 'viscero-somatic' neurons. In fact, recordings from spinal neurons indicate that afferents from thoracic and abdominal viscera project primarily to spinal neurons that also receive somatic input [93]. Relatively few cells have been reported to be 'viscero-specific'. Recent studies involving bladder distension and stimulation of hypogastric nerves indicate that pelvic visceral afferents also project to spinal neurons with somatic input [94,95].

Sympathectomy, by transecting afferents from pelvic viscera, is likely partially to denervate some viscero-somatic spinal neurons (and/or to alter their synaptic input significantly). Projections to these neurons from somatic afferents would remain functional. Because of the central processes described above, these somatic afferents, if excitatory, could become hypereffective in exciting the partially 'deafferented' viscero-somatic neurons.

Studies of spinal neurons in monkeys indicate that viscero-somatic neurons receive somatic afferents from *proximal* areas, e.g. the thigh, rather than from more distal somatic sites [94–96]. Thus, lumbar sympathectomy would be expected to denervate partially neurons with proximal, not distal, receptive fields – the very region to which patients refer post-sympathectomy pain.

Studies of spinal innervation from thoracic and rostral abdominal viscera indicate that most viscero-somatic spinal neurons are WDR neurons, i.e. they receive both nociceptive and non-nociceptive input [93,97,98]. There is no reason to suspect that neurons receiving pelvic visceral afferents differ in this regard. Thus the viscero-somatic spinal neurons proposed to become hyperexcitable following lumbar sympathectomy are probably most often pain-related WDR neurons. The importance of these neurons and particularly their sensitization (or in this case their hyperactivity) has been developed fully in the section on reflex sympathetic dystrophy syndrome.

Following development of hyperactivity, these pain-related viscero-somatic spinal neurons would respond strongly to moderate levels of input from their remaining (somatic) afferents. The afferents themselves could be activated as follows: (1) by normal mechanical stimuli such as touch or deep pressure; or (2) in some cases, by sympathetic efferent activation of non-nociceptive primary afferents, as discussed in the RSDS section. The latter input would be particularly strong when abnormally high levels of efferent sympathetic activity occurred, as has been reported to occur in the painful post-sympathectomy thigh [84].

A relatively long delay in the onset of pain after sympathectomy is consistent with the proposed involvement of denervation hypersensitivity. Rapid and complete cessation of post-sympathectomy pain in some patients following administration of the anti-epileptic drugs phenytoin and carbamazepine [82] also supports the possible involvement of this process. Work by McGregor *et al.* [99] and by Wall and Woolf [100] suggests that other central processes, not involving degeneration of central processes but related to post-transection hyperactivity, require a period of 4–14 days to develop, a period similar to that in which pain first appears after sympathectomy.

Sympathetic activation of low-threshold mechanoreceptors

Low-threshold mechanoreceptors that innervate the proximal painful area may contribute to pain through the mechanisms described in the section on RSDS. In essence, these afferents would be activated by sympathetic post-ganglionic neurons projecting to the painful area and would, in turn, excite spinal WDR neurons. Sympathetic activation of these afferents would contribute to the 'spontaneous' pain of post-sympathectomy neuralgia, whereas mechanical stimulation of the same low-threshold afferents would be responsible for skin and muscle 'tenderness'

Other considerations

Clinical reports indicating that the post-sympathectomy pain develops in tissues *adjacent* to the sympathectomized area make it very unlikely that the pain results from changes in primary afferent fibers subsequent to loss of sympathetic innervation, as proposed by Schon [101], because the painful area is not sympathetically denervated.

Janig and Kollmann [51] have proposed that post-sympathectomy pain may result from ephaptic conduction between non-nociceptive and nociceptive afferents secondary to degeneration of post-ganglionic sympathetic axons and subsequent changes in Schwann cells. This degeneration would be maximal in the sympathectomized region of the limb, which is not painful. It would not explain post-sympathectomy pain localized proximal to the sympathectomized area.

Raskin *et al.* [82] have also proposed an explanation of post-sympathectomy pain based on ephaptic transmission – in this case, between transected postganglionic efferents and presumably nociceptive (vascular?) afferents in the paravertebral chain. Presumably these would be afferents that normally innervate the painful region.

The hypothesis proposed here and that proposed by Raskin *et al.* [82] both assume that the initiating event is transection of afferents in the lumbosacral trunk; however, the hypotheses differ in regard to the consequences of that transection. In this hypothesis the consequence is proposed to be denervation-induced hyperactivity in spinal neurons; in the hypothesis of Raskin *et al.* [82] the consequence is proposed to be ephaptic conduction between sympathetic efferent and primary afferent neurons. The mechanisms proposed in both hypotheses could operate simultaneously, and both may be valid; however, the proximal localization of the pain provides strong support for the denervation hypothesis. More information is needed on the origin of afferents projecting through the sympathetic trunk to determine whether the ephaptic mechanism would produce pain predominantly in proximal regions.

Raskin *et al.* [82] also noted that their hypothesis provided no explanation for the rapid and complete elimination of post-sympathectomy pain in some patients following administration of anti-epileptic drugs. The efficacy of anti-epileptic medication is understandable, however, if post-sympathectomy pain depends upon hyperactivity of central neurons, as proposed here.

Summary

Post-sympathectomy neuralgia is reported to occur in many patients who undergo surgical sympathectomy. The physiologic basis for the disorder is not known, but a possible mechanism based on clinical and basic animal studies is proposed here. Pain-related viscero-somatic spinal neurons are proposed to become hyperactive in response to somatic input following their 'visceral deafferentation' by the sympathectomy. The peripheral origin of the somatic input to the 'deafferented' viscero-somatic neurons is the site to which patients project the post-sympathectomy pain. This mechanism has been discussed in relation to lumbar sympathectomy, but would apply also to cervical sympathectomy.

OVERALL SUMMARY

Clinical findings clearly indicate that sympathetic activity is causally related to pain in several syndromes.

In these syndromes, sympathetic involvement may be mediated by one or more of several possible mechanisms. Two of these mechanisms, although not widely recognized, are well substantiated by clinical and experimental evidence. These are: (1) *activation* of *non-nociceptive* mechanoreceptors by sympathetic efferents, and (2) *sensitization* of *nociceptors* by sympathetically induced release of prostaglandins. Regardless of mechanism, sympathetically related pain appears not to be initiated by sympathetic activity, but rather appears to be maintained or exacerbated by it.

Experimental data indicate that sympathetic activation of *non-nociceptive* mechanoreceptors results in pain because the elicited afferent activity intensely activates certain pain-related spinal neurons – WDR neurons made *hyperexcitable* by previous nociceptive input. The validity of this mechanism is strongly substantiated by clinical demonstrations that spontaneous pain can be abolished by *selective* blockade of *non-nociceptive* afferents. .

In contrast to the mechanism above, sympathetically induced release of prostaglandins involves *nociceptive* rather than non-nociceptive afferents. The effect is one of *sensitization* rather than excitation and the prostaglandins contribute to pain only if noxious stimulation, e.g. active tissue injury, occurs to activate the sensitized receptors. Thus, this mechanism would be relevant during acute herpes zoster, but would not be relevant in reflex sympathetic dystrophy syndrome occurring in the absence of current trauma.

Other mechanisms that might causally relate sympathetic activity to pain are known, but their significance is difficult to ascertain from the available evidence. For example, sympathetic efferent activity does activate regenerating primary afferent fibers under certain experimental conditions. However, questions remain as to the pertinence of this mechanism to certain clinical findings, e.g. to the occurrence of allodynia (pain elicited by non-noxious stimulation) distal to the locus of nerve injury.

Similarly, sympathetically induced pathologic conditions such as ischemia or dystrophy may contribute to pain in certain disorders, as has been proposed in the 'vicious circle' explanation of reflex sympathetic dystrophy. However, in the acute stages of reflex sympathetic dystrophy, the correlation between ischemia or dystrophy and pain is poor.

Regardless of the peripheral mechanism of sympathetic involvement, sensitization of spinal WDR neurons by nociceptive input is probably an important process in the development of sympathetically related (or any other) pain, especially when pain is persistent. Previous sensitization seems essential if pain is to occur via sympathetic activation of non-nociceptive afferents.

References

1. Schultzberg, M., Hokfelt, T., Lundberg, J. M., Dalsgaard, C. J. and Elfvin, L. G. Transmitter histochemistry of autonomic ganglia. In *Autonomic Ganglia* (ed. L. G. Elfvin), John Wiley & Sons, New York, pp. 205–233 (1983)
2. Leriche, R. De la causalgie envisagée comme un nevrite du sympathetique et de son traitement par la denudation et excision des plexus nerveux perarteriels. *Presse Medicale*, **24**, 178–180 (1916)
3. Hannington-Kiff, J. G. *Pain Relief*, J. B. Lippincott, Philadelphia (1974)
4. Loh, L. and Nathan, P. W. Painful peripheral states and sympathetic blocks. *Journal of Neurology, Neurosurgery and Psychiatry*, **41**, 664–671 (1978)
5. Loh, L., Nathan, P. W., Schott, G. D. and Wilson, P. G. Effects of regional guanethidine infusion in certain painful states. *Journal of Neurology, Neurosurgery and Psychiatry*, **43**, 446–451 (1980)
6. Bonelli, S., Conoscente, F., Movilia, P. G., Restelli, L., Francucci, B. and Grossi, E. Regional intravenous guanethidine vs. stellate ganglion block in reflex sympathetic dystrophies: a randomized trial. *Pain*, **16**, 297–307 (1983)
7. Fields, H. L. Sources of variability in the sensation of pain. *Pain*, **33**, 195–200 (1988)
8. Wiesenfeld-Hallin, Z. and Hallin, R. G. The influence of the sympathetic system on mechanoreception and nociception. A review. *Human Neurobiology*, **3**, 41–46 (1984)
9. Roberts, W. J. A hypothesis on the physiological basis for causalgia and related pains. *Pain*, **24**, 297–311 (1986)
10. Price, D. D. and Dubner, R. Neurons that subserve the sensory-discriminative aspects of pain. *Pain*, **3**, 307–338 (1977)
11. Maixner, W., Dubner, R., Bushnell, M. C., Kenshalo, D. R., Jr and Oliveras, J. L. Wide-dynamic-range dorsal horn neurons participate in the encoding process by which monkeys perceive the intensity of noxious heat stimuli. *Brain Research*, **374**, 385–388 (1986)
12. Heppelmann, B., Schaible, H. G. and Schmidt, R. F. Effects of prostaglandins E1 and E2 on the mechanosensitivity of Group III afferents from normal and inflamed cat knee joints. In *Advances in Pain Research and Therapy, Vol. 9* (ed. H. L. Fields *et al.*), Raven Press, New York, pp. 91–101 (1985)
13. Levine, J. D., Taiwo, Y. O., Collins, S. D. and Tam, J. K. Noradrenaline hyperalgesia is mediated through interaction with sympathetic postganglionic neurone terminals rather than activation of primary afferent nociceptors. *Nature*, **323**, 158–160 (1986)
14. Martin, H. A., Basbaum, A. I., Kwiat, G. C., Goetzl, E. J. and Levine, J. D. Leukotriene and prostaglandin sensitization of cutaneous high-threshold C- and A-delta mechanonociceptors in the hairy skin of rat hindlimbs. *Neuroscience*, **22**, 651–659 (1987)
15. Nakamura, M. and Ferreira, S. H. A peripheral sympathetic component in inflammatory hyperalgesia. *European Journal of Pharmacology*, **135**, 145–153 (1987)
16. Roberts, W. J. and Lindsay, A. D. Sympathetic activity shown to have no short-term effect on polymodal nociceptors in cats. *Society for Neuroscience Abstracts*, **7**, 227 (1981)
17. Shea, V. K. and Perl, E. R. Failure of sympathetic stimulation to effect responsiveness of rabbit polymodal nociceptors. *Journal of Neurophysiology*, **54**, 513–520 (1985)
18. Barasi, S. and Lynn, B. Effects of sympathetic stimulation on mechanoreceptive and nociceptive afferent units from the rabbit pinna. *Brain Research*, **378**, 21–27 (1986)
18a. Hu, S. J., Chen, M. and Tian, Q. L. Different effects of sympathetic stimulation on evoked and spontaneous discharges of the polymodal nociceptors in rat. *Acta physiologica sinica*, **38**, 232–242 (1986)
19. Edwall, L. and Scott, D., Jr. Influence of changes in microcirculation on the excitability of the sensory unit in the tooth of the cat. *Acta physiologica scandinavica*, **82**, 555–566 (1971)
20. Roberts, W. J. and Elardo, S. M. Sympathetic activation of A-delta nociceptors. *Somatosensory Research*, **3**, 33–44 (1985)
21. Wall, P. D. and Gutnick, M. Ongoing activity in peripheral nerves: the physiology and pharmacology of impulses originating from a neuroma. *Experimental Neurology*, **43**, 580–593 (1974)

22. Scadding, J. W. Development of ongoing activity, mechanosensitivity and adrenaline sensitivity in severed peripheral nerve axons. *Experimental Neurology*, **73**, 345–364 (1981)
23. Korenman, E. M. D. and Devor, M. Ectopic adrenergic sensitivity in damaged peripheral nerve axons in the rat. *Experimental Neurology*, **72**, 63–81 (1981)
24. Devor, M. and Janig, W. Activation of myelinated afferents ending in a neuroma by stimulation of the sympathetic supply in the rat. *Neuroscience Letters*, **24**, 43–47 (1981)
25. Habler, H. J., Janig, W. and Koltzenburg, M. Activation of unmyelinated afferents in chronically lesioned nerves by adrenaline and excitation of sympathetic efferents in the cat. *Neuroscience Letters*, **82**, 35–40 (1987)
26. Blumberg, H. and Janig, W. Discharge pattern of afferent fibers from a neuroma. *Pain*, **20**, 335–353 (1984)
27. Blumberg, H. and Janig, W. Activation of fibers via experimentally produced stump neuromas of skin nerves: ephaptic transmission or retrograde sprouting. *Experimental Neurology*, **76**, 468–482 (1982)
28. Burchiel, K. J. and Russell, L. C. Has the amount of spontaneous electrical activity in experimental neuromas been overestimated? *Somatosensory Research*, **5**, 63–75 (1987)
29. Nystrom, B. and Hagbarth, K. E. Microelectrode recordings from transected nerves in amputees with phantom limb pain. *Neuroscience Letters*, **27**, 211–216 (1981)
30. Burnstock, G. Do some nerve cells release more than one transmitter? *Neuroscience*, **1**, 239–248 (1976)
31. Burnstock, G. The changing face of autonomic neurotransmission. *Acta physiologica scandinavica*, **126**, 67–91 (1986)
32. Lundberg, J. M. and Hokfelt, T. Co-existence of peptides and classical neurotransmitters. *Trends in Neuroscience*, **6**, 325–333 (1983)
33. Pernow, J. Co-release and functional interactions of neuropeptide Y and noradrenaline in peripheral sympathetic vascular control. *Acta physiologica scandinavica* (Suppl. 568), **133**, 1–56 (1988)
34. Lundberg, J. M., Anggard, A., Terenius, L., Elde, R., Markey, K. and Goldstein, M. Organization principles in the peripheral sympathetic nervous system: Subdivision by coexisting peptides (somatostatin, avian pancreatic polypeptide and vasoactive intestinal polypeptide-like immunoreactivities). *Proceedings of the National Academy of Sciences of the United States of America*, **79**, 1303–1307 (1982)
35. Hokfelt, T., Fuxe, K. and Pernow, B., eds. *Coexistence of Neuronal Messengers – A New Principle in Chemical Transmission. Progress in Brain Research, Vol. 68*, Elsevier, Amsterdam (1986)
36. Lundberg, J. M., Anggard, A. and Fahrenkrug, J. Complementary role of vasoactive intestinal polypeptide (VIP) and acetylcholine for cat submandibular gland blood flow and salivary secretion. I. VIP release. *Acta physiologica scandinavica*, **113**, 317–327 (1981)
37. Lundberg, J. M., Rudehill, A., Sollevi, A., Theodorsson-Norheim, E. and Hamberger, B. Frequency- and reserpine-dependent chemical coding of sympathetic transmission: differential release of noradrenaline and neuropeptide Y from pig spleen. *Neuroscience Letters*, **63**, 96–100 (1986)
38. Bartfai, T., Iverfeldt, K., Fisone, G. and Serfozo, P. Regulation of the release of coexisting neurotransmitters. *Annual Review of Pharmacology and Toxicology*, **28**, 285–310 (1988)
39. Comb, M., Hyman, S. E. and Goodman, H. M. Mechanisms of trans-synaptic regulation of gene expression. *Trends in Neuroscience*, **10**, 473–478 (1987)
40. Stjarne, L. Prostaglandin E restricting noradrenaline secretion neural in origin. *Acta physiologica scandinavica*, **86**, 574–576 (1972)
41. Hedqvist, P. Basic mechanisms of prostaglandin action on autonomic neurotransmission. *Annual Review of Pharmacology and Toxicology*, **17**, 259–279 (1977)
42. Moore, P. K. *Prostanoids: Pharmacological, Physiological and Clinical Relevance*, Cambridge University Press, Cambridge (1985)
43. Ferreira, S. H., Moncada, S. and Vance, J. R. Prostaglandins and the mechanism of analgesia produced by aspirin-like drugs. *British Journal of Pharmacology*, **49**, 86–97 (1973)
44. Levine, J. D., Dardick, S. J., Roizen, M. F., Helms, C. and Basbaum, A. I. Contribution of sensory afferents and sympathetic efferents to joint injury in experimental arthritis. *Journal of Neuroscience*, **6**, 3423–3429 (1986)
45. Schott, G. D. Mechanisms of causalgia and related clinical conditions: the role of the central and of the sympathetic nervous systems. *Brain*, **109**, 717–738 (1986)
46. Ochoa, J. The newly recognized painful ABC syndrome: thermographic aspects. *Thermography*, **2**, 65–107 (1986)
47. Cline, M. A., Ochoa, J. and Torebjork, H. E. Chronic hyperalgesia and skin warming caused by sensitized C-nociceptors and antidromic vasodilatation. *Brain*, in press (1988)

48. Campbell, J. N., Raja, S. N., Meyer, R. A. and Mackinnon, S. E. Myelinated afferents signal the hyperalgesia associated with nerve injury. *Pain*, **32**, 89–94 (1988)
49. Sunderland, S. Pain mechanisms in causalgia. *Journal of Neurology, Neurosurgery and Psychiatry*, **39**, 471–480 (1976)
50. Nathan, P. W. Pain and the sympathetic system. *Journal of the Autonomic Nervous System*, **7**, 363–370 (1983)
51. Janig, W. and Kollmann, W. The involvement of the sympathetic nervous system in pain. *Arzneimittel-Forschung/Drug Research*, **34**, 1066–1073 (1984)
52. Wallin, G., Torebjork, E. and Hallin, R. Preliminary observation on the pathophysiology of hyperalgesia in the causalgic pain syndrome. In *Sensory Functions of the Skin in Primates with Special Reference to Man* (ed. Y. Zotterman), Pergamon Press, Oxford, pp. 489–502 (1976).
53. Reeh, P. W., Bayer, J., Kocher, L. and Handwerker, H. O. Sensitization of nociceptive cutaneous nerve fibers from rat's tail by noxious mechanical stimulation. *Experimental Brain Research*, **65**, 505–512 (1987)
54. Pierce, J. P. and Roberts, W. J. Sympathetically induced changes in the responses of guard hair and type II receptors in the cat. *Journal of Physiology*, **314**, 411–428 (1981)
55. Roberts, W. J., Elardo, S. M. and King, K. A. Sympathetically-induced changes in the responses of slowly-adapting type I receptors in cat skin. *Somatosensory Research*, **2**, 223–236 (1985)
56. Roberts, W. J. and Foglesong, M. E. II. Identification of afferents contributing to sympathetically evoked activity in WDR neurons. *Pain*, **34**, 305–314 (1988)
57. Roberts, W. J. and Foglesong, M. E. I. Spinal recordings indicate that wide-dynamic-range neurons mediate sympathetically maintained pain. *Pain*, **34**, 289–304 (1988)
58. Livingston, W. K. *Pain Mechanisms. A Physiologic Interpretation of Causalgia and its Related States*, Macmillan, New York (1943)
59. Schumacker, H. B., Jr. Causalgia. III. A general discussion. *Surgery*, **24**, 485–504 (1948)
60. Tahmoush, A. J., Mallet, J. and Jennings, J. R. Skin conductance, temperature, and blood flow in causalgia. *Neurology*, **33**, 1483–1486 (1983)
61. Nathan, P. W. On the pathogenesis of causalgia in peripheral nerve injuries. *Brain*, **70**, 145–170 (1947)
62. Devor, M. Nerve pathophysiology and mechanisms of pain in causalgia. *Journal of the Autonomic Nervous System*, **7**, 371–384 (1983)
63. Doupe, J., Cullen, C. and Chance, G. Post-traumatic pain and the causalgic syndrome. *Journal of Neurology, Neurosurgery and Psychiatry*, **7**, 33–48 (1944)
64. Grennan, D. M. and Jayson, M. I. V. Rheumatoid arthritis. In *Textbook of Pain* (ed. P. D. Wall and R. Melzack), Churchill Livingstone, Edinburgh, pp. 225–233 (1984)
65. Herfort, R. A. Extended sympathectomy in the treatment of advanced rheumatoid arthritis. *New York Journal of Medicine*, **56**, 1292 (1956)
66. Levine, J. D., Fye, K., Heller, P., Basbaum, A. I. and Whiting-O'Keefe, Q. Clinical response to regional intravenous guanethidine in patients with rheumatoid arthritis. *Journal of Rheumatology*, **13**, 1040–1043 (1986)
67. Yousufzai, S. Y. K., Gracy, R. A., Aboul-Khair, H. S. and Abdel-Latif, A. A. *In vivo* electrical stimulation of the sympathetic nerve of the eye increases inositol phosphate production and prostaglandin release in the rabbit iris muscle. *Journal of Neurochemistry*, **50**, 752–758 (1988)
68. Schaible, H. G. and Schmidt, R. F. Direct observation of the sensitization of articular afferents during an experimental arthritis. In *Pain Research and Clinical Management* (ed. R. Dubner, G. F. Gebhart and M. R. Bond), Elsevier, Amsterdam, pp. 44–50 (1988)
69. Schaible, H. G., Schmidt, R. F. and Willis, W. D. Convergent inputs from articular, cutaneous and muscle receptors onto ascending tract cells in the cat spinal cord. *Experimental Brain Research*, **66**, 479–488 (1987)
70. Woolf, C. J. and Wall, P. D. Relative effectiveness of C primary afferent fibers of different origins in evoking a prolonged facilitation of the flexor reflex in the rat. *Journal of Neuroscience*, **6**, 1433–1442 (1986)
71. Schaible, H. G., Schmidt, R. F. and Willis, W. D. Enhancement of the responses of ascending tract cells in the cat spinal cord by acute inflammation of the knee joint. *Experimental Brain Research*, **66**, 489–499 (1987)
72. Sato, A., Sato, Y. and Schmidt, R. F. Catecholamine secretion and adrenal nerve activity in response to movements of normal and inflamed knee joints in cats. *Journal of Physiology*, **375**, 611–624 (1986)
73. Baringer, J. R. and Townsend, J. J. Herpesvirus infection of the peripheral nervous system. In *Peripheral Neuropathy* (ed. P. J. Dyck *et al.*), W. B. Saunders Co., Philadelphia, pp. 1941–1954 (1984)
74. Loeser, J. D. Herpes zoster and postherpetic neuralgia. *Pain*, **25**, 149–164 (1986)

75. Colding, A. The effect of regional sympathetic blocks in the treatment of herpes zoster. *Acta anaesthesiologica scandinavica*, **13**, 133–141 (1969)
76. Olsen, E. R. and Ivy, H. B. Stellate block for trigeminal zoster. *Journal of Clinical Neuro-ophthalmology*, **1**, 53–55 (1981)
77. Toyama, N. Sympathetic ganglion block therapy for herpes zoster. *Journal of Dermatology*, **9**, 59–62 (1982)
78. Milligan, N. S. and Nash, T. P. Treatment of post-herpetic neuralgia. A review of 77 consecutive cases. *Pain*, **23**, 381–386 (1985)
79. Higa, K., Dan, K., Manabe, H. and Noda, B. Factors influencing the duration of treatment of acute herpetic pain with sympathetic nerve block: importance of severity of herpes zoster assessed by the maximum antibody titers to varicella-zoster virus in otherwise healthy patients. *Pain*, **32**, 147–158 (1988)
80. Chahl, L. A. and Iggo, A. The effects of bradykinin and prostaglandin E1 on rat cutaneous afferent nerve activity. *British Journal of Pharmacology*, **59**, 343–347 (1977)
81. Ferreira, S. H. Prostaglandins, pain, and inflammation. *Agents and Actions*, Suppl. **19**, 91–98 (1986)
82. Raskin, N. H., Levinson, S. A., Hoffman, P. M., Pickett, J. B. E. and Fields, H. L. Postsympathectomy neuralgia. *American Journal of Surgery*, **128**, 75–78 (1974)
83. Mockus, M. B., Rutherford, R. B., Rosales, C. and Pearce, W. H. Sympathectomy for causalgia. *Archives of Surgery*, **122**, 668–671 (1987)
84. Tracy, G. D. and Cockett, F. B. Pain in the lower limb after sympathectomy. *Lancet*, **i**, 12–14 (1957)
85. Hinsey, J. C. The anatomical relations of the sympathetic system to visceral sensation. In *Sensation: Its Mechanisms and Disturbances. Association for Research in Nervous and Mental Disease, Vol. XV* (ed. C. A. Patten, A. M. Franz and C. C. Hare), Williams and Wikins Co., Baltimore, pp. 105–180 (1935)
86. Kuntz, A. *The Autonomic Nervous System*, Lea and Febiger, Philadelphia (1953)
87. Pick, J. *The Autonomic Nervous System*, J. B. Lippincott Co., Philadelphia (1970)
88. Mendell, L. M. Modifiability of spinal synapses. *Physiological Reviews*, **64**, 260–324 (1984)
89. Pubols, L. M. and Sessle, B. J., eds. *Effects of Injury on Trigeminal and Spinal Somatosensory Systems*. Alan R. Liss, Inc., New York (1987)
90. Devor, M. and Wall, P. D. Reorganization of spinal cord sensory map after peripheral nerve injury. *Nature*, **276**, 75–76 (1978)
91. Devor, M. and Wall, P. D. Plasticity in the spinal cord sensory map following peripheral nerve injury in rats. *Journal of Neuroscience*, **1**, 679–684 (1981)
92. Fields, H. L. *Pain*, McGraw-Hill, New York (1987)
93. Cervero, F. and Tattersall, J. E. H. Somatic and visceral sensory integration in the thoracic spinal cord. In *Visceral Sensation. Progress in Brain Research* (ed. F. Cervero and J. F. B. Morrison), Elsevier, Amsterdam, pp. 189–206 (1986)
94. Foreman, R. D., Hobbs, S. F., Chandler, J. J. and Bolser, D. C. Differences in viscerosomatic inputs to spinothalamic (ST) cells projecting to VPLc and VPLo thalamus in monkeys. *Society for Neuroscience Abstracts,*, **14**, (Part 1) 121 (1988)
95. Hobbs, S. F., Bolser, D. C., Chandler, M. J. and Foreman, R. D. Could spinothalamic tract (STT) transmit muscle afferent input to primary motor cortex (MI) in monkeys? *Society for Neuroscience Abstracts*, **14**, Part 1, 181 (1988)
96. Milne, R. J., Foreman, R. D., Giesler, G. J., Jr and Willis, W. D. Convergence of cutaneous and pelvic visceral nociceptive inputs on to primate spinothalamic neurons. *Pain*, **11**, 163–183 (1981)
97. Hancock, M. B., Foreman, R. D. and Willis, W. D. Convergence of visceral and cutaneous input onto spinothalamic tract cells in the thoracic spinal cord of the cat. *Experimental Neurology*, **47**, 240–248 (1975)
98. Cervero, F. Somatic and visceral inputs to the thoracic spinal cord of the cat: effects of noxious stimulation of the biliary system. *Journal of Physiology*, **337**, 51–67 (1983)
99. McGregor, C. P., Gibson, S. J., Sabate, I. M., Blank, M. A., Christophides, N. D., Wall, P. D., Polak, J. M. and Bloom, S. R. Effect of peripheral nerve section and nerve crush on spinal cord neuropeptides in the rat: increased VIP and PHI in the dorsal horn. *Neuroscience*, **13**, 207–216 (1984)
100. Wall, P. D. and Woolf, C. J. The brief and the prolonged facilitatory effects of unmyelinated afferent input on the rat spinal cord are independently influenced by peripheral nerve section. *Neuroscience*, **17**, 1199–1205 (1986)
101. Schon, F. Postsympathectomy pain and changes in sensory neuropeptides: towards an animal model. *Lancet*, **ii**, 1158–1160 (1985)

5
Reflex sympathetic dystrophy syndrome: diagnosis and treatment

Richard Payne

CLINICAL FEATURES OF CAUSALGIA AND REFLEX SYMPATHETIC DYSTROPHY

Introduction

'Reflex sympathetic dystrophy (RSD)' and 'causalgia' are generic terms that are used to describe a cluster of symptoms and signs that follow injury to bone, soft tissue, and nerve. The terms are synonymous with a variety of other terms, such as ·'Sudeck's atrophy', 'major and minor causalgia', 'mimocausalgia', 'shoulder–hand syndrome', 'post-traumatic pain syndrome', 'sympathalgia', 'chronic traumatic edema', that describe pain occurring in association with swelling and dystrophic changes in skin, bone and connective tissue following trauma [1,2]. Although this chapter emphasizes RSD complicating trauma or injury to the limbs, sympathetically maintained pain may complicate injury to the face, thorax or abdomen as well.

RSD may have a variety of causes including: (1) blunt trauma (which may be trivial) [3]; (2) inflammatory disorders; (3) immobility associated with myocardial and cerebral infarction; (4) cervical osteoarthritis and other degenerative joint diseases; (5) frostbite; (6) burns; (7) drugs, especially phenobarbital [4,5]; (8) malignancy and associated paraneoplastic effects [6]. However, in about 35% of cases the cause of RSD is unknown.

Pain may begin within minutes or hours after injury, is usually burning in quality, often disproportionately intense with respect to the nature or extent of the injury, and persists after presumed healing of the injury. Initially, pain may be confined to a peripheral nerve or vascular distribution, but usually spreads beyond the local area of injury, particularly if not treated early or effectively. The syndrome is divided, somewhat arbitrarily, into three phases, but one must recognize that RSD represents a spectrum and almost no patient exhibits all of the symptoms and signs in the sequence as described below [7].

The *acute stage* lasts several weeks starting from the time of injury and is characterized by *spontaneous pain* which is aching and burning in nature, restricted to a vascular or peripheral nerve or root territory, and usually associated with *hyperpathia*. Hyperpathia is 'a painful syndrome, characterized by increased reaction to a stimulus, especially a repetitive stimulus, as well as an increased threshold', and often coexists with *allodynia* or 'pain due to a stimulus which does not normally provoke pain' [8]. The skin may be warm and red early in the course of the disorder, but later it is typically cold and cyanotic. Excessive sweating is also a well-known feature, and is often associated with swelling. Hair and nail growth may be increased. Dependent rubor and decreased range of motion in the extremity may also be seen at this stage.

The *dystrophic stage* begins about 3 months after injury if RSD has not been treated effectively. At this stage, pain may occupy a wider area than originally, and often extends outside the initial dermatome or vascular region of injury (*see* Figure 5.1a,b). Hyperpathia and swelling may be more pronounced than in the acute stage. There is increased joint thickness and tenderness and the range of motion of the joints may become more restricted. Muscle wasting and osteoporosis are also evident by this stage (*see* Figure 5.2).

The *atrophic stage* is the end-stage of RSD and usually occurs > 6 months after the injury. Pain often remains severe, but in some instances may be less prominent than in the earlier stages. The skin is usually cool, pale and cyanotic in appearance, and prominent irreversible trophic changes in the skin and subcutaneous tissues are evident. This is manifested as smooth, glossy appearance of the skin with loss of the usual skin wrinkles and folds. If the hands or feet are affected, there is tapering of the ends of the digits (*see* Figure 5.3) and the distal and proximal joints may be stiff and contracted. Frank osteoporosis and joint contractures may be evident.

The signs and symptoms listed above define the RSD syndrome, regardless of the cause, but not all are present in every patient. The mechanisms of these signs and symptoms are not known in all instances, but some relate to sympathetic nervous system activity (e.g. vasoconstriction, increased sweating, and perhaps allodynia and pain) because they improve after sympathetic blockade. Hypotheses relating to mechanisms of pain and hyperpathia in RSD are listed in Table 5.1 and are discussed in detail by Raja *et al.* (Chapter 2) and Roberts and Kramis (Chapter 4). The mechanisms producing the dystrophic changes are more problematic, however, and are not as clearly related to sympathetic hyperactivity. Some authors have suggested that many, if not all, of the dystrophic changes simply reflect disuse of the painful extremity and are not related to sympathetic hyperactivity *per se*. In favor of this argument is the observation that these changes are most evident in the late stages of the disease, and are less likely to improve with sympathetic blockade than are pain and hyperpathia. None the less, the dystrophic changes in skin, subcutaneous tissues, bone, joints and muscles are so characteristic of RSD, even in

Table 5.1 Proposed pain mechanisms in RSD and causalgia

Peripheral mechanisms	Central mechanisms
Abnormal discharges in sympathetic afferent fibers	Sensitization of nociceptive neurons in the spinal cord following trauma
Sensitization and/or activation of peripheral sensory receptors by sympathetic activity	
Ephaptic interactions between sympathetic efferent and nociceptive afferent fibers	

For detailed discussion of these hypotheses *see* chapters 2 and 4 (this volume) and Payne [9]

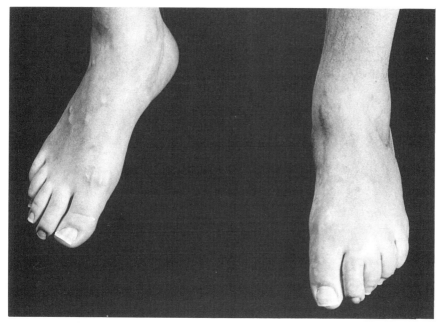

a

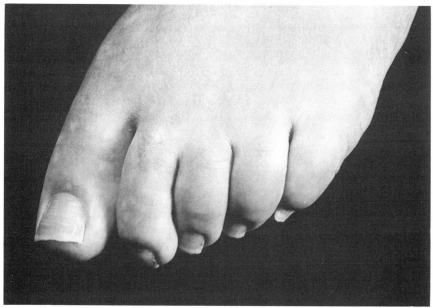

b

Figure 5.1 a, Swollen left lower extremity in patient with burning pain and hyperpathia of left foot following a fall from a ladder causing bilateral heel fractures. The injury had occurred more than one year before. b, Close-up view of left foot demonstrating the swollen and mottled appearance typical of the brawny edema seen in RSD

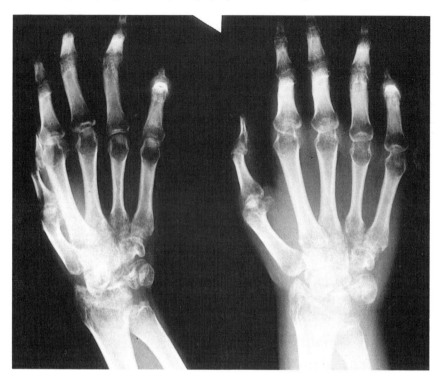

Figure 5.2 Bilateral osteoporosis affecting the hands in a patient with RSD complicating toxic epidermal necrolysis following a hypersensitivity reaction to phenytoin. Note the diffuse bone loss in the wrists and the subepiphysial bone lost in the metacarpal joints

in the early stages, that it is difficult to consider the diagnosis in their absence. It does appear that, in sum, these dystrophic changes are greater than one would expect from simple disuse of the extremity, but the mechanisms by which sympathetic activity may play a part in their appearance are not clear.

Causalgia: sympathetically maintained pain following nerve injury

Causalgia may be considered to be a special type of RSD [1,2,9]. Causalgia differs from other RSD in that it is associated with *peripheral nerve injury* and pain may be quite severe, even without striking vasomotor and sudomotor changes. In fact, one investigator has suggested that causalgia and RSD may be produced by different mechanisms [10,11]. As defined by the IASP subcommittee on taxonomy, causalgia is 'a syndrome of sustained, burning pain after a traumatic nerve injury combined with vasomotor and sudomotor and later trophic changes' [8]. The term causalgia was used by Weir Mitchell [12] to identify a continuous severe 'burning pain' of long duration which followed peripheral nerve injury (classically battlefield missile injuries). In addition to the severe burning pain, there were atrophic changes in skin, nails and subcutaneous tissue similar, if not identical, to the changes described above. Pain following traumatic nerve injury, particularly missile wounds involving the proximal nerve trunks, is typically referred to the distal portion of the extremity

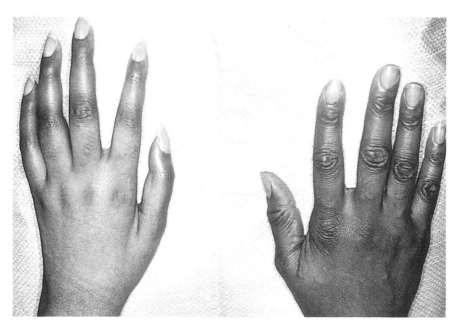

Figure 5.3 Subcutaneous atrophy with tapering of the digits and the appearance of 'sausage-shape' deformity of the fingers of the left hand following brachial plexus avulsion more than 3 years before. The patient complained of burning and aching pain in the shoulder and base of neck, and shooting, stinging pain radiating from the neck into all 5 digits. Myelography demonstrated avulsion of C5, C6, C7 and C8 nerve roots from the spinal cord. This was caused by an accident which is frequently associated with such injuries. The patient was struck by an automobile and thrown from her bicycle, landing in a position in which her head was turning violently to the right, and her shoulder was hyperextended. The shooting (but not the burning) pain was partially relieved by a stellate ganglion block

(i.e. the hand or foot). It is usually severe and although often described as burning in quality, very occasionally may not have this quality. Characteristically, the pain is aggravated by environmental or emotional stimuli. Most clinicians expect that pain will be persistent for several weeks, and the persistence of the pain serves to distinguish true causalgia from pain due to extensive non-neural tissue damage, which most often subsides within a few weeks in the absence of ongoing injury or sympathetic activity.

In order to *establish* the diagnosis, some would require that pain, mobility and joint function improve following sympathetic blockade; however, this is controversial. The interpretation of a positive response to sympathetic blockade may be difficult, as it is not always easy to determine if a truly selective sympathetic block has been performed (i.e. in the absence of somatic sensory blockade), and there are apparently some patients who have many of the clinical features of causalgia or RSD listed above, but who do not get pain relief with an unequivocally selective sympathetic block. Whether these patients truly have (or had) RSD and now do not respond to sympathetic blockade because the disease is to end-stage, or their pain is now primarily driven by secondary musculoskeletal complications of the disorder, is perhaps a semantic argument. However, it does not appear to be reasonable to assert that these patients now have 'sympathetically maintained' pain.

Weir Mitchell's classic descriptions of causalgia occurring in wounded Civil War soldiers described the onset of pain several days after battlefield injury in association with 'traumatic fevers' [12]. However, in modern series, pain begins within a few hours to one week after injury in > 80% of cases [13], although latencies of 10–30 days or longer have been reported [14]. The pain is usually so severe as to preclude usual daily activities, and promotes profound behavioral and personality changes. Intense pain and hyperpathia and their exaggeration by environmental stimuli and emotional distress (e.g. unexpected flashes of light; loud noises; the lighting of a common housefly on the skin) frequently lead the patient to withdraw into an isolated secluded environment and to protect the affected part cautiously. In one-half to two-thirds of patients, paroxysms of deep pain are superimposed on the continuous pain – these paroxysms may be described as 'stabbing' or 'crushing' [13]. Rarely, hyperpathia may be dissociated from burning pain [15].

The prognosis and duration of pain are variable. Pain persists for > 6 months in 85% and for > 1 year in 25% [13]. The clinical course of pain and dystrophy is not necessarily related to the degree of nerve injury, age of the patient or associated soft-tissue injury. Early aggressive treatment of pain, especially the use of sympathetic blockade, appears to be very important in improving pain and allowing aggressive physical therapy and rehabilitation early in the course of the disorder, and perhaps prevents the progression to end-stage RSD, although controlled prospective studies to prove this assertion are non-existent.

Causalgia is a relatively rare complication of peripheral nerve injury. Estimates from World War II are that persistent pain complicated about 2–5% of all peripheral nerve injuries; this incidence was somewhat less in the Vietnam War [13]. Although classically caused by penetrating missile wounds which produce partial injury to proximal nerve trunks, it may be associated with a variety of traumatic etiologies [11,16]. The common feature of most trauma associated with causalgia involves stretching and partial tearing or shearing of nerve, without complete severance of the nerve (*see* Figure 5.4). Causalgia has been recognized as an increasingly common complication of civilian and iatrogenic injuries – motor-cycle accidents with avulsion of roots of the brachial plexus [17], surgical retraction of bone and soft tissues, intramuscular injections and even venipuncture [16].

In battlefield injuries, about 90% of peripheral nerve lesions associated with causalgia are above the elbow and the knee [18]. Injuries of the median nerve, the medial cord of the brachial plexus, and the sciatic nerve are the most likely to produce causalgia [18]. The sciatic nerve is involved in 40% of all cases of causalgia; the median nerve in 35%; the medial cord of the brachial plexus in 12%; other nerves (greater occipital, intercostal, cauda equina, etc.) are involved 13% of the time [3,18]. The median and sciatic nerves carry the majority of the post-ganglionic sympathetic afferent fibers to the upper and lower extremities, respectively, and this may be the anatomic basis for their propensity to be associated with this complication of nerve injury [18].

At the time of injury there may be numbness and paresis coexisting with severe pain. This occurs because there is partial nerve damage and the injury has caused a conduction block. As motor and sensory fibers regenerate, a clinically complete lesion may be converted into an incomplete lesion, but the degree of recovery may be difficult to ascertain because the associated hyperpathia and swelling may preclude adequate clinical examination, and dystrophic connective tissue changes may produce secondary restrictive joint changes which limit mobility.

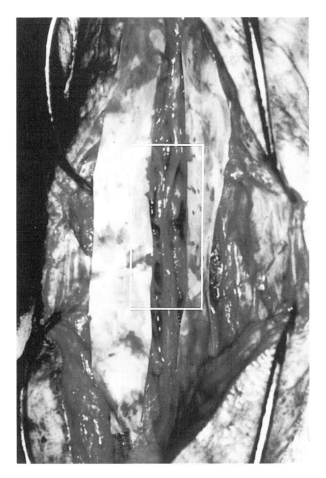

Figure 5.4 Intra-operative photograph of the tibial nerve in a patient who suffered a partial traumatic amputation on his leg in an automobile accident. Note (rectangle) that the nerve has been pushed backward and has been stretched (by a bone fragment which is not pictured). This patient suffered severe burning pain in the entire leg below the knee. Shooting pain could be elicited from a 'trigger point' by palpation just below the popliteal fossa. The burning and shooting pain was relieved with a lumbar sympathetic block

CLINICAL ASSESSMENT AND DIAGNOSIS

Clinical criteria for the diagnosis of RSD

The history of burning pain occurring hours or days after soft-tissue injury, and the finding of hyperpathia with smooth glossy skin and cutaneous vasoconstriction and subcutaneous atrophy, are virtually diagnostic of the RSD syndrome. As noted above, the precipitating injury may be trivial or not even remembered.

Kozin *et al.* [19] have proposed that patients be classified as 'definite', 'probable', 'possible' or 'doubtful' RSD, based on the following clinical criteria:

1. *Definite RSD*. Pain and swelling in an extremity with signs and symptoms of vasomotor instability, and swelling (dystrophic skin changes are *usually* also present).
2. *Probable RSD*. Pain and swelling in an extremity and either symptoms or signs of vasomotor instability or swelling (dystrophic skin changes are *often* present).
3. *Possible RSD*. Symptoms and signs of vasomotor instability and swelling are present. Pain is not a feature, but often tenderness is present.
4. *Doubtful RSD*. Unexplained pain in extremity. No vasomotor instability or swelling is present, and often no tenderness is present.

These criteria have been used to assess the sensitivity and specificity of bone scintigraphic and radiologic abnormalities in RSD, and to assess the efficacy of a variety of therapeutic interventions, particularly the use of corticosteroids (*see below*).

A recent report suggests that pain characteristics, the amount of edema in the extremity, and the loss of joint motion may be quantified in patients with RSD [20]. The methods by which this is accomplished include: (1) grading of the amount of pain to joint palpation; (2) volumetric measurements of the limb by determining the volume of water displaced by the affected extremity; (3) measurement of skin temperature in the hand and foot; (4) goniometric measurements of ankle motion to assess active range-of-motion (ROM), and (5) the use of the McGill Pain Questionnaire (MPQ) and a visual analog scale (VAS) to assess the sensory-affective qualities and intensity of pain.

These investigators evaluated 17 patients who met Kozin's criteria for definite or probable RSD, and reported that there was a statistically significant correlation between limb volume, active range of motion in the lower extremity, and the VAS reports of pain intensity [20]. It is noteworthy that skin temperature did not correlate with changes in joint pain, range of motion, limb volume or pain measures on the MPQ or VAS, although all of these scales were internally consistent. This attempt to quantify signs and symptoms occurring in RSD is important and apparently simple. As suggested by the authors, protocols such as this should be a part of clinical studies which attempt to assess the natural history of RSD and the efficacy of therapeutic interventions.

Use of diagnostic tests in RSD

Laboratory tests that are useful in confirming the diagnosis or following the response to treatment are based on measuring abnormalities of sympathetic 'tone' and on radiologic imaging of soft tissue and bony lesions. These are listed in Table 5.2 and are described in more detail below and by Löfström and Cousins [21].

Assessment of sympathetic function

Skin blood flow and temperature can be estimated by direct palpation of the skin (differences of > 2°C can be palpated). Skin temperature can be directly measured

Table 5.2 Some useful diagnostic tests in patients with RSD

Assessment	Test or procedure
Sympathetic function	Sweat tests (ninhydrin, starch iodine, cobalt blue)
	Skin plethysmography
	Skin galvanic resistance
Skin blood flow	Xenon-133 clearance
	Skin thermoprobe
	Thermography
Radiological examination	Plain X-rays
	Bone scintigraphy
Sympathetic blockade	Stellate
	Paravertebral
	Celiac plexus
	Continuous epidural infusion
	Intravenous regional
Pain	McGill Pain Questionnaire
	Visual analog and categorical scales of pain intensity

by a thermoprobe, and a qualitative 'map' of thermal skin changes can be measured by thermography (*see below*). Skin blood flow can be measured by the plethysmographic and xenon clearance methods [21]. Sudomotor function may be assessed by measuring the sympathogalvanic response (which is an indirect measure as it determines electrical resistance of the skin that is related to the degree of moisture), or more directly by a sweat test using ninhydrin, cobalt blue or starch–iodide (*see* Table 5.2).

Radiologic examination and bone scintigraphy in RSD

Radiologic examination is helpful to determine the presence of osteoporosis. Both extremities should be in the same exposure to avoid problems in interpretation of the radiographic changes which occur in Sudeck's atrophy, i.e. diffuse and patchy bony demineralization, particularly subepiphysial and periarticular demineralization (*see* Figure 5.2). Kozin reported the presence of osteoporosis in 69% of patients with definite, possible or probable RSD. However, osteoporosis is not specific for RSD, even when it occurs within four weeks of the onset of symptoms, although patients put in casts or who suffer paralysis generally require longer periods of immobilization (8 weeks or more) before osteoporosis is apparent [19].

Bone scintigraphy is often performed in patients with suspected RSD [19,22,23] (*see* Figure 5.5). Kozin *et al.* [19] reported that 60% of patients with RSD had abnormalities on bone scintigraphic imaging following intravenous administration of 15 mCi Tc-methylene diphosphonate (MDP) or Tc-ethane-1-hydroxy-1-1-diphosphonate (EDHP). After injection of these nucleotides, rapid sequence perfusion scans were obtained to assess regional blood flow, and delayed static images were obtained 3 h after injection. Positive scans were defined as those

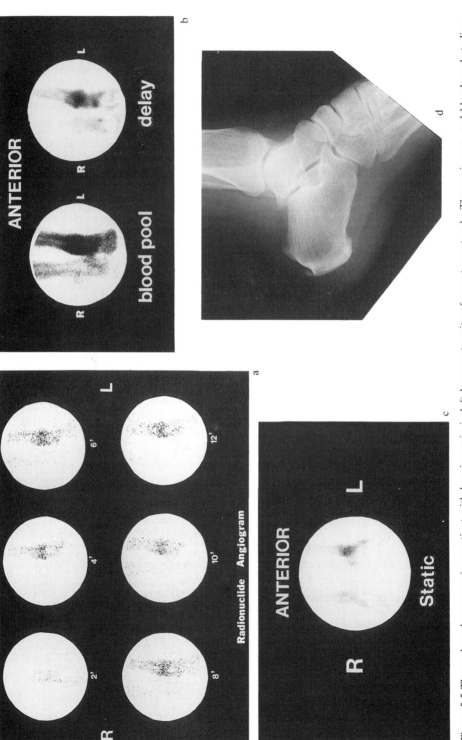

Figure 5.5 Three-phase bone scan in a patient with burning pain in left lower extremity of recent onset. a,b, The angiogram and blood pool studies demonstrate increased blood flow and increased uptake of radionuclide in the left foot and ankle. c, Delayed (3–4 h) images of feet demonstrate increased uptake in the left ankle. d, Plain radiographs of the left foot are normal. The three-phase bone scan may be more sensitive in detecting abnormalities of blood flow and bone than the plain X-ray

showing either asymmetric blood flow or increased periarticular activity in multiple joints of the affected distal extremity on the delayed images. The bone scan shown in Figure 5.5 demonstrates these findings. The increased activity of the radiopharmaceutical is a possible reflection of the 'vasomotor instability' so often commented upon in RSD, as it may represent increased uptake in bone as a consequence of altered blood flow [19].

These same investigators also noted that bone scintigraphy is as sensitive as plain radiographs, but is more specific in detecting abnormalities in RSD. This is so, in part, because the osteoporosis seen on plain radiographs may be caused by any painful disorder which produces immobilization. It is interesting that Kozin *et al.* [19] suggested that serial bone scans may allow one to correlate 'activity' of the disorder, and also noted that 90% of patients with positive bone scans had 'good' or 'excellent' responses when treated with systemic corticosteroids, whereas 64% of patients with negative bone scans had a 'poor' or 'fair' response.

Recently, Demangeat *et al.*,[23] have reported that RSD involving the hand may be staged on the basis of three phase bone scintigraphic imaging techniques. They studied 181 patients. Criteria for diagnosis of RSD were similar to those described by Kozin *et al.* [19]. Bone scintigraphy was accomplished following a bolus injection of 0.2 μCi/kg technetium-99m (^{99m}Tc) methylene diphosphonate, and the hand was imaged as follows: (1) an immediate radionuclide angiogram was done (Phase I); (2) an early static phase, also called a blood pool or tissue phase, was done 3–5 min after injection (Phase II), and a delayed high-resolution image was obtained 2–3 h after injection (Phase III). They reported that the patterns of abnormalities in the three phases differed, depending on the duration of symptoms of RSD. Thus, patients who were imaged 0–20 weeks after onset of symptoms (Stage I) had abnormal blood flow, blood pool and delayed images. Patients studied 20–60 weeks after onset of symptoms (Stage II) had normal blood-flow scans, but increased uptake on delayed images. Finally, patients with symptoms from 60 to 100 weeks in duration (Stage III) had decreased blood flow images and normal delayed static images [23].

In the acute stage (I), all radionuclide parameters are increased on the affected side, but during the later stages, normalization of blood flow occurred (Stage II), and then bone hypofixation (Stage III). It was speculated that the reduced blood flow in Stage III may be secondary to disuse or modification of the bone tissue as a result of RSD. Finally, these investigators suggested that differing descriptions of bone scintigraphic abnormalities in RSD may be reconciled by correcting for the duration or stage of the disorder. For example, Mackinnon and Holder [22] have reported that diffuse increase in the phase III bone scan was virtually 'diagnostic' for RSD, with a sensitivity of 96% and a specificity of 98%, whereas phase I and II scans were positive in only 45% and 52%, respectively.

Although the ultimate usefulness of bone scans in RSD is still not clear, this author recommends that a three-phase bone scan be performed in all patients in whom the diagnosis of RSD is considered, and the images compared with plain radiographs. It is possible that serial bone scans may allow one to assess the effectiveness of therapy (as suggested by Kozin [19] and Demangeat [23]), but proof of this concept awaits a formal study.

Thermography

Thermography has been used to provide qualitative and semi-quantitative information about temperature changes occurring in a variety of chronic pain conditions, including RSD [24]. Thermographic imaging is also helpful in assessing the effectiveness of sympathetic blockade. Although the specificity and sensitivity of thermographic changes occurring in RSD have not been widely studied, Uematsu *et al.* [24] reported that thermography was positive in 89% of patients suspected of having RSD or causalgia where there was corroborating clinical and electromyographic evidence of peripheral nerve injury. Clearly, the role of thermography in RSD requires further study.

Response to sympathetic blockade

Many investigators have suggested that a positive response to sympathetic blockade is essential for the diagnosis [25]. However, the response to sympathetic blockade appears not to be 100%, even in otherwise classic cases of causalgia [18], and there may be false-positive and false-negative responses to sympathetic blockade. The effectiveness of sympathetic blockade should be assessed by one of the measures discussed above [21]. Assuming that one has obtained an adequate sympathetic block, false-positive responses may occur when somatic sensory nerves are rendered anesthetic in addition to, or instead of, the sympathetic nerves. This may occur because the sympathetic nerves often lie in close proximity to somatic sensory nerves. In this circumstance, the patient usually reports pain relief associated with a subjective sense of 'numbness', or sensory loss may be demonstrated on physical examination. Therefore, the patient must be directly questioned about, and examined for, the presence of sensory loss before one can assume that there has been a selective sympathetic block.

On the other hand, in theory, patients may not report pain relief if the secondary musculoskeletal changes are major factors producing pain, even though sympathetic mechanisms may have been important contributors to their pain initially. This may be an important cause of failure of sympathetic blocks done in the late stages of RSD.

A full discussion of the techniques of sympathetic blockade and a detailed discussion concerning the assessment of sympathetic function following anesthetic blockade are beyond the scope of this chapter, but are presented by Löfström and Cousins [21].

THERAPY

Sympathetic interruption

Interruption of efferent sympathetic fibers is the mainstay of therapy in the reflex sympathetic dystrophies and may be accomplished by temporary or permanent anesthetic blockade of sympathetic ganglia, surgical lesions of the sympathetic trunk, intravenous injection of guanethidine or reserpine, or by oral administration of adrenergic blocking drugs.

Sympathetic blocks with local anesthetic agents

Sympathetic blocks may be done at the stellate ganglion (for head, trunk and upper extremity pain), celiac plexus (for abdominal pain), or the lumbar sympathetic ganglia (for lower extremity and pelvic pain). Local anesthetics are used for diagnostic and short-term therapeutic blocks. Mepivacaine (0.5%) or bupivacaine (0.25%) have durations of action of 1.5–3 and 3–4 h, respectively, and may be mixed with contrast medium to identify the site of injection by radiography. In general, volumes of 1–5 ml are injected for stellate or lumbar sympathetic blocks [21]. The duration of pain relief is expected to outlast the duration of action of the anesthetic agent, especially if the block is performed within days after the onset of pain. Success rates of up to 90% in RSD and 50–60% in causalgia have been reported [3,9]. The response rate is a function of : (1) the timing of the block in relation to the onset of pain; (2) the skill of the physician, and (3) the completeness of sympathetic blockade.

A recent series reported that 70% of patients (23 of 33) demonstrated improvement in pain relief over three years if sympathetic blocks were initiated within six months of onset of symptoms of RSD [26]. However, only 50% (5 of 10 patients) treated 6–12 months after initial symptoms reported improvement at three years follow-up. The most common sign of sympathetic blockade is an immediate rise in skin temperature ipsilateral to the side of the block. An ipsilateral Horner's syndrome (pupillary miosis, ptosis and loss of facial sweating) usually occurs immediately after blockade of the stellate ganglion, but if there is physical non-union of the cervical sympathetic ganglia, one may get a Horner's syndrome without skin temperature change. The onset of pain relief usually occurs within minutes of the block and may persist for days or weeks [27] even without persistent increase in skin temperature. Pain relief is usually accomplished by increased mobility and function in the extremity.

Continuous sympathetic blockade may be accomplished by use of a catheter placed in the epidural space and the slow infusion of dilute concentrations of local anesthetic drugs. The catheter location may be verified radiographically, or by the administration of 2-chloroprocaine (2 ml of a 3% solution) to provide a transient sensory block. In the lumbar epidural space, bupivacaine (0.2–0.3%) may be infused from 6 to 10 ml/h to produce a continuous sympathetic block. The concentration of bupivacaine and the rate of infusion (as well as catheter placement) can be adjusted to provide an optimum effect, i.e. sympathetic block in the absence of significant weakness or sensory loss. Other potential side-effects of this procedure include hypotension, nausea, vomiting, urinary retention and convulsion. This procedure should only be done by anesthesiologists familiar with regional anesthesia techniques, and in situations where the patient can be closely watched.

Complications of sympathetic blockade are listed in Table 5.3 and are discussed more fully by Löfström and Cousins [21].

Neurolytic or surgical sympathectomy

More permanent sympathectomy is indicated for patients with unquestioned but temporary pain relief from local anesthetic blocks. For neurolytic blocks, 7–10% phenol may be injected in contrast medium or 50–100% alcohol may be used. A full

Table 5.3 Complications associated with sympathetic blockade

Procedure	Complication	Presumed cause
Stellate and/or thoracic ganglionic block	Hoarseness and inability to cough	Recurrent laryngeal nerve block (needle placement superficial to pre-cervical fascia)
	Paresthesia, sensory loss or weaknesss in upper extremity and/or hand	Brachial plexus block (if needle is anterior to C6 vertebra)
	Bradycardia	Carotid sinus block
	Paraplegia or quadriplegia	Epidural or subarachnoid
	Pneumothorax	Penetration of pleura
	Seizures	Vertebral artery injection
Lumbar sympathetic block	Leg weakness	Block of somatic lumbar nerve roots
	Hypotension	Profound sympathetic (usually bilateral) block
	Back pain	Irritation of lumbar periosteal surface and/or perforation of disc
	Hematuria	Perforation of kidney
	Retroperitoneal hemorrhage	Perforation of aorta or vena cava
Continuous epidural infusion	Leg or arm weakness	Block of somatic lumbar or cervical nerve roots
	Hypotension	Bilateral sympathetic block
	Urinary retention	Parasympathetic block
	Epidural abscess	Bacterial infection of catheter

discussion of neurolytic and surgical techniques of sympathectomy are beyond the scope of this chapter, but are fully described in Löfström and Cousins [21], and White and Sweet [25], respectively.

Post-sympathectomy pain ('sympathalgia') may occur in 20–44% of patients who have either a surgical or chemical sympathectomy [28,29]. This complication is more frequent after lumbar sympathectomy, and typically begins abruptly 10–14 days after the procedure. It is described as dull, boring, cramping and occasionally as sharp pain, and is usually localized to within the area of sympathetic denervation (i.e. anterior thigh and knee after lumbar sympathectomy). This pain often ends spontaneously after a few weeks but persistent pain may be managed with analgesics or anticonvulsants [28].

The response rate for surgical sympathectomy in RSD is in the range of 12–97% [25]. Differences in response rates reflect differences in timing of the procedure, different criteria for the diagnosis of causalgia and reflex sympathetic dystrophy, varying skills in performing the procedures, and the length of follow-up. Recurrences of pain may occur in as many as one-third of patients following sympathectomy, in follow-up periods ranging from 3 to 8 years, although many of the patients will still report improvement over their pre-operative status despite recurrent pain [30–32]. One reason for failure of sympathectomy, marked by the return of pain and dystrophy, after an initially successful procedure may be collateral re-innervation of post-ganglionic sympathetic efferent fibers [15,32a].

Recently, radiofrequency lesions of the upper thoracic sympathetic chain have yielded satisfactory sympathetic interruption in 15 patients with RSD, and good pain relief in one of two patients with causalgia [33]. This procedure has the advantage of being safe, less costly and technically easier to do than open sympathectomy, and can be performed on an outpatient basis.

Intravenous regional sympathetic blockade

After isolation of the extremity from the circulation by application of a tourniquet applied at 50–100 torr (mmHg) above systolic blood pressure, one can inject guanethidine (10–20 mg), reserpine (1–2 mg), or phentolamine (10 mg), intravenously (i.v.), to produce regional sympathetic blockade [21,34,35]. These drugs deplete norepinephrine from synaptic vesicles in sympathetic efferent fibers by either blocking its pre-synaptic re-uptake and/or uncoupling the release of norepinephrine caused by the arrival of the action potential at the synapse. In addition, chronic guanethidine administration may destroy sympathetic neurons in the primate [36]. The extremity is isolated from the circulation for at least 10 min to allow the drug to fix to tissues [21]. This procedure is indicated when patients are poor candidates for surgery or needle injections (i.e. patients receiving anticoagulents); as an alternative to paravertebral blocks with local anesthetics for patients with hypersensitivity reactions to these agents, or when a longer duration of analgesia is desirable.

Hannington-Kiff [37] reported up to 80% pain relief in 10 patients at 15-week follow-up. Guanethidine is not currently approved by the FDA for this indication – reserpine may be used instead and is effective [35], although it may be associated with more side-effects [21]. Other potentially effective agents that require study are prazosin and prostaglandins I_2 and E_1 (not yet available for i.v. administration), and hydralazine, diazoxide, and calcium-channel-blocking drugs such as verapamil, diltiazem and nifedipine (although available for i.v. administration they have not yet been studied by this technique).

Pharmacologic management of pain in RSD

Drug therapy for RSD, causalgia and other neuropathic pain states include corticosteroids, tricyclic antidepressants, narcotic analgesics, anticonvulsants, calcium-channel blocks, adrenergic blocking drugs, and non-steroidal anti-inflammatory drugs [9,38] (Table 5.4).

Oral sympatholytic agents

Propranolol (a β-adrenergic blocker), guanethidine, prazosin and phenoxybenzamine (α-adrenergic blockers), have been used to manage the pain in causalgia [9]. Isolated case reports have reported pain relief when propranolol was given to patients with causalgia in doses up to 320 mg/day [39], although a controlled double-blind crossover trial showed no benefit [40].

Prazosin, an α-1 blocker, has produced pain relief in a patient with causalgia in oral doses of 2 mg b.i.d. [41]. Phenoxybenzamine, also an α blocker, has also been used to manage pain in causalgia. In an uncontrolled study Ghostine *et al.* [42] treated 40 consecutive patients with causalgia (secondary to battlefield missile or shrapnel wounds) with phenoxybenzamine in doses of 40–120 mg/day for 6–12

Table 5.4 Pharmacologic therapies for RSD

Category	Drug	Usual dose ranges
Oral sympatholytics	Propranolol	80 mg b.i.d.–q.i.d.
	Prazosin	2 mg b.i.d.
	Phenoxybenzamine	40–120 mg/day
Corticosteroids	Prednisone	60–80 mg/day*
Non-steroidal anti-inflammatory drugs[†]		
Tricyclic 'antidepressants'	Amitriptyline	10–150 mg/day
	Doxepin	10–150 mg/day
	Nortriptyline	25–200 mg/day
Calcium-channel blockers	Nifedipine	10–30 mg t.i.d.
Anticonvulsants	Carbamazepine	200 mg t.i.d.–q.i.d.
	Phenytoin	100 mg t.i.d.–q.i.d.
	Clonazepam	4–8 mg/day
Narcotic analgesics[†]		

* Dose usually given over 2-week period and then discontinued
† Many drugs are available in the class. No good studies of their efficacy (*see* text).

weeks. All had resolution of pain in follow-up periods ranging from months through six years, with no recurrences of pain after treatment. Side-effects included orthostatic hypotension and ejaculatory dysfunction, as well as a decreased amount of seminal fluid. The authors asserted that these adverse effects were transient and did not stop therapy in any instance. This study requires corroboration. It was not a controlled study, and the 100% response rate after only 6–12 weeks of treatment is surprising. The absence of clinically significant (particularly orthostatic) hypotension after administering phenoxybenzamine in doses > 1 mg/kg is also surprising, although the patients being treated in this study were all young and presumably otherwise healthy soldiers. In the author's experience, the use of phenoxybenzamine in this dose range is usually associated with significant light-headedness and orthostasis, and often requires discontinuation of the medication. Thus, the role of phenoxybenzamine in management of causalgia is still unsettled.

Anti-inflammatory agents

Corticosteroid therapy may be very helpful, especially when joint involvement is marked [43]. The typical regimen is a pulse dose of prednisone 60–80 mg during 2 weeks, with a taper over a 2-week period. In addition, dexamethasone may suppress spontaneous nerve discharges in acute and chronic experimental neuromas, although its mechanism of action is not clear [44]. This finding may provide the rationale for the beneficial effects of corticosteroid injection for the treatment of painful trigger points and amputation stump neuromas, which may complicate traumatic peripheral nerve injury.

Non-steroidal anti-inflammatory drugs (NSAIDs) are 'general purpose analgesics' [45] that may be helpful in managing secondary (particularly musculoskeletal) pain so often complicating RSD. No controlled studies demonstrating their efficacy in RSD have been done, however.

Tricyclic 'antidepressants'

Amitriptyline and other tricyclic antidepressants have been used as adjuvant analgesics in the management of neuropathic pain [38,46]. The mechanism of action may involve blockade of serotonin re-uptake in the CNS, thereby augmenting the antinociceptive actions of the descending inhibitory pain-modulating pathways, and the analgesic effects appear to be independent of antidepressant effects [47]. Tricyclics also potentiate the effects of morphine analgesia [48]. Although there are no controlled clinical trials to determine their efficacy in post-traumatic neuralgias or causalgia, anecdotal experience suggests that tricyclic antidepressants may be useful, particularly for the management of aching and burning (rather than paroxysmal sharp, sizzling or shooting) pain.

Narcotic analgesics

The use of narcotic analgesics in the management of chronic pain unrelated to cancer is controversial [49], including their use in causalgia and other neuropathic pain syndromes. Horowitz [16] reported that definite or suspected narcotic 'addiction' occurred in four of 11 patients treated for causalgia associated with iatrogenic injuries, although he did not define his use of the term 'addiction', so it is not clear if the patients were simply physically dependent. Magora *et al.* [50] used epidural morphine in four patients with causalgia and reported fair pain relief in one patient and poor pain relief in the other three. A recent investigation reported the lack of efficacy of opioids in neuropathic pain [51] and in general, this is consistent with most clinical experience which supports the notion that narcotic analgesics are only marginally, if at all, helpful in the management of RSD [52].

Anticonvulsants

Anticonvulsant drugs may provide pain relief in patients with neuropathic pain [38,53]. Swerdlow [53] reported that carbamazepine, clonazepam, phenytoin, sodium valproate or nitrazepam were effective in relieving 'shooting or stabbing pain' in 23 of 28 patients with post-traumatic neuralgia. There was a correlation between the mean plasma levels of these drugs and pain relief. Albert [54] reported pain relief in three of four patients treated with carbamazepine (200 mg t.i.d.) for management of dysesthesia and shooting pain following gunshot wounds to the sciatic nerve. Pain returned after 3–4 days and responded to increased doses of carbamazepine (up to 1200 mg/day) in two patients. A third patient responded to phenytoin 100 mg q.i.d. and one patient did not respond to either anticonvulsant. Although follow-up results were not reported, these studies provide support for the use of anticonvulsants in the management of causalgia.

Post-sympathectomy pain also may be managed with anticonvulsants. Raskin *et al.* [28] reported temporary pain relief in two patients given 400 mg phenytoin intravenously for management of post-sympathectomy pain. Two other patients responded to oral phenytoin in doses of 400 mg/day, and seven of nine patients responded to carbamazepine in doses of up to 600 mg/day.

Calcium-channel blockers

Nifedipine, a calcium-channel blocker, relaxes smooth muscles, increases peripheral blood flow, and antagonizes the effects of norepinephrine on arterial and venous smooth muscle. Theoretically, nifedipine may also interfere with ectopic impulse formation in regenerating neurites by blocking calcium conductance; Devor [55] has demonstrated the appearance of new calcium-channel protein on regenerating neurites (*see* Chapter 3). These pharmacologic actions and experimental observations provide a rationale for its use in RSD including causalgia. Prough *et al* [56] recently reported that seven of 11 patients with RSD had complete relief of pain using nifedipine in doses ranging from 10 to 30 mg t.i.d. Three patients remained pain free after cessation of nifedipine and six others required continued medication with 60% to complete relief of pain at 6 months. Three patients withdrew from therapy because of headache and another failed to respond. These results suggest that nifedipine or other calcium-channel-blocking drugs may have a role in the management of RSD but, as the authors noted, this was an uncontrolled study and the results should be confirmed with a formal double-blind, placebo-controlled clinical trial.

Other therapies

Physical therapy (PT)

PT is essential for effective treatment [2,9]; it counteracts dystrophic changes in muscles and joints. However, it may be necessary to do sympathetic blocks and trigger-point injections before initiating physical therapy. The therapist should do repeated and standardized assessment of muscle strength and range of motion to quantify progression or improvement with therapy. Patients should be instructed in home PT; this has the added benefit of allowing the patients to be actively involved in therapy.

Electrical stimulation of the nervous system

Broesta *et al.* reported good pain relief in eight patients with causalgia treated with epidural dorsal column stimulation. Although it has been used to manage deafferentation pain, including causalgia, there is no consensus that chronic brain stimulation (i.e. periaqueductal or periventricular gray or thalamic stimulation) is effective, especially in pain related to nerve injury, so-called 'deafferentation pain' [58].

Transcutaneous electrical nerve stimulation (TENS) applied proximal to the site of nerve injury may be effective in managing pain in causalgia: Meyer and Fields [59] reported pain relief (which generally outlasts the brief stimulus trials) in six of eight patients, two of whom did not require sympathectomy. The advantages of TENS are that it is non-invasive, has no systemic side-effects, and is simple to use. It should be tried in all patients, and is especially attractive in children and in adults in whom invasive therapies are relatively contraindicated.

Trigger-point injections

Myofascial trigger points are a 'focus of hyperirritability in muscle or fascia that cause . . . pain' [60]. Myofascial trigger points may complicate many types of musculoskeletal syndromes, are frequently associated with nerve and soft-tissue injury and are common in reflex sympathetic dystrophy [3,13,18]. Pain arising from the area of trigger points may be treated by local injections of anesthetic agents. Treatment of trigger points can be an important adjunct to other therapies in causalgia, especially physical therapy.

Psychologic therapies

Distraction by work or hobbies is a helpful strategy in all chronic pain states. The complete management of pain in patients with RSD and other peripheral nerve pain syndromes requires attention to the invariable psychologic complications associated with chronic pain [61]. This is particularly true in causalgia in which there is a suggestion that certain personality profiles (e.g. passive dependent personality disorder DSM III, category 301.60) may predispose to this complication of peripheral nerve injury [16]. In addition, patients with causalgia are particularly likely to become isolated and socially withdrawn because social encounters may exacerbate their pain. Interventions such as biofeedback, hypnosis and relaxation training have been helpful adjuncts in the management of chronic pain in general, and have been shown to be effective in pain associated with peripheral nerve injury [62–64]. This is particularly intriguing given recent microneurographic data in man demonstrating increased sympathetic firing with stress and/or arousal [65] and suggests a physiologic basis for the usefulness of these interventions.

RECOMMENDATIONS FOR MANAGEMENT

An approach to the diagnosis and treatment of RSD is depicted in Figure 5.6. It may be necessary to admit the patient to a pain unit to proceed with diagnostic tests and therapy. This allows the physician and staff to become more familiar with the nature and extent of behavior and psychosocial dysfunction in the specific patient circumstances. Consultation with a psychologist or psychiatrist competent in the evaluation and management of chronic pain is almost always helpful, although rarely is it necessary to make it the primary focus of treatment. Patients with reflex sympathetic dystrophy, especially causalgia, should be treated as early as possible because early treatment is the single most important variable in determining effective outcome. Sympathetic blockade should be initiated promptly (if one has

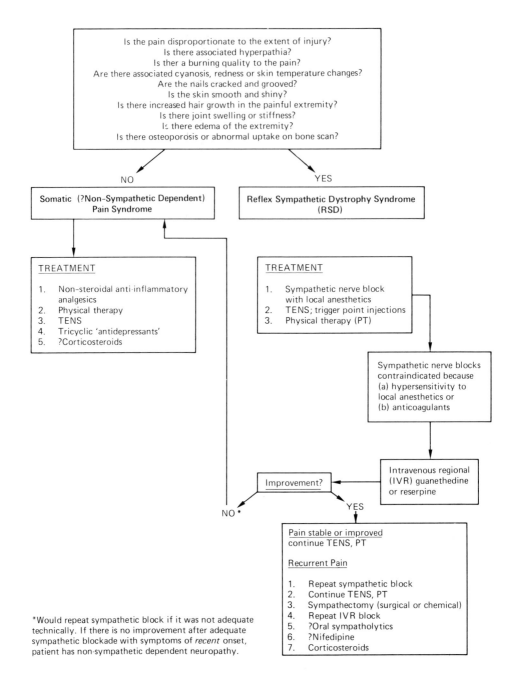

Figure 5.6 Pain following injury (which may be trivial) to bone, soft tissue or peripheral nerve; an approach to the diagnosis and treatment of the reflex sympathetic dystrophy syndrome (modified from Payne, R., Neuropathic pain syndromes with special reference to causalgia and reflex sympathetic dystrophy. *Clinical Journal of Pain*, **2**, 59–73 (1986) with permission).

the expertise available) as this will provide diagnostic as well as therapeutic information, even if there is no pain relief from the procedure. The type of sympathetic blockade is determined by the chronicity and intensity of pain and hyperalgesia and the degree of experience of the physician with a specific procedure. For RSD or causalgia of recent onset, cervical or lumbar sympathetic block with local anesthetic agents is the treatment of choice. Patients who have a coagulopathy or have experienced a hypersensitivity reaction to local anesthetic agents, so that nerve blocks are contraindicated, may be managed with regional i.v. guanethidine or reserpine, oral sympatholytic agents, or perhaps calcium-channel-blocking drugs. Physical therapy, trigger-point injections and TENS are important adjuncts and should be instituted simultaneously with sympathetic blockade. Occasionally, some patients may respond permanently to TENS or physical therapy or i.v. guanethidine and will not need further sympathetic blocks. Epidural dorsal column and thalamic stimulation should be reserved for the exceptional patient in whom the above therapies have been unsuccessful and the pain has not remitted by one year or more. Since the effectiveness of these invasive interventions are unknown, they should be reserved for those patients willing to participate in clinical studies to determine their efficacy. Therefore these procedures should be done in centers familiar with their potential problems, and by physicians who have experience in selecting the most appropriate patients.

References

1. Fields, H. L. *Pain*, McGraw-Hill, New York (1988)
2. Schwartzman, R. J. and McLellan, T. L. Reflex sympathetic dystrophy: a review. *Archives of Neurology*, **44**, 555–561 (1987)
3. Rowlingson, J. C. The Sympathetic Dystrophies. *International Anesthesiology Clinics*, **21**, 117–129 (1983)
4. Horton, P. and Gerster, J. C. Reflex sympathetic dystrophy syndrome and barbiturates. A study of 25 cases treated with barbiturates compared with 124 cases treated without barbiturates. *Clinical Rheumatology*, **3**, 493–500 (1984)
5. Taylor, L., Payne, R., Young, D., Stern, R. and Posner, J. Phenobarbital rheumatism in primary brain tumor patients. *Annals of Neurology*, **22**, 117–118 (1987)
6. Michaels, R. M. and Sorber, J. A. Reflex sympathetic dystrophy as a probable paraneoplastic syndrome: case report and literature review. *Arthritis and Rheumatism*, **27**, 1183–1185 (1984)
7. Rizzi, R., Visentin, M. and Maxetti, G. Reflex sympathetic dystrophy. In *Advances in Pain Research, Vol. 7* (ed. C. Benedetti, C. R. Chapman and G. Morrica), Raven Press, New York, pp. 451–464 (1984)
8. Merskey, H. (1986) Ed. *Classfication of Chronic Pain: Descriptions of Chronic Pain Syndromes and Definitions of Pain Terms. Pain, Supplement 3.* S217–S219
9. Payne, R. Neuropathic pain syndromes, with special reference to causalgia and reflex sympathetic dystrophy. *Clinical Journal of Pain*, **2**, 59–73 (1986)
10. Tahmoush, A. J. Causalgia: redefinition as a clinical pain syndrome. *Pain*, **10**, 187–197 (1981)
11. Tahmoush, A. J., Malley, J. and Jennings, R. D. Skin conductance, temperature, and blood flow in causalgia. *Neurology*, **33**, 1483–1486 (1983)
12. Mitchell, W. S. *Injuries of Nerves and Their Consequences*, Smith Elder, London (1872)
13. Bonica, J. J. *Sympathetic Nerve Blocks for Pain Diagnosis and Therapy, Vol. 1*, Breon Laboratories, New York, pp. 27–38 (1980)
14. Baker, A. G. and Wingarner, F. G. Causalgia. A review of twenty-eight treated cases. *American Journal of Surgery*, **117**, 690–694 (1969)
15. Hoffert, M. J., Greenberg, R. P., Wolskee, P. J. *et al.* Abnormal and collateral innervations of sympathetic and peripheral sensory fields associated with a case of causalgia. *Pain*, **20**, 1–12 (1984)
16. Horowitz, S. H. Iatrogenic causalgia: classification, clinical findings, and legal ramifications. *Archives of Neurology*, **41**, 821–824 (1984)

17. Parry, C. B. W. Pain in avulsion lesions of the brachial plexus. *Pain*, **9**, 41–53 (1980)
18. Sunderland, S. *Nerves and Nerve Injuries*, Second edn., Churchill Livingstone, New York, pp. 377–420 (1978)
19. Kozin, R., Soin, J. S., Ryan, L. M., Carrera, G. F. and Wortmann, R. L. Bone scintigraphy in the reflex sympathetic dystrophy syndrome. *Radiology*, **138**, 437–443 (1981)
20. Davidoff, G., Morey, K., Amann, M. and Stamps, J. Pain measurements in reflex sympathetic dystrophy. *Pain*, **32**, 27–34 (1988)
21. Löfström, J. B. and Cousins, M. J. Sympathetic neural blockade of upper and lower extremity. In *Neural Blockade in Clinical Anesthesia and Management of Pain*, Second edn (ed. M. J. Cousins and P. O. Bridenbaugh), J. B. Lippincott, Philadelphia, pp. 461–500 (1988)
22. Mackinnon, S. E. and Holder, L. E. The use of three-phase radionuclide bone scanning in the diagnosis of reflex sympathetic dystrophy. *Journal of Hand Surgery*, **9A**, 556–563 (1984)
23. Demangeat, J-L., Constantinesco, A., Brunot, B., Foucher, G. and Farcot, J-M. Three-phase bone scan in reflex sympathetic dystrophy of the hand. *Journal of Nuclear Medicine*, **29**, 26–32 (1988)
24. Uematsu, S., Hendler, N., Hungerford, D., Long, D. and Ono, N. Thermography and electromyography in the differential diagnosis of chronic pain syndromes and reflex sympathetic dystrophy. *Electromyography and Clinical Neurophysiology*, **21**, 165–182 (1981)
25. White, J. C. and Sweet, W. H. *Pain and the Neurosurgeon*, Charles C. Thomas, Springfield, Illinois (1969)
26. Wang, J. K., Johnson, K. A. and Ilstrup, D. M. Sympathetic blocks for reflex sympathetic dystrophy. *Pain*, **23**, 13–17 (1985)
27. Loh, L. and Nathan, P. W. Painful peripheral states and sympathetic blocks. *Journal of Neurology, Neurosurgery and Psychiatry*, **41**, 664–671 (1978)
28. Raskin, N. H., Levinson, S. A., Hoffman, P. M., Pickett, J. B. E. and Fields, H. L. Postsympathectomy neuralgia: amelioration with diphenylhydantoin and carbamazepine. *American Journal of Surgery*, **128**, 75–78 (1974)
29. Tracy, G. D. and Crockett, F. B. Pain in the lower limb after sympathectomy. *Lancet*, **i**, 12–14 (1957)
30. Mayfield, F. H. *Causalgia*, Charles C. Thomas, Springfield, Illinois (1951)
31. Schumaker, H. B. A personal overview of causalgia and other reflex dystrophies. *Annals of Surgery*, **201**, 278–289 (1985)
32. Sweet, W. H. and Poletti, C. E. Causalgia and sympathetic dystrophy (Sudeck's atrophy). In *Evaluation and Treatment of Chronic Pain* (ed. G. M. Aronoff), Urban and Schwarzenberg, Baltimore, pp. 149–165 (1985)
32a. Wirth, F. P. and Rutherford, R. B. A civilian experience with causalgia. *Archives of Surgery*, **100**, 633–638 (1970)
33. Wilkinson, H. A. Percutaneous radiofrequency upper thoracic sympathectomy: a new technique. *Neurosurgery*, **15**, 811–814 (1984)
34. Hannington-Kiff, J. G. Intravenous regional sympathetic block with guanethidine. *Lancet*, **i**, 1019–1020 (1974)
35. Benzon, H. T., Chomka, C. M. and Brunner, E. A. Treatment of reflex sympathetic dystrophy with regional intravenous reserpine. *Anesthesia and Analgesia*, **59**, 500–502 (1980)
36. Burnstock, G., Evans, B., Gannon, B. J. Helath, J. W. and James, V. A new method of destroying adrenergic nerves in adult animals using guanethidine. *British Journal of Pharmacology*, **43**, 295–301 (1971)
37. Hannington-Kiff, J. G. Relief of causalgia in limbs by regional intravenous guanethidine. *British Medical Journal*, **2**, 367–368 (1979)
38. Maciewicz, R., Bouckoms, A. and Martin, J. B. Drug therapy of neuropathic pain. *Clinical Journal of Pain*, **1**, 39–49 (1985)
39. Pleet, A. B., Tahmoush, A. J. and Jennings, J. R. Causalgia: treatment with propranolol in post-traumatic neuralgia. *Pain*, **14**, 283–292 (1976)
40. Scadding, J. W., Wall, P. D., Parry, C. B. W. and Brook, D. M. Clinical trial of propranolol in post-traumatic neuralgia. *Pain*, **14**, 283–292 (1982)
41. Abram, S. E. and Lightfoot, R. W. Treatment of longstanding causalgia with prazosin. *Regional Anesthesia*, **6**, 70–81 (1981)
42. Ghostine, S. Y., Comair, Y. G., Turner, D. M., Kassel, N. F. and Azar, C. G. Phenoxybenzamine in the treatment of causalgia: report of 40 cases. *Journal of Neurosurgery*, **60**, 1263–1268 (1984)
43. Kozin *et al.* 1976 (p. 19)
44. Devor, M., Govrin-Lippman, R. and Raber, P. Corticosteroids suppress ectopic neuronal discharge originating in experimental neuromas. *Pain*, **22**, 127–137 (1985)

45. Kantor, T. G. Control of pain by nonsteroidal anti-inflammatory drugs. *Medical Clinics of North America*, **66**, 1053–1059 (1982)
46. Pilowsky, I., Hallett, E. C., Bassett, D. L., Thomas, P. G. and Penhall, R. K. A controlled study of amitriptyline in the treatment of chronic pain. *Pain*, **14**, 169–179 (1982)
47. Feinmann, C. Pain relief by antidepressants: possible modes of action. *Pain*, **23**, 1–8 (1985)
48. Botney, M. and Fields, H. L. Amitriptyline potentiates morphine analgesia by a direct action on the central nervous system. *Annals of Neurology*, **13**, 160–164 (1983)
49. Portenoy, R. K. and Foley, K. M. Chronic use of opioid analgesics in nonmalignant pain: report on 38 cases. *Pain*, **25**, 173–186 (1986)
50. Magora, F., Olshwang, D., Eimerl, D. *et al*. Observations on extradural morphine analgesia in various pain conditions. *British Journal of Anaesthesia*, **52**, 247–252 (1980)
51. Arner, S. and Meyerson, B. A. Lack of analgesic effect of opioids on neuropathic and idiopathic forms of pain. *Pain*, **33**, 11–23 (1988)
52. Parry, 1983 (p. 21)
53. Swerdlow, M. Anticonvulsant drugs and chronic pain. *Clinical Neuropharmacology*, **7**, 51–82 (1984)
54. Albert, M. L. Carbamazepine for painful post-traumatic paresthesia. *New England Journal of Medicine*, **290**, 693 (1974)
55. Devor, M. Nerve pathophysiology and mechanisms of pain in causalgia. *Journal of the Autonomic Nervous System*, **7**, 371–384 (1983)
56. Prough, D. S., McLeskey, C. H., Boehlin, C. G. *et al*. Efficacy of oral nifedipine in the treatment of reflex sympathetic dystrophy. *Anesthesiology*, **62**, 796–799 (1985)
57. Broesta, J., Roldan, P., Gonzalez-Darder, J., Bordes, V. and Barcia-Solorio, J. L. Chronic epidural dorsal column stimulation in the treatment of causalgic pain. *Applied Neurophysiology*, **45**, 190–194 (1982)
58. Levy, R. M., Lamb, S. and Adams, J. E. Treatment of chronic pain by deep brain stimulation: long term follow-up and review of the literature. *Neurosurgery*, **21**, 885–893 (1987)
59. Meyer, G. A. and Fields, H. L. Causalgia treated by electric large fiber stimulation of peripheral nerve. *Brain*, **95**, 163–168 (1972)
60. Simmons, K. G. and Travell, J. G. Myofascial pain syndromes. In *Textbook of Pain* (ed. P. D. Wall and R. Melzack) Churchill Livingstone, New York, pp. 263–276 (1984)
61. Fordyce, W. E. *Behavioral Methods for Chronic Pain and Illness*, C. V. Mosby, St. Louis (1976)
62. Dogherty, 1980 (p. 24)
63. Turner, J. A. and Romano, J. M. Evaluating psychological interventions for chronic pain: issues and recent developments. In *Advances in Pain Research and Therapy, Vol. 7* (ed. C. Benedetti, C. R. Chapman and G. Moricca), Raven Press, New York, pp. 257–297 (1984)
64. Witherington and Parry, 1984 (p. 24)
65. Wallin, B. G. Newer aspects of sympathetic function in man. In *Clinical Neurophysiology* (ed. E. Stalberg and R. Young), Butterworths, London, pp. 145–167 (1981)

6
Pain in generalized neuropathies
Arthur K. Asbury

INTRODUCTION

Pain is one of the major features of generalized neuropathies, as are motor weakness, atrophy of muscle, attenuation of reflexes and sensory loss. Not all persons with generalized neuropathy experience the symptom of pain, but for those who do, suffering may be extreme and the anguish may dominate their existence. Medical management of pain in generalized neuropathies is mostly unsatisfactory from the standpoint of patient expectations and the wish of the physician to be helpful. This unfortunate situation reflects the partial and inadequate understanding of fundamental mechanisms through which symptoms of pain are produced and the lack of specific and effective methods with which to intervene.

Medical terminology used to characterize pain is entirely descriptive and has been arrived at mainly by convention. Pain that is labeled as neuropathic is so designated because of its particular clinical features (*see* Table 6.1) and because it is usually, but not always, associated with other symptoms and signs of nervous system involvement. Neuropathic pain is therefore thought to arise from damage to, and consequent dysfunction of, peripheral or central somatosensory pathways, or both. Dysesthesia is the general term used to denote all types of abnormal somatic sensations, whether induced by apparent stimulus or not. Not all dysesthetic sensations are experienced as painful, but they are almost always considered to be unpleasant. Hyperpathia is also a general term: it refers to painfulness following a stimulus in which the pain felt is out of proportion to the stimulus applied. Specific types of hyperpathia include hyperesthesia (pain in response to touch), hyperalgesia (severe pain in response to a mild noxious stimulus) and allodynia (pain perceived after non-noxious stimulation such as light stroking of the skin). When one type of hyperpathic pain is present in a given case of generalized neuropathy, the other types tend to be present also.

Like all pain, neuropathic pain is a positive symptom. As such, it reflects neural hyperactivity in afferent peripheral and central pathways, and probably an abnormal pattern and unusual frequency of impulses arriving at the dorsal horn and further centrally. Although this degree of afferent dysfunction is frequently associated also with symptoms and signs of sensory deficit, the association is not obligatory. In brief, states of neuropathic pain may occur without demonstrable sensory or autonomic deficit, even subclinically.

CLINICAL FEATURES OF PAIN IN GENERALIZED NEUROPATHIES

For purposes of this discussion, generalized neuropathies are taken to mean polyneuropathies or multifocal neuropathies involving two or more non-contiguous nerve trunks. Pathogenesis of damage to nerve fibers in generalized neuropathies includes such diverse processes as metabolic abnormalities, amyloid deposition, widespread occlusion and narrowing of vasa nervorum with consequent nerve trunk ischemia, and inflammatory demyelination. Any of these may result in neuropathic pain. Although diverse, these bases for nerve damage in generalized neuropathies differ from the usual causes for a lesion of a single nerve trunk, root or ganglion that is associated with neuropathic pain. In the latter (mononeuropathy), frequent causes of localized mononeuropathic pain are external physical trauma to a nerve trunk or root or virus-induced inflammatory destruction of a dorsal root or trigeminal ganglion (postherpetic neuralgia).

Despite dissimilarities in the basis for nerve fiber damage between generalized neuropathies and painful mononeuropathic pain syndromes, the nature of pain experienced in both is quite similar and differs only in extent and distribution. Dysesthetic pain and hyperpathia, the range of severity of painful experience, and its tenacity, are similar for generalized neuropathies and the more restricted neuropathic pain syndromes. This implies that particular patterns of nerve fiber damage, regardless of how the damage is incurred, will result in neuropathic pain. We do not yet know what the essential features of this particular pattern might be.

In peripheral nerve disorders, whether generalized or not, two major types of pain may be distinguished – namely dysesthetic pain and nerve trunk pain. The features of each are listed in Table 6.1. It should be emphasized that either type of pain rarely occurs in pure form; most neuropathies, either generalized or restricted, associated with pain will manifest some mixture of these two types of painful experience. Dysesthetic pain, because it has such arresting and never-before-experienced features, may predominate in the descriptions of symptoms given by patients. The hypothetical bases for dysesthetic and nerve trunk pain are more fully discussed in a subsequent section.

PATHOPHYSIOLOGIC MECHANISMS OF PAIN IN GENERALIZED NEUROPATHIES

Study of pain and pain mechanisms in generalized neuropathies has not been as intensive as in focal neuropathies and traumatic neuromas. Most current ideas about the pathophysiologic mechanisms of pain have come from investigation of focal neuropathy, either experimental or clinical. From such studies come the current concepts of hyperexcitability of (and ectopic generators in) nociceptive afferents, heightened mechanical and chemical sensitivity of either damaged or regenerating nociceptors, more proximal secondary changes ocurring in dorsal root ganglia neurons and in the dorsal horn of the spinal cord, involving increased frequency and altered pattern of firing in neural pathways thought to be nociceptive, and other central changes consequent on sustained activity in pain pathways. The evidence for these is amply reviewed elsewhere in this volume, but observations in generalized neuropathies add to our knowledge.

Clinical pathologic studies of generalized neuropathies carried out over the last two decades [3–7] support the idea that painfulness and cutaneous hypesthesia are

Table 6.1 Characteristics of two major forms of neuropathic pain[*]

Characteristics	Dysesthetic pain	Nerve trunk pain
Descriptors	Burning, tingling, raw, searing, jabbing, crawling, drawing, band-like, tightening, swelling, electric, shooting, needle-like	Aching, boring, gnawing, occasionally knifelike, tender
Recognition	Unfamiliar, never experienced before	Familiar, 'like a toothache'
Distribution	(a) Cutaneous or subcutaneous usually (b) In the cutaneous area innervated by the nerve (c) Generally more distal	(a) Deep (b) The nerve trunk itself (c) Generally more proximal
Constancy	Variable, may be intermittent, jabbing or lancinating	Usually continuous, but waxes and wanes
Better/worse	Little makes it better; worse following activity	Better with rest or optimal position; worse with movement, nerve stretch or palpation
Hypothetical basis	Increased firing of damaged or abnormally excitable nociceptive fibers, particularly sprouting, regenerating fibers	Increased firing due to physiologic stimulation of nociceptive afferents that innervate the nerve sheaths themselves (nervi nervorum)
Examples	(a) Causalgia (b) Small-fiber polyneuropathy, as in diabetes mellitus (c) Toxic polyneuropathies	(a) Spinal root compression (b) Brachial neuritis (c) Neuritis of leprosy reactions

[*] Modified from Asbury and Gilliatt [1] and Asbury and Fields [2]

observed with disease that mainly affects small myelinated and unmyelinated fibers, but predominant affection of large myelinated fibers does not result in pain. Thomas [8,9] has argued cogently that neuropathic pain may in part relate to abnormalities of nervi nervorum providing afferent input from the nerve sheaths, and Asbury and Fields [2] have further suggested that involvement of nervi nervorum may account for nerve trunk-type pain. Dyck and his colleagues [10], using teased nerve fiber techniques in combination with electrophysiologic studies *in vitro* of excised sural nerves, found that active axonal degeneration was the best correlate of painfulness in polyneuropathies. They also found that in chronic neuropathies the ratio of large to small persisting nerve fibers in distal sensory nerves was not a significant factor in determining painfulness.

A range of investigations in diabetic polyneuropathy provides some insight into putative pathophysiologic mechanisms of pain in generalized neuropathies [11]. Small-fiber neuropathies occurring in the setting of diabetes mellitus are characteristically associated with painfulness [7,12] although the nerve fiber changes responsible for painfulness could not be precisely identified. Brown and colleagues

[7] and later Asbury and Fields [2] hypothesized that overactivity in regenerating sprouts of nerve fibers subserving nociception was important in painfulness in diabetic polyneuropathy, and this suggestion is lent weight by the more recent observations of Llewelyn and coworkers [13]. These authors noted a profusion of regenerating neurites in a diabetic patient with acute painful polyneuropathy following upon initiation of insulin treatment. There is also evidence that active axonal degeneration may be important in pain mechanisms in acute painful neuropathy with diabetes mellitus [14].

Diabetic patients with polyneuropathy have poorer glycemic control both before and at onset of neuropathy than do otherwise matched diabetic patients without neuropathy [15]. It has been shown [16] that pain thresholds can be lowered acutely in normal individuals receiving large infusions of glucose and, similarly, that patients with diabetes mellitus manifest hyperalgesia in comparison to normal subjects. Thus, the glycemic state may be an additional factor in determining the degree of painfulness perceived for a given amount of nerve fiber abnormality. Assiduous correction of chronic hyperglycemia in diabetic patients using a continuous insulin infusion may be associated with dramatic improvement of painfulness in neuropathy [17]. Other factors, such as peripheral blood flow, may also affect the perception of pain in diabetic neuropathy [18].

PAINFUL NEUROPATHIC SYNDROMES

As mentioned previously, the quality and nature of neuropathic pain experienced in generalized neuropathies is usually similar to that experienced with single nerve trunk or root lesions, although the distribution differs widely. Nevertheless, the clinical features of neuropathic pain syndromes associated with a host of generalized neuropathies vary enough to warrant individual consideration.

Diabetic neuropathies

By far the commonest neuropathy occurring in the setting of diabetes mellitus is distal symmetrical primarily sensory polyneuropathy, which is commonly painful. Characteristically, the pain is dysesthetic in nature, frequently with a burning quality, distal and symmetrical. There is a tendency for it to be worse in the evening and night, and for hyperpathia to be present. From a clinical standpoint, diabetic patients exhibit either a pansensory deficit in the distal extremities or, on occasion, show mainly small-fiber deficit as marked by loss of temperature and pinprick sensation of the skin but with relative preservation of proprioception, vibratory sensation and deep tendon reflexes [19]. A study of sural nerves biopsied from such patients shows extensive axonal degeneration, sometimes involving all fiber types [20], or sometimes involving primarily small myelinated and unmyelinated fibers [7]. Once painfulness of distal symmetrical polyneuropathy of diabetes is established, it does not easily yield. In a 5-year follow-up study, Boulton and colleagues [21] showed that fewer than one-third of diabetics with painful polyneuropathy improved over that period, while the remainder either stayed the same or worsened from the standpoint of painfulness. For the distal symmetrical polyneuro-pathy of diabetes, painfulness once established tends to persist, in contrast to a number of other neuropathic syndromes in diabetes in which pain that heralds the onset of the condition is severe at first, ameliorates and disappears entirely within months to about one year (*see* Table 6.2).

Table 6.2 Classification of diabetic neuropathies

Symmetrical
1. Distal primarily sensory polyneuropathy
   (a) Mainly large fibers affected
   (b) Mixed
   (c) Mainly small fibers affected*
2. Autonomic neuropathy
3. Chronically evolving proximal motor neuropathy*

Asymmetrical
1. Acute or subacute proximal motor neuropathy* †
2. Cranial mononeuropathy†
3. Truncal neuropathy*†
4. Entrapment neuropathy in the limbs

* Usually with neuropathic pain
† Recovery, partial or complete, is likely
  Modified from Asbury [22]

A particular type of symmetrical diabetic polyneuropathy has been termed 'acute painful neuropathy' [11,14]. It occurs mainly in middle-aged or older men, often with poor glycemic control. First symptoms are often rapid and severe weight loss ($\geq$ 20–50 lb $\approx$ 9–22.5 kg), with appearance of severe constant burning pain of the feet and sometimes of the hands. Pain is maximal on the soles of the feet, is often associated with lancinations, is worse with weight bearing and at night, and is usually accompanied by a severe deep ache in the limbs and hyperpathia, including allodynia. Mental depression is usually present, together with anorexia during the period of most precipitous weight loss. Although severe in terms of pain, the syndrome is generally self-limited, runs its course and both the pain and the weight loss remit. This syndrome has also been called diabetic neuropathic cachexia, the term introduced by Ellenberg [23]. Management should focus on ruling out an occult malignancy, judicious use of tricyclic antidepressant medications and im-proved glycemic control.

Another self-limited paresthetic painful polyneuropathy, mainly sensory with few motor manifestations, may occur in diabetics first receiving insulin treatment. A recent sural nerve biopsy study of such a patient [13] demonstrated predomi-nantly loss of small fibers and a profusion of regenerating sprouts. The basis for painfulness was thought possibly to be related to excessive ectopic firing in regenerating fibers, a possibility first raised in diabetic neuropathy by Brown *et al.* [7], extrapolating from the experimental observations of Wall and his colleagues [24].

Pain is also frequent with the focal and multifocal diabetic neuropathies. About one-half of patients with diabetic ophthalmoplegia (third nerve palsy) experience some type of premonitory pain, generally from one to several days before the onset

of extra-ocular muscle weakness. Discomfort may be limited to prickling dysesthesias of the upper lid, but usually is an aching pain within, behind or just above the
eyeball [25]. Occasionally, a more diffuse frontal headache occurs [26]. Pain usually
lasts only a few days, and the ocular palsy itself has usually cleared or is clearing by
3 months. Possible explanations for the pain have included concurrent involvement
of the ophthalmic division of the trigeminal nerve, or both the ophthalmic and
maxillary divisions [25]. Another possibility is that the process affecting the third
nerve fibers also affects the afferent nervi nervorum in the sheath of the third nerve
as it traverses the cavernous sinus, thus activating nociceptive endings [27]. This
hypothesis is similar to the one more recently suggested for the basis of nerve trunk
pain [2].

Proximal motor neuropathy, sometimes called diabetic amyotrophy, tends to
occur in diabetics over the age of 50 years, the severity and duration of diabetes
being quite variable. This syndrome can be viewed as a spectrum, both in terms of
rate of evolution (from just a few days to up to several months) and in terms of its
symmetry or asymmetry [28]; proximal motor neuropathy of diabetes can be
further subdivided into meaningful sub-groups on the basis of the presence or
absence of concurrent distal polyneuropathy [29]. In all these sub-groupings of
proximal motor neuropathy pain occurs frequently – indeed, is rarely absent. It is
characteristically aching, persistent with nocturnal worsening, and may be noted
for a burning and raw quality. The pain may be unilateral, favoring the leg that is
becoming weak, and frequently involves also the low back, buttocks and perineum.
Pain may be bilateral even when the motor deficit is mainly unilateral. Although
pain may be the dominant symptom in proximal motor neuropathy of diabetes, the
physician can always remain optimistic about its eventual subsidence, although it
may take 12–18 months to do so.

In recent years, a multifocal diabetic neuropathy of the torso has been recognized [30–34]. This has generally been called diabetic truncal neuropathy, and
involves one or more intercostal nerves or lumbar nerves, generally on one side,
and the pattern of sensory deficit is quite patchy and often overlaps the areas of
innervation of several nerves [34]. A severe girdling pain, often similar to that
heralding herpes zoster of the trunk, is the first and often the only symptom and the
sensory deficit may be difficult to demonstrate. Unilateral weakness of muscles of
the abdominal wall may also be present, and electromyographic study of the
appropriate levels of torso muscles is often helpful in reaching the diagnosis.
Diagnostically, confusion with malignancy involving a vertebra or adjacent tissues
may arise. As with many of the diabetic neuropathies, the pain is severe, constant,
with both dysesthetic qualities, frequently burning, raw, stinging in quality along
with more deep aching and boring painfulness. As with the pain of other focal
diabetic neuropathies, the syndrome is limited in time: optimism can be maintained
about its eventual subsidence.

Toxic and nutritional neuropathies

The prototypical generalized neuropathy associated with an exogenous toxin or
nutritional deficiency is subacute axonal degeneration (axonopathy). In many toxic
states in which damage occurs in peripheral nerve, painfulness is either minor or
absent, even though sensory deficit may occur. When painfulness is a feature, it
often appears early, and is accompanied by paresthesias. Painful sensations are

usually a combination of dysesthetic and nerve trunk pain. Lancinations may also be experienced.

Another feature of many systemic intoxications that affect peripheral nerve is that they also affect the central nervous system, producing so-called central–peripheral distal axonopathy [35]. This raises the possibility that some of the sensory features, including painfulness, in some of these intoxications might be of central rather than peripheral origin. A possible example of this phenomenon is the profuse limb paresthesias experienced in clioquinol intoxication, referred to as subacute myelo-optico-neuropathy [36]. In this condition, no evidence of peripheral neuropathy exists, but the somatosensory pathways in the spinal cord clearly are affected and this damage is the probable source of the paresthesias and sensory deficit.

For most toxins and nutritional deficiency states the process is almost purely axonal, but with some toxins, for example perhexilene and amiodarone, an admixture of demyelination may occur [22]. In hexacarbon neuropathies, segmental axonal enlargement may cause secondary nodal changes, but painfulness is not an outstanding feature of any of these neuropathies in which axonal degeneration and demyelinating changes coexist.

Alcoholic and nutritional deficiency neuropathies are difficult to disentangle. One school of thought suggests that alcoholic neuropathy is simply a specialized form of nutritional deficiency [37]. Although precise figures are not available, painfulness is only present in a modest proportion of nutritional deficiency neuropathies, and is usually accompanied by dysesthesias. Although burning dysesthesias are a prominent and a particularly uncomfortable part of this syndrome (hence the term 'burning feet syndrome'), a number of other sensory abnormalities coexist, including lancinations and nerve trunk pain. The relief experienced by cooling the feet, for example by immersing them in cold water, suggests that polymodal fibers serving thermoreception (warm) and nociception may be damaged [38]. Although burning feet may be an early feature of deficiency neuropathy, by the time that pain appears there is often cutaneous sensory deficit, mainly to pinprick and to temperature.

Although several heavy metals are neurotoxic, including lead, mercury, arsenic and thallium, only thallium and arsenic consistently produce neuropathies with prominent painfulness. With both, dysesthetic pain appears as an early feature of evolving neuropathy, and neuropathic pain with hyperpathia is often severe, persisting for many months before eventual resolution.

A number of organic compounds, including the hexacarbon solvents, acrylamide, carbon disulfide and others, are neurotoxins that produce central–peripheral distal axonopathy; however, it is mainly large fibers that are at risk in the peripheral nervous system and dysesthesias are usually relatively mild and neuropathic pain is infrequent. This is in spite of relatively prominent sensory and motor loss in these toxic states.

Similarly, although many drugs are known to cause motor sensory polyneuropathy (for a list, *see* Asbury [22]), severe neuropathic pain is relatively uncommon, even though some degree of dysesthesia and sensory loss is the rule. Many drugs have more sensory than motor effects, such as *cis*-platin toxicity or pyridoxine megavitaminosis, and each may be associated with a degree of dysesthetic pain. Many other neurotoxic drugs announce their neurological effects with paresthesias, often quite uncomfortable: examples include isoniazid, thalidomide, misonidazole, hydralazine, nitrofurantoin and disulfiram.

Guillain–Barré syndrome and chronic inflammatory demyelinating polyneuropathy

Although acute and chronic forms of inflammatory demyelination of peripheral nerves are not ordinarily classed as painful neuropathies, pain is a frequent occurrence during their evolution. In Guillain–Barré syndrome (GBS) over one-half of all patients experience a particular type of aching discomfort in their proximal muscles and back during the early stages of illness, sometimes as the heralding symptom [39]. The symptom is usually likened to muscular pain experienced after unusually heavy or unaccustomed exertion [39]. Similar discomfort early in the course of poliomyelitis has long been recognized. Along the same lines, clinicians have long known that acutely denervated muscle is tender to palpation. Severe dysesthetic pain occurring during the course of GBS is highly unusual.

With chronic inflammatory demyelinating polyneuropathy, positive sensory symptoms (dysesthesias) are the rule, and in most cases accompany detectable sensory deficits [40]. Although such dysesthesias are considered to be painful ('burning, aching, raw, like a tight band, shooting') in about 15% of the cases [40], severe neuropathic pain is unusual [41].

Leprous neuritis

Mycobacterium leprae appears to favor early infestation of Schwann cells associated with intracutaneous unmyelinated nerve fibers [42]. For all forms of leprous neuritis (tuberculoid, dimorphous and lepromatous), the cardinal neurological manifestation is hypesthesia for cutaneous sensory modalities and not pain. None the less, pain may be prominent as a result of organ involvement such as orchitis or iridocyclitis. Nerve trunk pain may be severe and dramatic in erythema nodosum leprosum, a complication of lepromatous leprosy. The complication is thought to be due to a humoral immune response consisting of excessively released mycobacterial antigen, antigen–antibody complex formation and deposition in cutaneous vessel walls and consequent vasculitis [43]. Clinically, the key features are nodular inflammation of the skin, constitutional symptoms and painful swollen tender nerve trunks with rapidly appearing motor-sensory deficit. Corticosteroids and, surprisingly, thalidomide are the mainstays of management of erythema nodosum leprosum [42].

Vasculitic neuropathy

The vasculitides associated with connective tissue diseases characteristically involve small arteries, arterioles and venules in the size range of vasa nervorum. As a consequence, extensive damage to vasa nervorum results in multifocal ischemia of nerve trunks and patchy, partial clinical deficits (mononeuritis multiplex). Shooting pains in the affected nerve trunk distribution may be an early feature of ischemic neuropathy, and dysesthetic neuropathic painfulness of focal distribution may punctuate the course of vasculitis. In a recent case seen by the author, of polyarteritis nodosum with mononeuritis multiplex, classic causalgia in one foot was the major residue once the systemic illness was brought under control and other manifestations of the neuropathy had subsided. Such cases must be rare.

Hereditary neuropathies

An hereditary neuropathy in which pain has an important role is Fabry's disease (angiokeratoma corporis diffusum), which is a sex-linked recessive disorder characterized by burning pain and dysesthesias in the feet and legs, purplish maculopapular rash over the lower torso, corneal opacities and eventual renal failure and hypertension [44]. Pain may be severe enough to render sufferers unable to stand or bear weight. Deficiency of ceramide trihexosidase, the metabolic defect [45], allows accumulation of lipids in many tissues, including nerve trunks and ganglia. Ohnishi and Dyck [5] showed convincingly a loss of small myelinated and unmyelinated axons and sural nerve and corresponding loss of small neuron cell bodies in lumbar dorsal root ganglia. Some sprouting of unmyelinated fibers was present, as indicated by the presence of microfibers < 0.2 μm in diameter, and could represent the basis for painfulness.

In other hereditary neuropathies, pain is uncommon. Hereditary sensory neuropathies of either the dominantly or recessively inherited types may be marked by lancinations in the limbs, usually as a transient phase. In addition, burning feet syndrome is occasionally encountered as the main manifestation of a relatively mild dominantly inherited neuropathy [46].

MANAGEMENT OF PAIN IN GENERALIZED NEUROPATHIES

Control of pain can be one of the most vexing and frustrating problems in clinical medicine, for both patient and physician alike. For painfulness encountered as part of the clinical syndrome in generalized neuropathies, the primary measure in reducing pain is the management of the primary process. For instance, in toxic or metabolic neuropathies, the most important measure is to remove the patient from exposure or to correct the metabolic defect. Strict glycemic control, therefore, is the key to management of diabetic neuropathy, including the neuropathic pain that may accompany it. Other more specific pain measures in diabetic neuropathy that have been suggested are the use of aldose reductase inhibitors and myo-inositol supplementation (for a recent review of these, *see* Thomas and Scadding [11]), but neither aldose reductase inhibitors nor myo-inositol supplementation has been proven to have efficacy in the management of pain in diabetic neuropathy.

Other than the specific management directed at the primary underlying cause for generalized neuropathies with neuropathic pain, the mainstay of symptomatic treatment is tricyclic antidepressants [47–50 and Chapter 11]. Other agents that non-specifically modulate neuropathic pain, particularly if there is a lancinating component, are the anticonvulsants phenytoin and carbamazepine; their use and effectiveness were reviewed recently by Mucke and Maciewicz [51] and are discussed in Chapter 11.

References

1. Asbury, A. K. and Gilliatt, R. W. The clinical approach to neuropathy. In *Peripheral Nerve Disorders* (ed. A. K. Asbury and R. W. Gilliatt), Butterworths International Medical Reviews, London, pp. 1–20 (1984)
2. Asbury, A. K. and Fields, H. L. Pain due to peripheral nerve damage: an hypothesis. *Neurology*, **34**, 1587–1590 (1984)
3. Kocen, R. S. and Thomas, P. K. Peripheral nerve involvement in Fabry's disease. *Archives of Neurology*, **22**, 81–88 (1970)

4. Dyck, P. J., Lambert, E. H. and Nichols, P. C. Quantitative measurement of sensation related to compound action potential and number and sizes of myelinated and unmyelinated fibers of sural nerve in health, Friedreich's ataxia, hereditary sensory neuropathy and tabes dorsalis. In *Handbook of Electroencephalography and Clinical Neurophysiology* (ed. W. A. Cobb), Elsevier Publishing Co., Amsterdam, pp. 83–118 (1972)

5. Ohnishi, A. and Dyck, P J. Loss of small peripheral sensory neurons in Fabry's disease. Histologic and morphometric evaluation of cutaneous nerves, spinal ganglia and posterior columns. *Archives of Neurology*, **31**, 120–127 (1974)

6. Thomas, P. K. The anatomical substratum of pain. *Canadian Journal of Neurological Sciences*, **1**, 92–97 (1974)

7. Brown, M. J., Martin, J. R. and Asbury, A. K. Painful diabetic neuropathy – a morphometric study. *Archives of Neurology*, **33**, 164–171 (1976)

8. Thomas, P. K. Painful neuropathies. In *Advances in Pain Research and Therapy, Vol. 3* (ed. J. J. Bonica), Raven Press, New York, pp. 103–110 (1979)

9. Thomas, P. K. Pain in peripheral neuropathy: clinical and morphological aspects. In *Abnormal Nerve and Muscle as Impulse Generators* (ed. W. J. Culp and J. Ochoa), Oxford University Press, London, pp. 553–567 (1982)

10. Dyck, P. J., Lambert, E. H. and O'Brien, P. C. Pain in peripheral neuropathy related to rate and kind of fiber degeneration. *Neurology*, **26**, 461–466 (1976)

11. Thomas, P. K. and Scadding, J. W. Treatment of pain in diabetic neuropathy. In *Diabetic Neuropathy* (ed. P. J. Dyck, P. K. Thomas, A. K. Asbury, A. Winegrad and D. Porte), W. B. Saunders Company, Philadelphia, pp. 216–222 (1987)

12. Said, G., Slama, G. and Selva, J. Progressive centripetal degeneration of axons in small fiber-type diabetic polyneuropathy: a clinical and pathological study. *Brain*, **106**, 791–807 (1983)

13. Llewelyn, J. G., Thomas, P. K., Fonseca, V., King, R. H. M. and Dandona, P. Acute painful diabetic neuropathy precipitated by strict glycemic control. *Acta Neuropathologica*, **72**, 157–162 (1986)

14. Archer, A. G., Watkins, P. J., Thomas, P. K., Sharma, A. K. and Payan, J. The natural history of acute painful neuropathy in diabetes mellitus. *Journal of Neurology, Neurosurgery and Psychiatry*, **46**, 461–499 (1983)

15. Boulton, A. J. M., Worth, R. C., Drury, J. *et al.* Genetic and metabolic studies in diabetic neuropathy. *Diabetologia*, **26**, 15–19 (1984)

16. Morley, G. K., Mooradian, A. D., Levine, A. L. and Morley, J. E. Mechanisms of pain in diabetic peripheral neuropathy: effect of glucose on pain perception in humans. *American Journal of Medicine*, **77**, 79–82 (1984)

17. Boulton, A. J. M., Drury, J., Clarke, B. and Ward, J. D. Continuous subcutaneous insulin infusion in the management of painful diabetic neuropathy. *Diabetes Care*, **5**, 386–390 (1982)

18. Archer, A. G., Roberts, V. C. and Watkins, P. J. Blood flow patterns in painful diabetic neuropathy. *Diabetologia*, **27**, 563–567 (1984)

19. Brown, M. J. and Asbury, A. K. Diabetic neuropathy. *Annals of Neurology*, **15**, 2–12 (1984)

20. Behse, F., Buchthal, F. and Carlsen, F. Nerve biopsy and conduction studies in diabetic neuropathy. *Journal of Neurology, Neurosurgery and Psychiatry*, **40**, 1072–1082 (1977)

21. Boulton, A. J. M., Armstrong, W. D., Scarpello, J. H. B. and Ward, J. D. The natural history of painful diabetic neuropathy – a four-year study. *Postgraduate Medical Journal*, **59**, 556–559 (1983)

22. Asbury, A. K. Disorders of peripheral nerve. In *Diseases in the Nervous System* (ed. A. K. Asbury, G. M. McKhann and W. I. McDonald), WB Saunders Co., Philadelphia, Chapter 24, pp. 321–336 (1986)

23. Ellenberg, M. Diabetic neuropathic cachexia. *Diabetes*, **23**, 418–423 (1974)

24. Wall, P. D. and Gutnick, M. Ongoing activity in peripheral nerves: the physiology and pharmacology of impulses originating from a neurone. *Experimental Neurology*, **43**, 580–593 (1974)

25. Zorilla, E. and Kozak, G. Ophthalmoplegia in diabetes mellitus. *Annals of Internal Medicine*, **67**, 968–975 (1967)

26. Jackson, W. P. U. Ocular nerve palsy with severe headache in diabetes. *British Medical Journal*, **2**, 408–409 (1955)

27. Asbury, A. K., Aldredge, H., Hershberg, R. and Fisher, C. M. Ocular motor palsy in diabetes mellitus: A clinicopathological study. *Brain*, **93**, 555–566 (1970)

28. Asbury, A. K. Proximal diabetic neuropathy. *Annals of Neurology*, **2**, 179–181 (1977)

29. Subramony, S. H. and Wilbourn, A. J. Diabetic proximal neuropathy: clinical and electromyographic studies. *Journal of the Neurological Sciences*, **53**, 293–304 (1982)

30. Ellenberg, M. Diabetic truncal mononeuropathy – a new clinical syndrome. *Diabetes Care*, **1**, 10–13 (1978)

31. Longstreth, G. F. and Newcomer, A. D. Abdominal pain caused by diabetic radiculopathy. *Annals of Internal Medicine*, **86**, 166–168 (1977)
32. Sun, S. F. and Streib, E. W. Diabetic thoracoabdominal neuropathy: clinical and electrodiagnostic features. *Annals of Neurology*, **9**, 75–78 (1981)
33. Kikta, D. G., Breuer, A. C. and Wilbourn, A. J. Thoracic root pain in diabetes: the spectrum of clinical and electromyographic findings. *Annals of Neurology*, **11**, 80–85 (1982)
34. Stewart, J. D. Diabetic truncal neuropathy. *Annals of Neurology*, **25**, 233–238 (1989)
35. Schaumburg, H. H. and Spencer, P. S. Clinical and experimental studies of distal axonopathy – a frequent form of brain and nerve damage produced by environmental chemical hazards. *Annals of the New York Academy of Sciences*, **329**, 14–28 (1979)
36. Tsubaki, T., Honma, Y. and Hoshi, M. Neurological syndrome associated with clioquinol. *Lancet*, **i**, 696–697 (1971)
37. Victor, M. Polyneuropathy due to nutritional deficiency and alcoholism. In *Peripheral Neuropathy* 2nd edn (ed. P. J. Dyck, P. K. Thomas, E. H. Lambert and R. P. Bunge), W. B. Saunders Company, Philadelphia, pp. 1899–1940 (1984)
38. Ochoa, J. The newly recognized painful ABC syndrome: thermographic aspects. *Thermology*, **2**, 65–107 (1986)
39. Ropper, A. H. and Shahani, B. T. Pain in Guillain–Barré syndrome. *Archives of Neurology*, **41**, 511–514 (1984)
40. Dyck, P. J., Lais, A. C., Ohta, M., Bastron, J. A., Okazaki, H. and Groover, R. V. Chronic inflammatory polyradiculoneuropathy. *Mayo Clinic Proceedings*, **50**, 621–637 (1975)
41. Dyck, P. J. and Arnason, B. G. W. Chronic inflammatory demyelinating polyradiculoneuropathy. In *Peripheral Neuropathy*, 2nd edn (ed. P. J. Dyck, P. K. Thomas, E. H. Lambert and R. P. Bunge), W. B. Saunders Co., Philadelphia, Chapter 91, pp. 2101–2114 (1984)
42. Sabin, T. D. and Swift, T. R. Leprosy. In *Peripheral Neuropathy*, 2nd edn (ed. P. J. Dyck, P. K. Thomas, E. H. Lambert and R. P. Bunge), W. B. Saunders Co., Philadelphia, Chapter 84, pp. 1955–1987 (1984)
43. Wemambu, S. N. C., Turk, J. L., Waters, M. F. R. and Rees, R. J. W. Erythema nodosum leprosum: a clinical manifestation of the Arthus phenomenon. *Lancet*, **ii**, 933–935 (1969)
44. Brady, R. O. Fabry disease. In *Peripheral Neuropathy*, 2nd edn (ed. P. J. Dyck, P. K. Thomas, E. H. Lambert and R. P. Bunge), W. B. Saunders Co., Philadelphia, Chapter 73, pp. 1717–1727 (1984)
45. Brady, R. O., Gal, A. E., Brady, R. M. *et al.* Enzymatic defect in Fabry's disease: ceramide trihexosidase deficiency. *New England Journal of Medicine*, **276**, 1163–1167 (1967)
46. Dyck, P. J., Low, P. A. and Stevens, J. C. 'Burning feet' as the only manifestation of dominantly inherited sensory neuropathy. *Mayo Clinic Proceedings*, **58**, 426–429 (1983)
47. Turkington, R. W. Depression masquerading as diabetic neuropathy. *Journal of the American Medical Association*, **243**, 1147–1150 (1980)
48. Langohr, H. D., Stohr, M. and Petrich, F. An open and double-blind cross-over study on the efficacy of clomipramine (Anafranil) in patients with painful mono- and polyneuropathies. *European Neurology*, **21**, 309–317 (1982)
49. Watson, C. P., Evans, R. J., Reed, K. *et al.* Amitriptyline versus placebo in postherpetic neuralgia. *Neurology*, **32**, 671–673 (1982)
50. Max, M. B., Culnane, M., Shafer, S. C. *et al.* Amitriptyline relieves diabetic neuropathy pain in patients with normal or depressed mood. *Neurology*, **37**, 589–596 (1987)
51. Mucke, L. and Maciewicz, R. Clinical management of neuropathic pain. *Neurologic Clinics*, **5**, 649–663 (1987)

7
Management of nociceptive, deafferentation and central pain by surgical intervention
Ronald R. Tasker

INTRODUCTION

The surgical treatment of intractable pain is a demanding exercise. There are no panaceas, so that both surgeon and patient must be realistic about their expectations. There is often a plethora of recommended procedures with a dearth of objective outcome data for the treatment of individual pain syndromes. Although it is essential for intelligent planning of treatment strategy, the accurate diagnosis of the type of intractable pain syndrome may be difficult, and complicated by the frequent coexistence of more than one type. Finally, the pathophysiology of so many pain syndromes, as well as the mechanisms of many of the surgical procedures used to relieve them, is often poorly understood, making the matching of symptoms with treatment uncertain.

The decision to embark on surgical treatment of pain is governed by several considerations. The pain must be intractable, meaning that all practical primary therapy has been exhausted. All non-invasive modes of therapy must have been tried. Disability for which relief is sought must be from the pain, not other consequences of the causative disease, including psychological ones. The degree of pain must warrant the procedure being considered with its limitations and risks and should be assessed by semi-quantitative techniques such as analog rating, measuring drug intake, evaluating interference with work, avocations and sleep. The pain syndrome must then be dissected into its component parts against which surgical techniques must be matched, using the simplest techniques first.

CLASSIFICATION OF THE PATIENT'S PAIN SYNDROME

It is helpful to regard the normal state – absence of pain – as a state of homeostasis between pain input and modulating activity that suppresses it. Pain can theoretically result from excessive input or modulatory failure. Whether the latter alone ever causes pain is uncertain but several types of excessive pain input are known.

Pain syndromes may be divided into four basic types: chronic nociceptive; psychogenic, muscle tension, and deafferentation or nerve injury pains.

Chronic nociceptive pain, such as that caused by cancerous destruction of long bones or chronic osteoarthritis, is the result of continual peripheral input from primary afferent nociceptors with continual transmission in central pain pathways, particularly the spinothalamic tract. The pain generated is sharp, aching, throbbing, knife-like, crampy, or crushing, and can be related one-to-one with causative stimuli. Also nociceptive and of similar quality is the pain of sciatica or of cancerous compression (not destruction) of brachial or lumbosacral plexus, although the pathophysiology is obscure, possibly the stimulation of nociceptors in nervi nervorum or arteriorum [1], as nociceptors have not been demonstrated along nerve trunks themselves. Certain vascular pain syndromes, such as migraine, are also felt to be nociceptive in origin, presumably dependent upon the nociceptor innervation of the intracranial blood vessels.

Psychogenic pain, including the rare hysterical or schizophrenic pain syndromes and the commonly observed psychogenic magnification of existing organic pain syndromes, have presumably a central cortical input. Muscle tension pain is presumably dependent upon stimulation of nociceptors in muscle, arising, in this author's opinion, from muscle contraction. This could be of psychogenic origin.

Most difficult to understand are deafferentation and central pain syndromes, related to lesions of the peripheral and central nervous systems, respectively. Included are major causalgia and other painful states associated with lesions of peripheral nerves. The latter are sometimes referred to as minor causalgia and often confused with RSD (reflex sympathetic dystrophy), a term that ought to apply to the sympathetic hyperfunction that can accompany central or deafferentation pain [2]. When the peripheral nerve lesion is complete and the painful region is anesthetic, the associated pain syndrome is often referred to as anesthesia dolorosa. There are also pain syndromes associated with lesions of brachial or lumbosacral plexus, such as those resulting from iatrogenic causes, radiation necrosis, destruction by cancer, or stretch injury. Deafferentation pain may also result from damage to dorsal roots. Incisional pain, including post-thoracotomy pain, and post-traumatic syndrome, is often of this type. The commonest central pain syndromes are those associated with cord lesions. Although these usually result from trauma, they may also be caused by such diverse processes as neoplasm, myelitis, infarction or cordotomy. Finally, some central pain syndromes are associated with supraspinal lesions, those caused by supratentorial stroke being the commonent. However, lateral medullary syndrome, hemorrhage, neoplasm and surgical procedures such as tractotomy, can also result in central pain.

Although Livingston [3] and others [4–24] were impressed by the peculiar features of such pain and speculated on the pathophysiology, such perceptions were not widely shared until recently.

Our attention was attracted to the unusual nature of central and deafferentation pain in 1975 while reviewing our experience with percutaneous cordotomy [25] and ignorant of Livingston's work, leading to a series of clinical studies [26–39]. These suggested that deafferentation and central pain shared common clinical features and possibly, therefore, common pathophysiologic substrates distinct from those of nociceptive pain. These studies also give rise to a number of theories, some amply supported by clinical observations, others still in need of further scrutiny, as outlined in Table 7.1.

Evoked pain (allodynia, hyperpathia and hyperesthesia), which sometimes accompanies deafferentation and central pain, is dependent upon peripheral input through receptors, which is abnormally processed centrally, as proposed by Lindblom [40].

Table 7.1 Features of deafferentation, central and nociceptive pain

Nociceptive pain	Deafferentation and central pain
Not idiosyncratic; lesions characteristically produce pain	Idiosyncratic; not all patients with given lesion develop pain
Immediate onset	Onset may be delayed after causative event
Caused by adequate stimulation of nociceptors	Usually does not require stimulation of nociceptors – results from abnormal somatosensory function
Pain not related to somatosensory loss	Pain usually related somatotopographically to somatosensory malfunction
Sympathetic dysfunction not a feature	In unusual cases, sympathetic dysfunction may accompany pain and when present is usually relieved by sympathectomy
Pain may be evoked and/or spontaneous	Pain may be evoked and/or spontaneous
Evoked pain can occur as hyperesthesia from stimulation of receptors	Evoked pain, in the form of hyperesthesia, hyperpathia, or allodynia, can occur in areas of partial somatosensory function
Spontaneous pain is usually sharp, aching, crampy, stabbing, knifelike, crushing, etc., suggesting tissue damage and may be steady or intermittent	Spontaneous pain may be steady or intermittent, usually in similar but not identical sites related somatotopographically to somatosensory malfunction
	Intermittent pain, (rare in isolation), consisting of localized sharp, often shooting, jabbing and lancinating elements may accompany steady pain. When present it is usually more intense than the steady pain it accompanies
	Steady pain is nearly always present and burning and/or tingling in quality
Usually relieved by opiates, proximal somatosensory local anesthetic blockade, slow rates of neural stimulation, chronic stimulation of periventricular-periaqueductal gray, and interruption of all somatosensory or (selective) spinothalamic transmission	Evoked and spontaneous intermittent elements respond to same strategies as nociceptive pain
	Spontaneous steady burning pain does not usually respond to the same strategies as nociceptive pain but often is temporarily relieved by small i.v. doses of thiopental sodium, by local anesthetic somatosensory blockade, and by rapid-rate electrical stimulation of somatosensory fibers subserving the painful area. Also occasionally relieved by temporary sympathetic interruption, when hyperpathia or allodynia are present. It is not usually relieved permanently by sympathectomy or somatosensory interruption

Intermittent spontaneous lancinating elements appear to depend upon peripheral mechanisms, perhaps arising from ectopic impulses generated at injury sites or ephapses or from the effects of central influences on damaged receptors or synapses.

Steady spontaneous burning and tingling elements are probably generated centrally, possibly through denervation neuronal hypersensitivity, somatotopic reorganization, alterations of transmitter balance, reorganization of synaptic input, loss of inhibitory input, or acquisition of new connectivity [3–40].

CLINICAL STUDIES OF CNS FUNCTION IN HUMAN SUBJECTS

We have exploited the necessary physiological exploration of the brain during stereotactic procedures to examine the pathophysiology of deafferentation and central pain, using macro- and microstimulation and microelectrode recordings [27,28,31,32,35,39,41–51]. The following abnormalities have been noted in patients with central and deafferentation pain:

1. Alterations of quality of response perceived by the patient in response to electrical stimulation of the brain.
2. Alterations of somatotopic organization in ventrobasal complex.
3. Alteration of neuronal firing patterns in thalamus.

Alterations of quality of stimulation-induced response

In the patient who does not suffer from central or deafferentation pain, either macro- or microstimulation of the dorsal columns, medial lemniscus, trigeminal tract and nucleus, and ventrobasal complex in the vicinity of tactile cells, results in highly somatotopically organized paresthesias that are nearly always contralateral. In the spinothalamic tract, similarly organized responses are induced, that usually are reported as feeling warm or cold. Stimulation in the vicinity of kinesthetic cells usually induces paresthesias similar to those seen with stimulation near tactile cells but occasionally induces sensations suggesting muscular contraction, although no muscular contraction actually occurs. Stimulation of the mesencephalon medial to the spinothalamic tract or the medial thalamus medial to the ventrobasal complex elicits no response, other than from volume conduction. Stimulation of the periventricular–periaqueductal gray induces non-somatotopographically organized warmth, a feeling of satiety or other autonomic effects.

Burning and pain are rarely elicited. However, in patients with deafferentation and central pain, we, and many other surgeons [27], have often elicited both burning and pain.

Eliciting pain

Unpleasant painful responses, often resembling the patient's deafferentation or central pain, are elicited in several sites nearly always somatotopographically related to the area of the patient's own pain: the mesencephalon medial to spinothalamic tract, the thalamus medial to ventrobasal complex, the spinothalamic tract, the ventrobasal complex, the thalamic radiations, and the somatosensory cortex.

In stimulating somatotopographically organized sites such as ventrobasal complex and sensory cortex, such abnormal responses occur only in those parts of the body where pain is perceived. Stimulation related somatotopographically to normal parts of the body results in the patient perceiving the non-painful paresthesias described above. Stimulation of non-somatotopographically organized structures such as the medial mesencephalon and medial thalamus, which usually does not elicit a response, induces diffuse contralateral non-somatotopographically organized feelings of burning or pain in patients with central or deafferentation pain.

A total of 39 patients, 20 suffering from central and 19 from deafferentation pain, underwent such macro- and/or microstimulation. Pain was induced in 17, 16 of whom (94%) suffered from allodynia or hyperpathia. Of the 22 patients in whom pain was not induced, 10 (45%) suffered from allodynia or hyperpathia. In other words, pain was induced in 16 (62%) of the 26 patients with hyperpathia or allodynia but only in 1 (8%) of the 13 with neither hyperpathia nor allodynia. Thus the induction of pain by CNS electrical stimulation may be a central marker for hyperpathia and allodynia – a central allodynia, as it were, mediated by the spinothalamic tract, ventrobasal complex and, presumably, the reticulothalamic system. The converse does not appear to be true: the presence of hyperpathia and allodynia does not necessarily imply that central allodynia is present.

In 17 patients in whom microelectric recordings were made at the sites where stimulation induced the perception of pain, tactile cells with receptive fields in the painful area were identified in 12 (71%).

Burning

The significance of eliciting burning by electrical stimulation of the brain is less clear. It is most prominently found in medial mesencephalon and medial thalamus, referred non-somatotopographically to large areas of the contralateral body, not always clearly referable to deafferented areas. When elicited in spinothalamic tract and ventrobasal complex, it is referred somatotopographically to a deafferented area. It is elicited equally in the presence or absence of allodynia and hyperpathia [39,50]. Of the 39 patients explored with macro- or microstimulation, burning alone, without pain, was elicited in nine, four of whom (44%) suffered from hyperpathia or allodynia. In the 26 patients with hyperpathia or allodynia, stimulation induced burning alone in four (15%) while in the 13 patients without hyperpathia or allodynia, burning occurred in 5 (38%). When neurons are identified at sites where microstimulation induces burning, they are usually tactile, occasionally kinesthetic, and their receptive fields are related to deafferented areas.

Alterations of somatotopic reorganization

Two types of somatotopic reorganization have been recognized in patients with central and deafferentation pain using microelectric recording. When a large part of the body has been deafferented, for example a leg following multiple rhizotomy or the lower half of the body after a cord lesion, neurons with tactile responses other than deafferented body parts have been found in parts of the ventrobasal complex where, normally, input from the deafferented body part is expected. Tactile neurons with unusual receptive fields at the margin of the deafferented zone may also appear here [48,49]. As the former type of alteration also appears in 'control' patients who have suffered from deafferentation but who do not have pain, it appears to be a marker of deafferentation rather than of pain.

Alterations of neuronal firing

Two types of altered neuronal firing pattern have been recognized. In a patient rendered totally quadriplegic at the third cervical level [48,49], it was noticed that tactile neurons with abnormal receptive fields of the type mentioned above fired in bursts and at higher rates than did adjacent trigeminal tactile cells that had not suffered clinical deafferentation. This observation would be in keeping with a deafferented tactile neuron with denervation hypersensitivity and which also acquired a new somatosensory input. It is possible that these changes might generate chronic pain, although such suggestions are conjectural.

The commoner abnormality of firing pattern seen in every patient with central and deafferentation pain explored with microelectrodes, is the occurrence of bursting cells. Cells firing in repetitive bursts have been widely recognized in animal studies of deafferentation. The author has found them throughout the thalamus as well as in the periventricular gray matter, not only in patients with central and deafferentation pain, but also in those suffering deafferentation without pain; they are more numerous in the former. Most bursting cells could not be classified further and stimulation at sites where they were recorded usually produced no identifiable response. Of the few bursting cells found to have receptive fields, most were tactile in type and the receptive fields were sometimes unusual, associated with alterations in somatotopy as mentioned above. Stimulation occasionally induced burning in the vicinity of such bursting cells.

While bursting cells in general appeared to be markers of deafferentation and not of pain, closer analysis identified a class of neurons with regular bursts of spikes. The bursts consisted of regular high-frequency spikes and occurred every 50.5 ± 52.3 ms. These neurons appeared to be peculiar to patients with central and deafferentation pain [51]. In contradistinction to other types of bursting cells that were more diffusely distributed, these regularly bursting cells tended to occur in ventrocaudal and immediately adjacent nuclei and were much more likely to have receptive fields in the deafferented part of the body.

Although it would be presumptuous to make conclusions based on these observations, they raise the following possibilities:

1. Somatotopographic reorganization is a response to deafferentation and not necessarily a marker for pain.

2. Certain sub-types of reorganization, such as the acquisition of unusual receptive fields, may be peculiar to patients suffering from pain.
3. Pain induced by electrical stimulation in certain CNS structures is a central marker for hyperpathia or allodynia and may predict a poor therapeutic result with chronic stimulation. Both the lemniscal and reticulothalamic pathways are implicated.
4. Stimulation-induced burning implicates reticulothalamic structures in deafferentation and central pain (presumably the steady burning tingling element). As the reticulothalamic tract is not known to be topographically organized, in order that pain be localized should it arise in reticulothalamic structures, a connection must exist with some topographically organized structure such as the spinothalamic tract. This would fit with the observation that burning in these patients is also elicited in spinothalamic tract, ventrobasal complex and somatosensory cortex.
5. Although bursting cells in general appear to be markers of deafferentation rather than pain, the regularly firing, regularly bursting cells may reflect a central process involved in pain production. It is tempting to consider such cells as markers of denervation neuronal hypersensitivity capable of producing pain. Such activity could arise in the reticulothalamic tract with cross-connections to the spinothalamic tract.
6. Abnormal firing rates may occur in tactile or other somatosensory neurons deprived of input, whether or not they acquire alternate input. Such a process may also generate pain.

CHOICE OF SURGICAL PROCEDURE

For nociceptive pain, interruption or inhibitory modulation of ascending pathways should bring relief. Ablative procedures and possibly spinothalamic modulation will also stop evoked pain and, if performed proximally, the spontaneous intermittent element in deafferentation and central pain syndromes. On the other hand, the spontaneous steady burning should only be expected to respond to procedures that eliminate or normalize central abnormal neuronal activity.

Table 7.2 lists the various surgical procedures available for the treatment of chronic intractable pain. N denotes those considered useful in treating nociceptive pain; S denotes those used to treat the steady spontaneous burning tingling element of deafferentation and central pain. Those marked with an asterisk are probably little used today [2,5,14,16–19,21,25,29,30,33–35,37,38,52,53].

SURGICAL TREATMENT OF NOCICEPTIVE PAIN

Destructive-interruptive procedures

Neurectomy and rhizotomy

Percutaneous neurotomy and rhizotomy are seldom appropriate in the treatment of intractable nociceptive pain because they sacrifice significant motor and/or sensory

Table 7.2 Surgical procedures used in the treatment of pain

Modulating		Destructive		Miscellaneous
I	Chronic stimulation	N†	Neurectomy	Neuroma resection
	S† (a) Nerves		Sympathectomy	Various neurolyses
	S (b) Dorsal cord (DCS)	N	Dorsal rhizotomy	and neural repair
	S (c) Medial lemniscus	N? S?	Dorsal root entry zone (DREZ)	procedures
	S (d) Ventrocaudal nucleus	N	Cordotomy	
	S (e) Internal capsule	N S?	Midline commissurotomy	
	S? N (f) Medial thalamus;	N S	Trigeminal tractotomy	
	other periventricular-	N	Mesencephalic spinothalamic	
	periaqueductal		tractotomy	
	structures	S N	Mesencephalic medial	
			tractotomy	
II	Chronic infusion of opiates			
	N (a) Epidural or	S N	Medial thalamotomy	
	intrathecal spinal	N *	Hypothalamotomy	
	N (b) Third ventricle	N *	Pulvinarotomy	
III	N Alcohol injection of	*	Psychosurgery	
	pituitary			

* Probably little used today
† N, used to treat nociceptive pain; S, used to treat steady spontaneous burning tingling element of deafferentation and central pain.

function and eventual regeneration with pain recurrence is probably the rule. Furthermore, such pains are rarely confined to the distribution of one or a few nerves or roots. In selected cases they may be helpful in avoiding the impact of more complex or extensive procedures.

The target structure is identified by imaging and accessed with a needle electrode with an appropriately sized bare tip under local or intermittent general anesthesia. Then, with an electronic backup such as the Owl Cordotomy System* or that provided by the Radionics Corporation†, threshold slow (2 Hz) and rapid (30–100 Hz) stimulation is used to elicit motor and sensory effects respectively, guiding the surgeon to avoid motor damage and to denervate the painful areas accurately with a graded radiofrequency lesion.

Facet rhizotomy
This procedure attempts to identify and interrupt the posterior rami of spinal nerves, including articular branches, to alleviate spondylogenic pain. It is usually employed bilaterally at the L3–4–5 levels for pain confined to the lumbosacral area, buttock and upper thigh, preferably that aggravated by activity and relieved by rest, and is performed particularly at sites where stimulation induces paresthesias or motor effects in the patient's area of pain but not extending below the knee.

The procedure was originally popularized by Rees [54], using a scalpel blindly; it is now usually done by the percutaneous radiofrequency technique introduced by Shealy [55], using anatomic and physiologic guidelines outlined by Fox and Rizzoli [56] and by Pedersen *et al.* [57]. Pain relief varies from 50 to 60% of patients

* Diros Technology Inc., 965 Pape Avenue, Toronto M4K 3V8, Canada
† Radionics Corporation, PO Box 43876, Cambridge Street, Burlington, Massachusetts 01803-0738, USA.

[34,38,58], and is better (63% relief) in patients who have not previously undergone open spinal surgery than in those who have (25% relief) [55]. Ouden-hoven [59] reported 74% excellent, 15% good results in 60 unoperated patients, and 35% excellent, 24% good results in 48 previously operated patients. Burton [60] found that only 42% of his 126 patients overall did well while 67% of the unoperated group enjoyed significant relief. McCulloch [61] also found 67% good results in 82 unoperated patients. Dunsker *et al.* [62], on the other hand, attained only 20% overall relief in previously operated patients but when previous diagnostic local blockade of the facet nerves relieved the pain, 40% did well. This author has found facet rhizotomy disappointing; however, it may occasionally be useful in the unoperated patient mainly with back pain related to degenerative disk disease.

Occipital neurectomy
Blume [63] and Blume and Fromm [64] have used percutaneous radiofrequency occipital neurectomy to relieve pain at the cervicocranial junction, locating the nerve by stimulation-induced paresthesias in the proper distribution. During a 1–4-year follow-up of 114 and 250 patients respectively, 75% derived significant relief.

The procedure can be used sparingly to relieve occipital neuralgia, either the result of bony pathology at the occiput–C1–C2 junction or of myofascial tension, when the pain is sharp, intermittent or lancinating. The procedure is not useful for the patient with steady burning occipital pain.

Intercostal neurectomy
Percutaneous radiofrequency intercostal neurectomy [32,34,65], performed using a curved needle electrode inserted under the trailing edge of the appropriate rib, is an easily performed procedure requiring only postoperative chest radiographs to rule out significant pneumothorax, and particularly useful in treating nociceptive pain cased by malignant involvement of the chest wall. It is useless in most cases of post-thoractomy pain – a deafferentation pain syndrome – only 25% of the author's patients having benefited, unless there is a major element of evoked or intermittent lancinating pain. It is also ineffective in intercostal neuralgia caused by thoracic disk disease because the technique does not allow the root to be sectioned proximal to the site of irritation. Furthermore, in the author's experience it is useful in postherpetic neuralgia only for the relief of hyperpathia.

Trigeminal neurectomy and rhizotomy
Although the medical treatment of tic douloureux is discussed in Chapter 11, the surgical techniques have a limited role in other types of chronic pain. On the basis of the original work of Kirschner [66] and Härtel [67], Sweet and Wepsic [68] introduced the percutaneous radiofrequency method, making destruction of the nerve safer because it facilitates both physiologic localization and controlled lesion size.

An appropriately insulated needle with a 3–4 mm bare tip is introduced into Meckel's cave via the foramen ovale under brief general anesthetic. The patient is awakened, stimulated at 20 Hz or more and the needle's position adjusted until paresthesias occur in the area of the patient's pain. A carefully graded, temperature-monitored radiofrequency lesion is then made under general anesthetic until the desired effect is achieved.

The selective technique [69–71], using a smaller curved electrode, although useful in tic, is not appropriate for the nociceptive pain of cancer, where the largest lesion possible should be made. Siegfried and Broggi [72] reported good enduring pain relief in ten of 20 patients with trigeminal pain caused by cancer. Maxwell [73] relieved all eight of his patients with chronic migrainous neuralgia. Watson *et al.* [74] reported relief of eight out of 13 patients with cluster headache, and Onofrio and Campbell [75] of 16 out of 26 patients.

Complications in tic [70,76] include usually transient masticatory weakness (22–27%), dysesthesia (14–27%), diplopia (2%) and keratitis (4%). Although not mentioned in the published list, meningitis, brain abscess and fatal intracranial hemorrhage due to hypertension induced by the process have all occurred.

Pain in the distribution of the lower cranial nerves can be similarly treated with the risk of dysphagia or vagal dysfunction [70,77–83].

The glycerol injection technique introduced by Håkansson [84] is probably indicated only for tic douloureux, as are the various trigeminal compression and decompression techniques [85–88]

Thus, trigeminal or lower cranial nerve destruction by the percutaneous radiofrequency technique is useful in selected cases of cancer pain. It may also have a limited role in managing otherwise intractable cases of migrainous facial pain. These procedures should be avoided in unexplained pain syndromes and are useful in deafferentation and central pain only to eliminate allodynia and hyperpathia.

Dorsal rhizotomy

Although dorsal rhizotomy was originally performed by open laminectomy, the introduction of the percutaneous radiofrequency technique [65,89] has greatly reduced the complications. An electrode similar to that used for trigeminal denervation is introduced into the dorsal aspect of the appropriate intervertebral foramen under radiographic control and is positioned so that its stimulation produces paresthesias without motor effects in the area of pain when a graded radiofrequency lesion is made.

McLaurin [90] found open rhizectomy useful in 28–56% of cases reported in the literature. Loeser [91] reported 28% long-term and 63% short-term relief in 46 patients with varied pain syndromes; 43% of his cancer patients enjoyed long-term relief and 54% short-term relief. Onofrio [92] found the procedure successful in five out of 18 (28%) patients with cancer pain and in 23% of 78 patients with lumbar disk disease. Saris *et al.* [93] reported 53% good results in 28 patients undergoing sacrococcygeal rhizotomy for cancer pain, followed for 3 years. Only 22% of patients suffering from coccydynia were relieved by the same procedure. Sindou *et al.* [94] reviewed 585 case reports in the literature of cancer pain treated by rhizotomy, 153 of whom were followed long term, and noted that 59% derived early, and 47% enduring, pain relief; mortality ranged from zero to 20%.

Smith [95] has advised dorsal ganglionectomy to improve the results of dorsal rhizotomy by eliminating possible ventral root afferents; however, in this author's opinion, the technique needs further study.

Using a percutaneous radiofrequency method, Uematsu [89] reported nine out of 17 (53%) useful results in a variety of pain syndromes, while Pagura [96] reported 76% overall pain relief in 13 patients with cancer and 37 with disk disease, two of whom suffered temporary paresis. This technique may be inappropriate for pain associated with intervertebral disk disease, as the lesion is made distal to the site of irritation. Moreoever, caution must be exercised in the T1–T4 and T11–L1 areas to avoid damage to the indispensable radicular arterial supply to the cord.

Percutaneous radiofrequency rhizotomy has an occasional application in treating nociceptive pain limited to one or several dorsal roots when the lesion can be made proximal to the irritative focus. It is also occasionally useful for relieving allodynia, hyperpathia or lancinating intermittent pain in deafferentation and central pain syndromes.

Miscellaneous techniques

The injection of phenol or alcohol (except to achieve sympathectomy) and that of other sclerosing agents, as well as the subarachnoid injection of cold or hypertonic saline for the relief of nociceptive pain are, in the author's opinion, inferior to the percutaneous radiofrequency techniques which are more permanent, allow physiologic localization and avoid indiscriminate spread of the agent [97–104].

Percutaneous cordotomy

Cordotomy was introduced by Spiller and Martin [105] as an open procedure and has remained one of the most useful surgical procedures for the treatment of pain. The introduction of the percutaneous radiofrequency technique by Mullan *et al.* [106] and Rosomoff *et al.* [107] has made open cordotomy virtually obsolete because of the reduced morbidity and risk, and the enhanced accuracy of physiologic localization that the percutaneous procedure allows, despite continued suggestions to the contrary [108]. This author considers percutaneous cordotomy by the lateral high cervical route to be the treatment of choice for cancerous nociceptive pain and some selected cases of central pain (*see* pages 170–172) [29,34,35,38]. It can be performed under general anesthesia if necessary; it can safely be done bilaterally if proper criteria are met. Absolute contraindications include pain above the C5 dermatome (where lasting analgesia cannot be achieved) and where there is the risk of producing cervical analgesia ipsilateral to the only adequately functioning lung; such lesions interrupt the only functional, unilaterally distributed, reticulospinal tract that activates unconscious respiration. In such situations, instillation of morphine into the third ventricle might be considered, or else Sindou's dorsal root entry lesion, both described below (pages 160 and 156-157, respectively). Percutaneous cordotomy is also unsuited to the relief of bilateral truncal (especially perineal) pain, when epidural or intrathecal morphine instillation is preferable (described below, page 160). The role of low anterior percutaneous cordotomy, in this author's opinion, is the avoidance of respiratory complications when high levels of analgesia are unnecessary, because the meticulous manipulation of electrode position required for percutaneous cordotomy is difficult when the electrode has first to be passed through a cervical disk.

A fine sharpened electrode with a 2 mm bare tip is introduced into the cord guided by myelography, usually in the C1–C2 interspace. Penetration of the cord is monitored with electrical impedance while the spinothalamic tract is recognized, with 100 Hz stimulation, by the contralateral topographically organized perception of warmth, cold or, occasionally, burning in the absence of any accompanying motor effect. When proper criteria have been met, a graded radiofrequency lesion is made, monitoring current flow and/or temperature. If the electrode has been introduced too anteriorly, into the ventral horn, tetanization of ipsilateral neck muscles occurs; if it lies too posteriorly, in the corticospinal tract, ipsilateral tetanization of muscles in any part of the body may occur.

In our experience with 380 consecutive percutaneous cordotomies [29,37], the procedure was technically completed in 99%, achieving initially adequate spinothalamic interruption. At the latest follow-up, 93.4% still showed evidence of spinothalamic interruption, although the degree varied, and 84.2% of patients enjoyed significant (but not always complete) relief of the pain for which the cordotomy was done. Inadequacies (in 15.8%) nearly always paralleled imperfections of level or degree of spinothalamic interruption.

Results after bilateral cordotomy follow the P* squared rule where significant relief bilaterally of the pain for which cordotomy was done was achieved in 72% of patients at last follow-up; 4.6% of patients developed new pain, above the original levels of analgesia, from progress of the disease, and 41% experienced new or worsened pain on the opposite side of the body. In our most recent 136 consecutive patients undergoing percutaneous cordotomy, 6.1% continued to suffer from the pain for which the cordotomy was done despite adequate levels of analgesia; this pain may have been of central or deafferentation origin. In 33.7%, new pain of a dysesthetic quality appeared, below solid levels of analgesia, for the most part attributable to clinically demonstrable progression of their cancer. This pain was deemed to be of a deafferentation type not amenable to relief by cordotomy. With increasingly aggressive and successful oncotherapy, patients are surviving longer with cancerous involvement of lumbosacral or brachial plexus and are at greater risk of suffering deafferentation pain in addition to their nociceptive pain; cordotomy dissects out the latter, leaving the former behind.

Complications in 380 consecutive cases when the procedure was done unilaterally included 0.3% mortality, 0.8% incidence of permanent paresis, 2.9% permanent worsening of bladder function, 16.8% transient paresis, 6.6% minor urinary problems and 33% usually transient Horner's syndrome. After bilateral cordotomy the mortality was 1.6%, permanent paresis affected 1.6%, significant bladder impairment 18.8%, transient paresis 28% and minor bladder complications 9.4%. Post-cordotomy dysesthesia was seen in 6% and was significant in 3%. Two patients died from their disease in the first postoperative month.

Rosomoff [109] found a similarly satisfactory experience in a review of 789 patients. Lipton [110] produced immediate complete analgesia and thermanalgesia in 80% of his patients but levels fell soon postoperatively in 4%. Mortality was 6.2% and 80% suffered from some degree of paresis, 20% with enduring disability. Ataxia occurred in 0.5%, post-cordotomy dysesthesia in 2%, Horner's syndrome in 100%. Bladder dysfunction was not seen after unilateral cordotomy but affected every patient undergoing bilateral surgery. Meglio and Cioni [111] reported 79%, Lahuerta *et al.* [112] 64%, Kühner [113] 59% and Siegfried *et al.* [114] 75% satisfactory pain relief. Lorenz [115], in a review of 3000 published cases, found 75–96% results that were good to excellent. Ischia *et al.* [116] reported complete pain relief in 47% and incomplete relief in 12.5% of the 36 patients that underwent bilateral operation out of his series of 540.

---

* If bilateral cordotomy is performed, the interval between the operations on the two sides is usually too short for the outcome on the first side to influence the decision to operate on the second. Therefore if the success rate for one side is 84.2%, that for both sides is $(84.2\%)^2$ or 70.9%

Ischia *et al.* [117] noticed that although 81% of 36 patients were relieved of the pain for which unilateral cordotomy was performed, 63% developed pain on the other side of the body and 14% developed or continued to suffer from pain below an adequate level of analgesia. In another report [118] the same authors noticed a 47.8% incidence of postoperative ipsilateral pain, 4.3% incidence of new pain below the level of analgesia and 8.7% of pain below adequate levels of analgesia. In 103 patients undergoing percutaneous cordotomy for cervicothoracic pain, 92.4% achieved adequate analgesia: of these, 56.3% suffered from ipsilateral pain and 3.9% pain above the level of analgesia postoperatively; 6.8% continued to suffer from pain below levels of adequate analgesia.

Complications of unilateral cordotomy reported in these publications [112,113,116,118,119] were mortality 0–6%, respiratory insufficiency 2.6–4.2%, transient – presumably ipsilateral – limb paresis ≤ 69% (permanent in 1–4%), contralateral limb paresis 0–6%, transient bladder dysfunction ≤ 19% (permanent in 3–8.7%) and post-cordotomy dysesthesia ≤ 20%. For bilateral cordotomy, mortality was 10%, respiratory insufficiency affected 20% of patients, limb paresis 36.1% (permanent in 1.8%), bladder dysfunction 12–58% and hypotension 36.1%.

Commissurotomy

Open spinal midline commissurotomy was introduced in 1927 by Armour [120] as a substitute for cordotomy, interrupting spinothalamic fibres as they decussated in the anterior commissure over three levels above the dermatomal level of the pain. Bilateral relief of pain was usually achieved, with transient bilateral analgesia at the appropriate levels; however, as the location of pain relief does not correlate with this analgesia, the mechanism of commissurotomy is obscure [121]. As the procedure requires a laminectomy, there seems little to recommend it today.

Wertheimer and Lecuire [122] reported 65% pain relief in 93 patients with various types of pain, at the expense of a 7.5% mortality. Piscol [108] although advocating a microscopic technique, nevertheless produced paresis in 26% of patients. Payne [123] achieved initial relief of perineal and lower trunk cancer pain in 75% of 24 patients, with leg paresthesias that were temporary in 71% and permanent in 8%; 50% of patients suffered from loss of position sense and 45% from pain recurrence. Adams *et al.* [124] achieved pain relief in 88% of 24 patients, most suffering from cancer, 12% of whom developed bladder dysfunction, 8% paresis and 6% persistent dysesthesia. McLaurin [90] achieved 47% long-term excellent pain relief with 3% mortality and 6% dysesthesia. Broager [125] reported 47% long-term excellent results in 34 patients, most of whom suffered from cancer, with a 3% mortality and a 4% incidence of dysesthesia. Sourek [126] relieved pain in 79% of 39 patients, with eight deaths, but pain relief was often temporary and most patients suffered from transient dysesthesia, bladder disturbances and difficulty in walking. Appropriate girdle anesthesia faded with time but loss of touch, vibration and position sense persisted.

Hitchcock [127] introduced a stereotactic percutaneous cervical radiofrequency commissurotomy technique in the occipital–C1 interspace with the patient seated. An electrode was advanced to a point 5 mm anterior to the dorsal cord margin, as outlined with contrast medium, in the mid-sagittal plane. When the electrode lay in the dorsal columns stimulation caused paresthesias in both feet. As the penetration proceeded towards the central canal, these paresthesias spread from the lower limbs to the face, the opposite limbs and both upper limbs; even burning in the trunk might be produced. Radiofrequency lesions similar to those made for percutaneous cordotomy were then made anterior to, or at the level of, lower limb responses. In 14 patients with nociceptive pain there were ten excellent and two good results, pain being relieved at any level in the body without clinically detectable sensory loss, even immediately postoperatively. Eiras *et al.* [128] found 100% initial pain relief, with a tendency to pain recurrence, at the expense of temporary dysmetria and an ataxic gait. Schvarcz [129] reported 78% relief in 79 patients with nociceptive pain, transient gait ataxia being a common postoperative complication. Papo [130] found that pain relief was transient, complications being dysmetria and ataxic gait.

It would appear to the author that commissurotomy has no advantage over percutaneous cordotomy, or over chronic morphine instillation (page 160).

Percutaneous lesions of the descending tract and caudal nucleus of trigeminal nerve

Stereotactic destruction of the descending tract and caudal nucleus of the trigeminal nerve can be done at both the medullary and upper cervical levels [131–139].

The former procedure is performed with the patient prone under local anesthesia, the floor of the fourth ventricle, obex and dorsum of the brain stem being outlined with contrast medium and used as landmarks to guide a No. 22 insulated bare-tipped needle under impedance control through a No. 18 thinwall lumbar puncture needle to the target. Here 50 Hz stimulation produces facial paresthesias when a graded radiofrequency lesion is made with serial neurological testing.

Fox [133] operated on eight patients with cancer, noting transient pyrexia and ipsilateral ataxia in most patients postoperatively; contralateral analgesia in the body occurred in three.

The cervical procedure is done under local anesthesia with the patient seated. The anterior–posterior aspect of the cord and cisterna magna are demonstrated with contrast medium and a 0.5 mm sharpened insulated needle with a 2 mm bare tip is advanced toward the expected position of the tract, using impedance monitoring and serial stimulation. Where facial paresthesias occur, a graded carefully monitored radiofrequency lesion is made. Schvarcz [137,138] reported 83.8% relief of cancer pain in 30 patients followed for 2–30 months; complications included contralateral hypalgesia and ipsilateral ataxia. This little-utilized technique deserves further attention for facial cancer pain.

Lesions in the region of the dorsal root entry zone

Hyndman [140] originally introduced open Lissauer tract section to raise the level of analgesia achieved by open cordotomy. Then, in 1972, Sindou [141–144] introduced the procedure of cutting the dorsal root entry zone to a depth of 2 mm at a 45 degree angle with a razor blade just lateral to the dorsal rootlets in an endeavour to treat nociceptive pain, particularly that associated with Pancoast's syndrome and spasticity. In cancer patients some 65% experienced relief, with a 5–15% mortality. By this means, global sensory loss and respiratory complications could be avoided and higher levels of analgesia achieved than possible with percutaneous cordotomy; lesions at C4 were not recommended. The main complication was hypotonia in the leg. Sindou *et al.* [144] reported significant reduction of spasticity in 88% of 16 hemiplegic patients, as well as total relief in nine and partial relief in two out of 12 patients who also suffered from pain; eight of these patients showed postoperative sensory loss.

Sindou's procedure may have a role in treating nociceptive pain when cordotomy is contraindicated for respiratory reasons.

Operations on the brain

Whereas, in the past, open medullary and mesencephalic tractotomy and other procedures were performed to relieve intractable nociceptive pain, particularly in the head and neck, these procedures have been replaced by stereotactic techniques with their lower morbidity and mortality, greater accuracy and, strangely, much lesser risk of post-operative dysesthesia.

Stereotactic pontine spinothalamic tractotomy

Hitchcock and his associates introduced pontine spinothalamic tractotomy [145–147] hoping to avoid the respiratory insufficiency, dysesthesia and sphincter disturbance of cordotomy. They introduce an electrode, using the imaged aqueduct, floor and fastigium of the fourth ventricle as landmarks, confirm the location physiologically and make a graded radiofrequency lesion. In seven out of eight patients, pain caused by cancer was completely relieved until the patient died, even though levels of analgesia tended to fade with time; one patient died. Barbéra *et al.* [148] obtained satisfactory relief in five cancer patients.

The limited experience makes it difficult to evaluate this operation.

Stereotactic mesencephalic tractotomy

In the upper mesencephalon, several important structures lie side by side. The periaqueductal-periventricular gray (PAG-PVG) lies in the wall of the aqueduct and third ventricle; the reticulothalamic tract extends laterally from PAG to about 7 mm from the midline; the spinothalamic tract extends from there to 9 mm lateral and the medial lemniscus from 10 to 12 mm lateral. The first stereotactic mesencephalotomy [149,150] aimed at interrupting the mesencephalic-spinothalamic tract, combined with dorsomedian thalamotomy to alleviate anxiety. The mesencephalic lesion was subsequently extended to include the reticulothalamic tract. Localization was achieved by macro-stimulation, the spinothalamic tract being identified by the induction of contralateral burning pain, prickling, and electrical sensations. Medial to these responses, diffuse, unusual induced effects often associated with a choking sensation referred to the chest, were reported. In early series, 72% of patients enjoyed immediate relief and 31% longer-term relief of pain caused by a mixed group of pain syndromes. Complications included a 7.4% mortality (compared with 24% for open mesencephalic tractotomy), 15% contralateral dysesthesia (compared with 70% for the open operation), 50% hearing loss, 7% paresis, 17% oculomotor palsies and 4% ataxia, effects that were mostly transient. Mazars and his coworkers [151, 152], who carefully plotted the somatotopic organization of the mesencephalic tract, noted encouraging results in cancer patients with a 1% mortality. Turnbull [153] advocated addition of cingulumotomy. Nashold and his group made many contributions [154–158]. They suggested, as Spiegel *et al.* had done [159] that the most medial part of the mesencephalic tract mediated suffering. They reported a different somatotopic arrangement of spinothalamic fibres to that of Walker [160]. Responses elicited in the most medial 5 mm of the mesencephalic tract were diffusely referred to central parts of the body and body cavities and were unpleasant and endowed with emotional and autonomic content. From 5 to 12 mm from the midline, sharply defined contralateral superficially referred effects, often painful, occurred. Stimulation 12 mm or more lateral in the medial lemniscus produced paresthesias. The procedure is done using standard stereotactic techniques, confirming the target by imaging and using macrostimulation for physiologic corroboration. Amano *et al.* [161] have described a technique for physiologic corroboration of targets in the mesencephalic tract, using microelectrodes.

In our experience [27,28,31,35,39,41], stimulation of PAG-PVG yields inconsistent responses, sometimes a diffuse feeling of warmth or satiety. Stimulation more caudally in PAG may produce unacceptable feelings of horror and fear, as well as oculomotor effects. Stimulation of the reticulothalamic tract produces conscious effects only in patients suffering from central and deafferentation pain. Stimulation of the spinothalamic tract produces somatotopically organized contralateral hot or cold sensations, organized as Walker had stated [160]. Paresthesias were produced in the medial lemniscus.

There is extensive experience with stereotactic mesencephalic tractotomy [149–158, 161–171], results in nociceptive and deafferentation–central pain syndromes being often intermixed. Persistent relief of nociceptive pain ranges from 67% to 100%, one author reporting 100% initial relief but 100% recurrence. Mortality varies up to 7%. Oculomotor complications range from 13% to 88% while dysesthesia affects 6.5–38%. Nashold [53] concluded that a mortality of 3–5% could be expected, with a morbidity of 37%. The latter, usually transient, was chiefly attributable to oculomotor disturbances which affected almost every patient in a small way, frank diplopia being reported in 1–5% and dysesthesia in 5%.

This author has reviewed the literature, selecting 92 published protocols sufficiently documented to conclude that the patients suffered from nociceptive pain. Of these patients, 80% enjoyed useful pain relief at the expense of a 15–20% incidence of dysesthesia, 15–20% of transient oculomotor disturbances and a mortality of 5–10%. We have performed 32 stereotactic mesencephalic tractotomies with a 9% mortality, achieving complete or nearly complete relief of nociceptive pain in 45% and partial relief in 23%. Major complication affected 9%; 32% suffered mild or transient disability.

Stereotactic mesencephalic tractotomy has a limited role in the treatment of nociceptive pain beyond the range of cordotomy or other simple procedures when the instillation of third ventricular morphine is not possible.

Ventrobasal thalamotomy
Ventrobasal thalamotomy was pioneered by Monnier and Fischer [172] and thoroughly studied by Mark and his associates [173–178]. It has been used frequently for the relief of pain, although the procedure is perhaps of mainly historic interest now, having been replaced by mesencephalic tractotomy or medial thalamotomy; these latter procedures have a lower risk of loss of position sense and dysesthesia. The same applies to lesions made in Hassler's parvicellular subnucleus of ventrobasal complex [179–181], thought by him to be the specific relay nucleus for the spinothalamic tract. The experience of Talairach and his associates, with

lesions made in the thalamic radiations passing to the second somatosensory cortex, has not been pursued [182].

Medial thalamotomy
At an early stage, attention switched from the ventrobasal complex to the other thalamic termination of pain fibres, in the medial thalamus. Although surgery is often directed towards the centre médian, in order to be succesful medial thalamic lesions should probably be made in parafascicular or central lateral nuclei which are the nociceptive terminals here, rather than the centre médian [183].

The procedure is performed as for any other functional thalamotomy. After approximate identification of the target by imaging, either macrostimulation or microstimulation and microrecording are carried out to identify the medial margin of the ventrobasal complex. Using this as a basis, the exploring electrode is now passed medially into the desired structure where, in this author's experience, identifiable stimulation-induced effects are difficult to achieve [27,41,42]. Sano and his group, however, have published protocols for localization here, using stimulation and recording [184–187].

Medial thalamotomy was pioneered by Monnier and Fischer [172] and by Hécaen *et al.* [188]. Mark and his associates, in an ongoing study of the effects of thalamotomy, clearly advocated their preference for medial versus ventrobasal lesions [173–178] because of superior pain relief, lower complication rate and the fact that lesions in medial thalamus produced no identifiable neurological defect. There is an extensive literature on the subject [17,30,33,181,184–209]. This author extracted 175 patient protocols from the literature, in which it was possible to identify the patient's pain as being nociceptive [30,33]. It appeared that 46% of this group of patients achieved good relief, 11% fair relief with, perhaps, a 50% recurrence rate. There were 10–20% complications, usually confusion or other cognitive difficulties. The data presented by Fairman and his colleagues are imprecise but cite a 70% incidence of pain relief, which is better than that of most other studies [210–212]. The author has made medial thalamic lesions in 21 patients with nociceptive pain, sometimes in addition to lesions made elsewhere: 62% achieved significant pain relief.

Thus, medial thalamotomy yields poorer pain relief than mesencephalic tractotomy, but the complication rate is less, particularly in sick patients with cancer of the head and neck. Furthermore, the complications differ, usually consisting of transient confusion or psychiatric disturbances, especially after bilateral lesions. The risk of mortality and dysesthesia are negligible.

Frank *et al.* [165] have compared the procedures in treating nociceptive pain usually caused by cancer. With medial thalamotomy they obtained 51.9% relief with 41% recurrence; 70% of patients suffered from transient confusion. There were few neurological effects other than a 1.9% incidence of aphasia and there was no mortality. In the mesencephalic tractotomy group, there was 83.5% persisting pain relief, at the expense of a 1.8% mortality rate and a 10.1% incidence of oculomotor and dysesthetic disturbances.

When destructive lesions are being considered for the treatment of nociceptive pain that cannot be managed by simpler means, the choice lies between stereotactic medial thalamotomy, with its lower efficacy and morbidity, and mesencephalic tractotomy, with its greater efficacy and morbidity.

Modulatory procedures

Two types of modulating procedures are in common use for the relief of nociceptive pain: morphine instillation into the spinal epidural or intrathecal space or third ventricle, and periventricular gray stimulation.

Morphine instillation

Pilon and Baker [212] first attempted to modulate pain pharmacologically using epidural instillation of local anesthetics. When opiates were shown to block nociceptive transmission at the dorsal horn level [214], Wang *et al.* [215] were prompted to instill morphine intrathecally at the spinal level for the relief of cancer pain. At first, spinal morphine injections became popular for the relief of acute and postoperative pain, then for the relief of chronic cancer pain [216], both in the cervical and lumbar areas. Epidural or intrathecal spinal cannulas, attached either to a programmable pump or a subcutaneous refillable reservoir, can be used [217–225].

   With epidural injections, dosages may begin as low as 2 mg every 8–12 hours, building up to 15–18 mg daily, achieving effective pain relief in 60% of patients. Complications include technical failures and urticaria. Respiratory depression is rare and escalation of dosage often does not occur. Before inserting an intrathecal cannula pump system, an epidural screening trial is first carried out to select patients who are more likely to respond. Any tolerance develops slowly: dosage in one study increased from 4.8 to 21 mg/day over a year; in another study it doubled in 3–9 months.

   In this author's opinion, morphine instillation should be considered in patients with nociceptive cancer pain where percutaneous cordotomy or some other simple destructive procedure is inappropriate. It is particularly useful in patients with bilateral truncal, especially perineal, pain.

Intraventricular morphine instillation
After the practical application of intraspinal morphine instillation, delivery into the third ventricle using a similar system was tried and proved effective, particularly for pain caused by cancer of the head and neck, and obviated the risks of major destructive operations.

   Some 50–88% (average 73%) of patients derived satisfactory relief, with few complications such as psychological disturbance, occasional respiratory depression and pruritus. Dosages typically start at 0.1–2 mg/day and often there is only modest dose escalation with time. Infection occurs in about 1%, respiratory depression in 2%, and 25–50% of patients suffer early transient side-effects [223,226,227].

Hypophyseal alcohol injection
Destruction of the pituitary gland for the relief of cancer pain was inspired by the beneficial endocrinologic effects of hypophysectomy on hormone-dependent cancer of breast and prostate, with concomitant relief of pain [228–231]. For example, Tindall *et al.* [231] reported 76% pain relief in hormone-dependent tumors after open hypophysectomy with a 5% mortality, a 4% incidence of meningitis, and a 14% incidence of CSF leakage.

   Among many strategies to avoid open hypophysectomy in relieving pain in these sick cancer patients, the percutaneous alcohol technique was popularized by

Morricca [232] who reported the unexpected observation that pain caused by endocrinologically independent tumors was also relieved.

Pain relief may initially be achieved in 41–95% of patients with hormonally dependent cancer and 69% of those with non-hormonally dependent cancer [233–240]. There is a tendency for pain to recur in 3–4 months. Mortality varies from 2% to 6.5%; rhinorrhea occurs in 3–20%, meningitis in 0.3–1%, visual and oculomotor disturbances in 2–10% and diabetes insipidus in 50–60%. Hypothalamic disturbances and headache are frequent, although most of the complications tend to be transient.

This is a procedure of unknown mechanism, the results of which are apparently unrelated to pituitary destruction, hypothalamic involvement or alteration of blood or CSF levels of any known substance, including endorphins; moreover, its effects are not reversed with naloxone [241–243]. Its great advantage is simplicity and independence from expensive equipment. It would appear, however, that percutaneous cordotomy, where feasible, is more effective and safer and, failing that, that chronic morphine instillation should be considered.

Chronic stimulation of periventricular gray (PVG)

On the basis of the work of Reynolds [244], Richardson and Akil [245,246] and Richardson [247] demonstrated that stimulation of the mid-brain periaqueductal gray or its rostral extension, the periventricular gray to the hypothalamus, relieved chronic pain. Presumably, this is attributable to the activation of the pain-modulating network discussed in Chapter 1. In man, stimulation was acceptable only in PVG near the posterior commissure, unpleasant concomitant stimulation-induced effects precluding its use elsewhere.

The operation is performed using CT or MR-guided stereotaxis, directly visualizing PVG 2 mm lateral to the wall of the third ventricle at the most medial limit of parafascicular nucleus. An electrode is introduced, stimulating every millimetre or two to the target site, and trial stimulation is carried out before internalization with a totally implantable or radiofrequency-coupled stimulating device. Stimulation-induced effects in PVG are unpredictable: sometimes no effect is produced, or else a feeling of pleasure, warmth, satiety, with relief of pain. Sites at which anxiety, fear, discomfort or oculomotor effects occur must be avoided.

Although most consider PVG stimulation treatment for nociceptive pain, as would be expected [246,248–257], there is also evidence for relief of non-nociceptive pain and sometimes its effects are not reversed by naloxone [248,250,256,258–260]. Relief of nociceptive pain occurs in up to 80% of patients, complications consisting of neural trauma (up to 11%), infection (4–15%), device failure (3–9%), lead breakage (11%) and electrode migration (7%). Duration of stimulation is often restricted to avoid the development of tolerance.

In recent publications, Young and Brechner [259] found virtually total relief of pain in 76% of patients with cancer, using PAG-PVG stimulation either alone or associated with stimulation in ventrobasal complex. Young and Chambi [260] noted that tolerance developed equally in patients stimulated in PVG-PAG or the ventrobasal complex and that there was no cross-tolerance between PVG-PAG stimulation and morphine. Hosobuchi [257] considered PVG stimulation to be effective in non-deafferentation pain if it was responsive to narcotics. Levy *et al.* [258] found 60% pain relief in 337 patients with nociceptive pain recorded in the literature, including data on 57 patients of their own. Stimulation was apparently carried out both in PVG-PAG and in the ventrobasal complex. Meyerson *et al* [249]. have avoided expensive stimulating equipment in cancer patients with short life expectancies by using transcutaneous stimulation long term without significant infection.

DEAFFERENTATION AND CENTRAL PAIN

As described above, deafferentation and central pain includes the following components:

1. Steady spontaneous burning-tingling pain.
2. Intermittent spontaneous lancinating pain.
3. Evoked pain.
4. Sympathetic hyperfunction.

Although the author regards the identification of these elements in a patient's pain protocol as essential in planning therapy, most previous reports have not made such distinctions, so evaluation of the literature is difficult. We have advanced the proposition that intermittent and evoked pain appear to respond to the same strategies as nociceptive pain. This section deals primarily with the relief of steady spontaneous burning-tingling pain, usually a difficult, frustrating and imperfect exercise. First the role of various operative procedures is summarized, followed by a brief discussion of surgical therapy in selected deafferentation and central pain syndromes.

Destructive procedures

Neurectomy and rhizotomy

The general ineffectiveness of denervating procedures in the treatment of the steady burning element of deafferentation pain has been noted, even though local anesthetic blockade proximal or distal to the causative lesion often affords temporary relief. It is as if such pain responded to changing of levels of somatosensory input, Condouris [261] having suggested that local anesthetic blockade acts as a modulating influence. The chief role of such denervating procedures is in the relief of hyperpathia or allodynia in the distribution of partially damaged nerves or roots, or the relief of intermittent lancinating pain.

Neurolysis, neuroma resection or nerve grafting may relieve evoked pain or the nociceptive pain associated with neural compression, but not the steady burning pain associated with deafferentation syndromes [262–266] and there appears to be no advantage in adding ganglionectomy to dorsal rhizotomy to interrupt possible ventral root afferents in these conditions [267–269].

Cordotomy

Cordotomy is also usually unsuccessful in relieving steady burning pain in deafferentation and central pain. Of 65 out of 244 of the author's patients undergoing percutaneous cordotomy for such pain, 70.6% reported complete and 78.4% significant if not complete, pain relief at discharge from hospital. By the time of longest follow-up these figures had fallen to 33.3% complete and 50% significant relief, respectively, despite an adequate level of sensory loss. When the data for the largest group of these patients – those with central pain of cord origin – were examined, it appeared that the patients enjoying relief tended to have lower incomplete cord lesions and chiefly intermittent lancinating pain (*see* section on Central Pain of Cord Origin, pages 170–172). Steady burning pain was usually not affected [25,26,29,31,32,35,37,39].

Cordectomy

The role of cordectomy appears to be similar to that of cordotomy (*see* section on Central Pain of Cord Origin, pages 170–172).

Percutaneous stereotactic destruction of the descending tract and caudal nucleus of the trigeminal nerve

Although this procedure would seem best suited to the treatment of nociceptive pain, reported experience suggests that it is also useful in deafferentation pain [133,137,138]. Schvarcz [137,138], in a series of 52 patients followed for 6 months to $5\frac{1}{2}$ years, reported relief in 87.5% of those suffering from postherpetic neuralgia, 56% with anesthesia dolorosa, and 74% with 'dysesthetic' pain.

Commissurotomy

Although this originally was performed for the relief of cancer pain, Hitchcock [127] reported that the percutaneous technique, and Fink [270] that the open procedure, was useful in relieving deafferentation pain.

Cord lesions in the vicinity of the dorsal root entry zone

This procedure and its indications are covered in Chapter 11.

Stereotactic mesencephalic tractotomy

From the beginning [149], this procedure has been used for the relief of deafferentation and central pain as well as nociceptive pain [5,14,17–19,33,35,52,53,150–153, 155–158,161–163,165,166,169,271–273]. It has a 30–84% chance of relieving central and deafferentation pain, but at the risk of frequent recurrence. Average mortality was 3–5%, morbidity 30–40%, mostly in the form of oculomotor dysfunction and dysesthesia. It is of interest that Nashold and Wilson [154] reported patients with central pain in whom an EEG focus in the medial mesencephalic tract fired in time with exacerbations of the patient's pain. In these patients, mesencephalic stimulation of the focus exacerbated, and radiofrequency destruction of the focus ameliorated, the pain. Nashold [53] concluded that stereotactic mesencephalic tractotomy afforded a 50% chance of relief of deafferentation and central pain. This author, in a similar review of 92 published protocols where central and deafferentation pain could be distinguished from nociceptive pain, found only 27% significant relief [33].

With levels of success no greater than that achieved by the considerably less invasive techniques such as chronic stimulation, stereotactic mesencephalic tractotomy must be looked on as a last resort, as stated by Pagni [17].

Thalamotomy

Stereotactic lesions in the lemniscal relay nucleus [188,189,271] or in Hassler's parvicellular portion of it that is thought to represent the spinothalamic relay, are probably of mainly historic interest in the treatment of different types of pain [180,181,197,274,275]. The results of Hitchcock and Teixeira [181] with 'basal thalamotomy' are, however, exceptional: they reported relief in two out of three patients with thalamic pain, four out of six with postherpetic neuralgia, five out of five with iatrogenic dysesthesia and three out of three with multiple sclerosis, at the expense of 48% transient and 18% permanent complications including cognitive and oculomotor dysfunction. Talairach *et al.* [182] reported relief in eight out of eight patients with deafferentation and central pain after lesions made in the thalamic radiations to the second somatosensory cortex.

Cassinari and Pagni [5] and Davis and Stokes [52] in reviewing published experience, concluded that, usually, ventrobasal thalamotomy offered a 50% chance of useful relief of central pain. This author [30], reviewing the published protocols of 56 patients that could be diagnosed as suffering from central or deafferentation pain, found 36% significant, 27% partial pain relief, with 34% complications.

Medial thalamotomy

Medial thalamotomy has been extensively employed in the treatment of deafferentation and central pain, after the pioneering work of Hécaen *et al.* [188] and Monnier and Fischer [172] with successful pain relief in 25–50% of patients [170,181,184–186,189,201,205–208]. Review of 46 published protocols in which it was possible to make a diagnosis of deafferentation or central pain [30], reveals that 29% of the procedures produced good and 38% fair pain relief, with complications in 4–21%, chiefly of a cognitive nature.

Procedures that modulate pain

There are three modulatory procedures, usually considered for the treatment of nociceptive pain, in which there is anecdotal evidence of relief of deafferentation and central pain as well: these are intrathecal morphine instillation, alcohol injection into the pituitary gland and PVG stimulation. Portenoy and Foley [276] reported relief of deafferentation pain syndromes by parenteral morphine, pointing the way to using spinal instillation. Penn *et al.* [220] reported 50% excellent, 50% good relief in patients with arachnoiditis, postherpetic neuralgia, radiation lumbar plexopathy and osteoporosis. Levin *et al.* have reported relief of central pain caused by stroke with the intrapituitary injection of alcohol [277].

The role of PVG stimulation is most controversial. Despite the assumptions (1) that PVG stimulation effects pain relief by activating a pathway that suppresses input into the spinothalamic tract and (2) that central and deafferentation pain are not dependent upon peripheral spinothalamic transmission, PVG stimulation is reported to relieve central and deafferentation pain [245,246,251–253,258,278–280]. The two obvious possibilities are (1) that PVG stimulation may activate other pain-inhibiting pathways not mentioned above, and (2) that central and deafferentation pain may be dependent in some way on spinothalamic transmission [249,281,282].

Implantation of stimulating electrodes in peripheral nerves

Chronic stimulation of peripheral nerves was proposed as a means of selectively activating large nerve fibres in order to suppress activity in small, presumably pain fibres, as postulated by the gate theory of pain [283]. However, such stimulation at 20–100 Hz producing paresthesias in the area of pain, seems to be more effective for deafferentation than for nociceptive pain [284]. It is possible that slow (say 2 Hz) TENS or mechanical acupuncture or slow-rate stimulation with implanted stimulators, may be more effective for nociceptive pain [38]

Chronic stimulation of peripheral nerves which requires open exposure of the nerve has a limited application. Early experience suggested a 30–50% incidence of relief of various types of pain with a general fall-off in efficacy over the first two years. There was a 1% risk of nerve damage, 3–5% of infection, 3% of tissue reaction, 3% of technical failure, 3% of electrode displacement and 16% failure of pain relief, despite continued effective technical performance of the device [285–289].

Trigeminal nerve stimulation

Trigeminal stimulation was proposed by Sheldon [290] and first done by Atkinson [291], then elaborated by Meyerson and Håkansson [292,293] using a bipolar electrode openly sutured to the dura over Meckel's cave after a successful trial of test transcutaneous stimulation via the foramen ovale. Steude [294] simplified the procedure by using a percutaneous foramen ovale electrode permanently attached to a receiver. Meyerson and Håkansson reported that 58% of their patients tested percutaneously experienced sufficient pain relief to warrant insertion of a permanent electrode in Meckel's cave and that 75% of this implanted group continued to do well. They subsequently reported long-term relief in 79% of 14 patients chronically implanted [295]. Steude found that 30% of his patients enjoyed pain relief during trial stimulation. Of the present author's patients treated by trial stimulation through the foramen ovale, 74% derived significant pain relief; nine of these suffered from deafferentation pain, six from central pain. Eight went on to permanent implantation of a stimulating system in Meckel's cave, two of which were converted to foramen ovale implants, and five through the foramen ovale in the first place, 60% continuing to derive long-term relief [296]

Dorsal cord stimulation

Following Wall and Sweet's pioneering experience with nerve stimulation [284], Shealy [297] carried the exercise one step further, openly implanting an electrode on the dorsal columns of the spinal cord at laminectomy. This technique did not allow pre-implantation testing for efficacy and a large number of authors reported 22–65% successful relief of a variety of pain syndromes, mostly of the deafferentation pain type. Relief tended to fall off with time, from 63% at 3 months to 30% at 5 years in one series, 59% at 1 year to 43% at 21 months in another, and 70% at 2 years to 43% at $2\frac{1}{2}$ years and 13% at 3 years in another. Complications included a 1–4% incidence of cord compression, 0.5–17% CSF leakage and 5–20% formation of seroma [256,297–303].

The percutaneous technique for chronic spinal epidural stimulation allowed trial stimulation before committal to implantation and avoided laminectomy; this was a major advance [304–306]. In most series some 40–50% (range 42–80%) of patients 'pass the test' of trial percutaneous stimulation and go on to implantation of either a radiofrequency-coupled or self-contained battery-powered stimulation pack. Of implanted patients, 60–84% continued to derive long-term relief. There is a certain steady decay of efficacy with time despite continued production of paresthesias in the area of pain. Complications with the percutaneous technique include electrode migration in up to 61%, infection in 1–7%, incisional pain in up to 58%, electrode breakage in 4–23%, receiver failure in 0.5%, transmitter failure in 5% and skin breakdown in 1–5% [256,304,305,307–311].

Of the author's patients with deafferentation and central pain, 42% passed the test of trial stimulation and 61% of those implanted derived long-term relief.

The amelioration of pain in peripheral vascular disease has stimulated a debate as to whether such effects are the result of pain modulation or amelioration of vascular insufficiency, as suggested by the microscopic studies of peripheral circulation by Jacobs *et al.* [312]; amelioration of angina pectoris has been described by Murphy and Giles [313].

Chronic stimulation of the ventrobasal complex

The final exploitation of stimulation for relief of chronic pain was the stereotactic insertion of stimulating electrodes into either medial lemniscus, ventrobasal complex or internal capsule (cortical–subcortical stimulation may cause seizures), as pioneered by Mazars *et al.* [314] and explored by many workers. The target area is explored by, usually, macrostimulation or else microstimulation and microelectrode recording, until a locus is found where stimulation produces paresthesias in the patient's area of pain. A suitable electrode is left at this site for a transcutaneous trial of stimulation and, if this is successful, the electrode is internalized. Again, 50–70% of patients pass the test of trial stimulation and 35–75% of those chronically implanted experience lasting relief. Complications include infection in 2–15%, brain damage in 2–15%, electrode migration in 2–27.5%, lead breakage or avulsion in 18–30%, receiver or transmitter failure in 7.9–18%, skin erosion in 3–6% and pain at the implant site in 3% [256,258,314–324]. Levy *et al.* [258] reviewed results in 628 patients reported in the literature, as well as 84 of their own, noting an overall 47% relief of pain using this technique.

To this author it seems that chronic stimulation should be the first step in attempts to treat the steady burning-tingling element of deafferentation and central pain, its effectiveness presumably depending upon some unknown central modulating activity. The fact that only 50% of candidates actually respond to trial stimulation is not only disturbing but puzzling, suggesting that there is some basic gap in our understanding of these pain problems and their treatment and pointing out the need for discovering more effective criteria for patient selection. The failure sometimes of pain relief with time, despite continuing technically adequate stimulation, is also difficult to understand; it may be a manifestation of central nervous plasticity. Nevertheless, in this author's opinion, chronic stimulation in these patients with pain is mainly useful in tiding them over a few critical years, until, it is hoped, their pain syndrome subsides; this is happening in an increasing percentage of patients, the longer they are followed.

TREATMENT OUTCOME IN SELECTED DEAFFERENTATION AND CENTRAL PAIN SYNDROMES

Unlike nociceptive pain, deafferentation and central pain syndromes may be readily divided into distinct clinical entities, often with distinct requirements for treatment. Unfortunately, published experience often pools different types of pain syndromes, making identification of specific strategies difficult.

Major causalgia

Major causalgia ·was described by Weir Mitchell [35] but is only rarely seen in civilian practice, usually resulting from incomplete gunshot lesions of the sciatic or median nerve or of the medial cord of the brachial plexus [2,15,16,21,39,326]. The condition is of extraordinary interest, however, in that, unlike other deafferentation pain syndromes, it is apparently often relieved by sympathectomy, as popularized by Leriche during World War I [10], although reported series show a range of 12–97% success [2,10,15,16,21,39,326–330]. It would appear that this success has led to the indiscriminate and largely unsuccessful use of sympathectomy to treat other deafferentation and central pain syndromes. This author has seen only two cases of major causalgia in partial lesions of the sciatic nerve, both relieved by lumbar sympathectomy in the 1960s.

Pain after peripheral nerve injuries other than major causalgia

Just as major causalgia is rare, pain from other peripheral nerve injuries, referred to by Homans [326a] as minor causalgia, are common in civilian practice. The condition is often confusingly equated with reflex sympathetic dystrophy (RSD), which term ought to refer to the sympathetic hyperfunction that sometimes accompanies neural injury pain [2,39]. For treatment, Sunderland [21] did not find neurolysis or posterior rhizotomy helpful. Saris *et al.* [331] found the dorsal root entry zone (DREZ) procedure disappointing in treating intractable sciatica related to chronic disk disease. Bernard *et al.* [332] found the trigeminal DREZ operation disappointing in trigeminal disturbances other than postherpetic neuralgia. Chronic peripheral nerve stimulation yields an initial 30–60% relief, results decaying with time as discussed above. Levy *et al.* (258) reported 75% success in 16 patients with neuropathy and 18% in 12 patients with trigeminal anesthesia dolorosa, using chronic stimulation of PVG and/or ventrobasal complex. Complications for their whole group of 141 patients treated with chronic brain stimulation included a 12.1% infection rate, 7.1% erosion of hardware, 5% foreign body reaction, 3.5% intracerebral hemorrhage and 2.1% psychosis. Of our 14 patients with deafferentation pain caused by nerve injuries, 57% improved during a percutaneous trial of dorsal cord stimulation, all continuing to benefit with long-term relief. Four out of six patients with trigeminal deafferentation pain passed a trial of stimulation, three of whom continued to derive long-term relief.

Post-thoracotomy pain

Treatment of post-thoracotomy and other chronic incisional pains is unsatisfactory, only short-term relief following local blockade, TENS, neurotomy, or scar resection [333]. Temporary relief was reported in 50% of 14 patients after cryoneurotomy [334], with pain aggravated in 33%. Percutaneous radiofrequency intercostal neurectomy relieved the pain in only 25% of the author's patients [32]. Onofrio [92] found dorsal rhizotomy unsuccessful in 23 patients with incisional pain. Smith [335] reported pain relief in eight patients after ganglionectomy; Carlsson *et al.* [333] relieved one patient in seven using dorsal cord stimulation. Of our 10 patients, 40% were relieved during trial dorsal cord stimulation while only 50% of these had long-term relief after implantation. Picaza and his group [286,289] reported 44% relief of a mixed group of postoperative pain syndromes using peripheral nerve stimulation, while Levy *et al.* [258] obtained relief with chronic brain stimulation in only one patient out of four.

Phantom and stump pain

Treatment of amputation-related pain is generally discouraging [335–337]. Sherman *et al.* [339] found that only 1% of his veterans had obtained useful pain relief by any means. Reviewing published series, he found that neurectomy, posterior rhizotomy and mesencephalotomy gave disappointing results, sympathectomy afforded a 10% enduring and 43% temporary relief, cordotomy 38%, thalamotomy 18% and DREZ 56% relief. Iacono *et al.* [340] also found the DREZ procedure encouraging but Saris *et al.* [341,342] found it disappointing in phantom and stump pain unless associated with brachial plexus avulsion. In six patients with brachial plexus avulsion before their amputation, 83% were relieved while three of 16 patients with amputations unassociated with brachial plexus avulsion did well. Five of these 16 patients had stump pain alone, all unrelieved; five had phantom pain alone, of whom two were relieved, and six had both, of whom one was relieved. Krainick and Thoden [343] relieved 43% of 61 amputees with dorsal cord stimulation, particularly of 'continuous background pain' but not of 'attacks of severe pain'. After 5 years, however, only half of their initially successful patients were still doing well [344]. Siegfried and Cetinalp [337] reported 39% pain relief with dorsal cord stimulation. Levy *et al.* [258] obtained 20% long-term relief in five patients with phantom pain treated with chronic brain stimulation. Of our 16 patients with phantom stump pain treated with dorsal cord stimulation, 56% passed the test of trial percutaneous stimulation but only 56% of these who underwent implantation continued to do well.

'Failed back surgery' pain

The pathogenesis of pain in chronic lumbar disk disease is varied. Assuming that treatable conditions such as instability, root irritation by disk and spinal stenosis have been appropriately dealt with, one is left with a group of patients with pain of uncertain origin referred to the region of the lumbosacral spine and legs, probably including musculoskeletal pathology, root irritation caused by scar or bony compression, and deafferentation associated with lesions of the lumbosacral roots.

Specific therapeutic reviews are infrequent. Onofrio [92] reported relief of 23% of 78 patients by dorsal rhizotomy. Delaporte and Siegfried [345] used dorsal cord stimulation to treat 94 patients who suffered from pain over wide areas of the trunk and lower limbs of mixed deafferentation and nociceptive origin: only 40% passed the test of trial stimulation and went on to implantation, of whom 95% enjoyed over 50% pain relief at first, 68% after 1 year, 57% after 2 years and 53% after 3 years. In a review of 1111 published cases they found that 64% enjoyed good to excellent relief from dorsal cord stimulation after varying periods of follow-up but, after 2 years, the success rate ranged from 33 to 35%. Levy *et al.* [258] reported 32% long-term relief of pain in 51 patients with low back and skeletal pain using chronic brain stimulation. Of our 24 patients treated with dorsal cord stimulation, 42% passed trial stimulation, 60% continuing to gain long-term relief. Saris *et al.* [331] reported poor results in patients with disk-related pain treated with the DREZ operation, the lesions being localized by recording evoked potentials from involved nerves. The results were good in two out of 12 patients but bad in ten, half of whom felt that their pain was worse after surgery by virtue of burning dysesthesia in a larger area of the body. Three developed postoperative shooting pains in their area of numbness.

Postherpetic neuralgia

This distressing condition, reviewed in Chapter 10 and by Loeser [346] requires more effective therapy.

Milligan and Nash [347] found that repeated stellate blocks, if started within one year of the onset of pain, resulted in pain relief in 40% of cranial cases. If the blocks began more than one year after the onset, only 22% did well. Denervating procedures were unsatisfactory [346,348]. Onofrio [92] relieved one of five patients with dorsal rhizotomy. Demierre and Siegfried [348] relieved 77% of patients with facial, and 63% with distal, postherpetic neuralgia out of a series of 21 patients, using chronic brain or cord stimulation. Only two of our four patients treated with dorsal cord stimulation passed trial stimulation and none gained long-term relief. Two more failed to pass a test of trial trigeminal stimulation. and two more of brain stimulation.

Nashold and his group were initially optimistic about the DREZ procedure in postherpetic neuralgia, finding that eight out of 12 patients gained relief [349]. Subsequently, only 50% relief was reported [350] while the most recent analysis

[351] noted that only 25% of 32 patients enjoyed ongoing pain relief, although 31% had partial relief. It appeared that, although the operation was very successful at first, recurrence was the rule, the recurrent pain often differing from the pre-operative pain; 69% of the patients suffered from motor dysfunction as a result of the DREZ procedure, 25% to a serious degree.

The outlook appears to be different with trigeminal postherpetic neuralgia treated with destructive lesions. Schvarcz [137] reported 88% pain relief after percutaneous lesions of the descending tract or caudal nucleus of trigeminal nerve, while Nashold and his associates [332,352] reported six out of nine cases of facial postherpetic neuralgia relieved by open radiofrequency lesions of the nucleus caudalis. In their overall experience with 27 patients undergoing this operation, there was one instance each of stroke, myocardial infarction, pneumonia and meningitis; 20 patients suffered from mild ipsilateral dysmetria, 12 in the upper limb, eight in both upper and lower limb, none to an incapacitating degree.

Brachial plexus lesions

A great variety of lesions affect the brachial plexus to produce deafferentation pain: gunshot wounds, laceration, stretch injuries, radiation necrosis, destruction by cancer, iatrogenic damage and actual avulsion from the spinal cord. The nature of the causative lesion is significant when it comes to discussing treatment. In closed stretch avulsion injuries, Wynn-Parry [353] found TENS useful but conventional deafferenting surgery disappointing. Demierre and Siegfried [354] relieved five out of seven patients with pain caused by radionecrosis of the brachial plexus using dorsal cord stimulation. Two out of five of the author's patients with various types of brachial plexus injuries were relieved in the long term by dorsal cord stimulation.

The interesting results are with Nashold's DREZ operation. This procedure is described in more detail in Chapter 8. Of Nashold's original 18 patients [355], 78% were relieved of pain. In a subsequent report, 67% of 21 patients did well [350]. Thomas and Sheehy [356] reported 75% or more persisting pain relief in 58% of 19 patients treated by them. Friedman and Bullitt [357] reported 39 patients followed for 1–8 years with 54% good, 13% fair and 33% unsatisfactory results. Sixty per cent suffered some neurological deficit postoperatively in the ipsilateral leg, none of which prevented ambulation. Both steady burning and twisting pain, as well as intermittent paroxysms, were relieved. Good results occurred only in actual cases of avulsion, not in other types of brachial plexus injury. Other reports and the author's own limited experience have generally indicated favorable results with DREZ for avulsion injury [358,359]. Moossy and Nashold [360] found the procedure also useful in seven out of eight patients with lumbosacral root avulsions.

Central pain of cord origin

Cord lesions, most of them traumatic, can result in a wide variety of pain syndromes which, for therapeutic purposes, need to be distinguished [35]. Botterell *et al.* [361] in a review of seven patients found cordotomy effective for the relief of sharp, stabbing, aching, cramp-like as well as evoked pain, but not for the steady burning dysesthetic pain or discomfort referred to the perineum. White [362], and White and Sweet [363] found cordotomy useful for 'radicular' and 'somatic' pain, particularly after lesions of the cauda equina, but not in lesions of the thoracic cord. Of our 72 patients with pain caused by cord lesions, 25 underwent percutaneous high cervical cordotomy. Of the ten patients with both steady and intermittent lancinating pain, 70% were relieved of the lancinating intermittent element which was their main problem, while only 53% of the 15 with steady pain alone experienced any improvement. Seventy per cent of 10 patients with lesions of the conus–cauda area and 40% of 15 patients with lesions higher in the cord were relieved of their major pain. Ninety-two per cent of 12 patients with incomplete lesions and 31% of 13 patients with complete lesions of the cord gained significant relief.

Results with cordectomy are similar. Although it is useless for the relief of steady pain, it offers a good chance of relieving evoked and spontaneous intermittent lancinating pain [17,361,364–367]. Jefferson [367], in reviewing 21 patients undergoing cordectomy, found that pain from lesions below T12 was likely to be relieved but that from lesions at T10 or above (four cases) was not, the results of lesions at T11 being variable. Good results were obtained with pain referred to the knees (relief in six out of six), thighs (three out of three), or diffusely through the leg (six out of six). Episodic pain was particularly likely to be helped. Pain in a bathing suit distribution did not respond (none out of five). In eight of our patients undergoing cordectomy, the two patients with intermittent pain were relieved of that element but not of their steady burning pain, while the six with steady burning pain were not helped at all. Nashold and Bullitt [368] reported that 77% of 13 patients with pain associated with paraplegia, all of them with lesions at the level of the conus–cauda, were relieved by the DREZ procedure. In a later report [369], 50% relief was reported in the (presumably) same 13 patients. Richter and Seitz [370] reported success in two of ten patients, Sweet and Poletti in one out of two [371]. Three of our 72 patients with central pain caused by cord lesions underwent the DREZ procedure unsuccessfully. Friedman and Nashold [372] reported 50% of 56 patients relieved using the DREZ operation, particularly when the pain was unilateral extending caudally from the level of injury. The operation was not helpful in sacral burning or diffuse pain. The most recent review of Nashold's experience [351] of 56 patients followed for 6 months to 6 years suggested 50% good pain relief overall. It suggests that 'end zone' pain, especially if it is stabbing and running a certain distance from the level of the cord lesion in a non-dermatomal fashion, is relieved in 80% (31 patients). Only 34% of 25 patients with diffuse pain had good or fair pain relief. Any recurrence of pain following the DREZ operation tended to occur within 5 months. Sixteen per cent developed spinal fluid leaks, 5% additional weakness to that present pre-operatively, and 4% developed new paresthesias.

Sweet and Wepsic [303] reported that three out of 21 patients were relieved using dorsal cord stimulation; Lazorthes and Verdie [300] reported two out of nine; Richardson *et al.* [373] reported five out of ten; Urban and Nashold [311] reported one out of three and Picaza *et al.* [289] reported that 45% were relieved. Pagni [19] found dorsal cord stimulation disappointing. Of 37 of our patients with central pain of cord origin treated by dorsal cord stimulation, 38% passed trial stimulation, 64% of these deriving ongoing relief. The failure was often technical, obliteration of the epidural space as a result of previous surgery or atrophy of the dorsal columns making the induction of paresthesias in the area of pain impossible. Success with dorsal cord stimulation depended upon the level and degree of cord damage. With lesions above the conus–cauda, only 19% passed trial stimulation, all of whom continued to benefit after implantation, whereas 83% with low lesions passed trial stimulation, 78% continuing to derive relief. None of our patients with clinically complete lesions passed trial stimulation, whereas 69% with incomplete lesions did so, 80% continuing to do well. Approximately 40% of patients with central pain of cord origin have been reported relieved by chronic brain stimulation in either ventrobasal complex or PVG [19,245,246,317,320,323,324]. Turnbull [324] considered brain stimulation disappointing in this condition. Levy *et al.* [258] failed to relieve pain in 11 patients with 'paraplegia' pain. They did succeed in relieving two (40%) of five patients with post-cordotomy dysesthesia. Of our 11 patients with central pain caused by cord injury, all of whom had failed in attempted treatment with dorsal cord stimulation, 36% passed a trial of brain stimulation, 75% with ongoing relief.

Central pain of brain origin

Although lesions of any pathology at many sites in the brain may cause pain, supratentorial occlusive stroke is the commonest cause [374]. Pain occurs in one out of 15 000 of all strokes. Treatment is frustrating [5,18,19]. The results of stereotactic procedures in deafferentation and central pain reviewed above apply equally well to central pain of supratentorial origin. Namba *et al.* [375] found stereotactic centre médian lesions produced only temporary relief in eight out of nine patients. Niizuma [376] relieved about one-half of 17 patients for periods of up to one year with medial thalamotomy. Shieff and Nashold (273) reported 67% long-term relief after mesencephalic tractotomy in 24 patients with thalamic pain at the expense of 7.4% mortality. Levin *et al.* [277] relieved thalamic pain in three patients with intrapituitary injection of alcohol. Eight of our 50 patients underwent stereotactic mesencephalic tractotomy with or without additional medial thalamotomy. In one patient, stereotactic medial thalamotomy alone was carried out. Three patients with intermittent pain and one with evoked pain were relieved, with some reduction of steady pain in three other patients. Sindou *et al.* [144] used the dorsal root entry zone (DREZ) lesion technique in 16 spastic hemiplegic cases. Not only was the spasticity and accompanying musculoskeletal pain relieved, but also the central pain of the 'thalamic syndrome' in those patients that suffered from it. Of 12 patients with this type of pain, nine obtained total relief, a rather remarkable observation.

When central pain of brain origin is confined to the face, trigeminal stimulation obviates the need for stereotaxis. Four out of six of our patients with trigeminal pain of brain origin passed trial trigeminal stimulation, 75% continuing to gain relief in the longer term. Nashold [14] reported relief in three cases using high cervical epidural trigeminal tract stimulation. Although dorsal cord stimulation may give initial relief when pain is limited to one limb, we, like Pagni [19], found the benefits transient. Two of eight of our patients passed trial dorsal cord stimulation, none with persisting relief.

Reported experience with chronic brain stimulation is mixed. Mazars and his colleages [377] and Turnbull [324] found it disappointing. Levy *et al.* [378] reported relief in 39% and Tsubokawa *et al.* [254] in five out of eight patients. In 54 published cases, 54% were relieved [317–319,322,323,375,379–382]. Although internal capsular stimulation [383] has been suggested as being superior to thalamic stimulation, there does not appear to have been a study of this matter. Four out of six of our patients passed a trial of brain stimulation, two continuing to gain relief.

Levy *et al*. [258] reported 24% long-term relief in 14 patients with 'thalamic pain' using chronic brain stimulation.

ILLUSTRATIVE CASE REPORTS

Patient No. 1

This diabetic woman (12 units regular insulin daily) born in 1932, underwent open reduction of a fractured left humerus in 1973 with removal of fixation devices in 1974. Immediately after insertion of a left elbow prosthesis in 1981, she noticed sensory and motor dysfunction in the left ulnar nerve distribution with hot burning tingling, worse with activity, in the same distribution as the sensory loss. This was associated with aching in the arm and forearm which was worse than the burning (Figure 7.1) – symptoms not relieved by ulnar nerve transposition in 1981. The pain

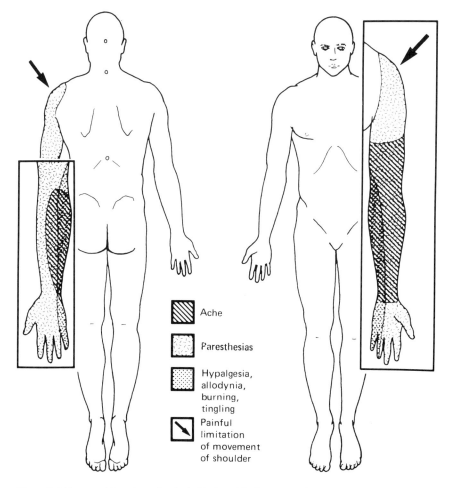

Figure 7.1 Type and location of pain in Patient 1 before operation

interfered with sleep, caused her to stop teaching in 1983, and was not relieved by six Tylenol 3 or Percodan tablets taken daily. She also had painful limitation of elevation and internal rotation of the left shoulder. Neither 125 mg thiopental sodium or 150 µg fentanyl given intravenously in aliquots altered her pain; a trial of monopolar percutaneous epidural dorsal cord stimulation was instituted on 8 February 1984. On 15 February 1984 the electrode was attached to a radiofrequency-coupled receiver. Stimulation at 50 Hz, 0.4 ms pulse width, several times daily, caused paresthesias down both upper extremities and diminished her pain from a level of 9 to 2–3 out of 10. Pain relief occurred within minutes and the effect outlasted stimulation for 1–1.5 h. On 23 March 1984 the device had to be removed because of infection and was replaced on 9 August 1984. Using 75 Hz stimulation at 0.4 ms, paresthesias were produced in the left shoulder and down the left upper extremity, again relieving her pain and allowing her to return to teaching on 1 March 1985, off all medication for pain. She used the device regularly until Janury 1986 when her pain had become so minimal that she felt that stimulation was unnecessary. She took no medication. This state continued until last seen, 8 July 1987, 3 years after the initial implantation. Despite the relief of the upper limb deafferentation pain, the painful limitation of shoulder movement was not affected by the stimulator, even though paresthesias were felt in the area of pain.

Comment

A case of deafferentation pain with chiefly a steady spontaneous burning element relieved by dorsal cord stimulation until it resolved. No relief of accompanying nociceptive pain in the left shoulder.

Patient No. 2

This man was born in 1945 and injured his left shoulder in a sports accident in 1965, suffering an unspecified injury to the skeleton. This required many operative procedures including a shoulder prosthesis complicated by wound infection, and leading in 1983 to forequarter amputation of, what was by that time, an anesthetic and functionless limb. Pain had been present in the left arm from the first, being replaced after amputation by phantom pain of a different quality. By 1986, when the patient was first seen, various painful sensations migrated about the phantom, which seemed to be constantly moving and 6 inches ($\approx$ 15 cm) shorter than normal. He had the illusory sensation of skin being avulsed from the hand, the arm being broken, the whole limb constantly and bizarrely being painfully twisted, and of various sites of tearing, burning or tightness, Jabs of excruciating pain shot down the phantom limb when he moved. When pain was severe, the phantom fist felt clenched. The clavicle felt as if it was being pulled inwards and there was aching pain in the left pectoral area (Figure 7.2). Various medications, TENS and multiple intercostal neurectomies, all failed to relieve his pain. On 21 November 1986, 200 µg fentanyl did not alter his pain, which remained at the 9.5 out of 10 level, although it made him feel more comfortable. Percutaneous monopolar chronic epidural cervical cord stimulation was instituted on 24 November 1986, the electrode requiring repositioning on 27 November 1986 before being attached to a

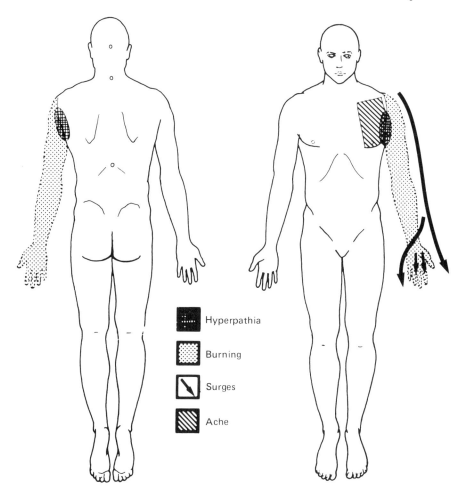

Figure 7.2 Type and location of pain in Patient 2 before operation

radiofrequency-coupled stimulator on 1 December 1986. Despite initial 75% reduction of pain using 30–50 Hz stimulation at 0.2 ms pulse width, inducing paresthesias in a band over the left scapular spine and down the ulnar aspect of the left extremity phantom as well as the right upper extremity, by 13 February 1987 he claimed he was experiencing no relief, was taking up to 600 mg Demerol (meperidine) daily and suffering from epileptic seizures which he attributed to his medications. He discussed suicide. By that time the pain had changed somewhat to a constant diffuse burning, with excruciating intermittent shocks running down the entire phantom. On 1 June 1987 a DREZ procedure was done at the levels of the normal-appearing C5–T1 rootlets, making some 30 lesions in all, 1.5–2 mm apart, each at 75 degrees for 15 s using the Owl Cordotomy System with somatosensory evoked potential monitoring. On 17 July 1987 the phantom was normal in proportion, folded comfortably across his chest where it moved slowly up and down. Stump jactitation was described but not witnessed. Phantom pain was relieved except for an occasional twinge. Initially he dragged the left foot, performed tandem and Romberg testing with difficulty, could not stand on the left leg alone, and complained of an aching constant pain down the left buttock and posterior aspect of the left lower extremity as far as the heel, aggravated by activity and straight leg raising; he walked with a cane. When last seen on August 1, 1989, two years postoperatively, these problems had all resolved, his only pain being left pectoral tightness and soreness over the upper dorsal spine. There was hypesthesia encircling the stump, induced by the DREZ operation; he was taking no medication and working as a volunteer in the local hospital (Figure 7.3).

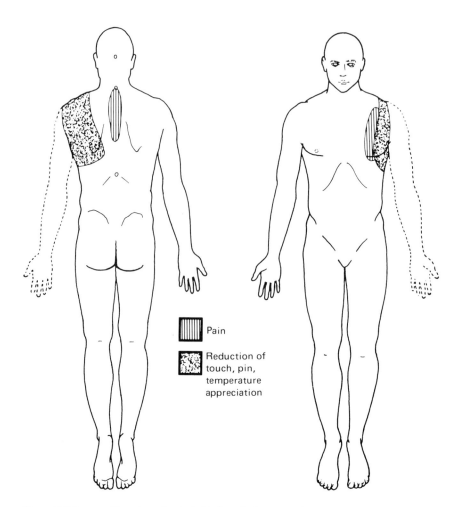

Pain

Reduction of touch, pin, temperature appreciation

Figure 7.3 Type and location of pain in Patient 2 after operation

Patient No. 3

This man, born in 1955, fell from a tree in 1981, being rendered completely quadriplegic at C5–6. He was treated by halo traction and open fusion; 2 weeks later he began to feel a bruise-like sensation in the right C5 distribution. This was associated with much more severe and disabling allodynia and hyperpathia in the same distribution, aggravated by clothes and movement. This steadily worsened and was accompanied by a much less severe, similar effect in both the right and the left C6 dermatomes. The pain was unaffected by drugs or sympathetic block, but was temporarily relieved by local anesthetic blockade of the brachial plexus. An open right C5 dorsal rhizotomy performed elsewhere produced relief of the lesser symptoms in the C6 dermatome at the expense of what residual position sense he had in the right fingers and wrist, and also abolished the sensation of touch in the right thumb, index and distal radial forearm. On 21 October 1983, the cord was explored with a possible C5 DREZ lesion operation in mind but a massive arachnoiditis prevented the procedure from being safely carried out. By January 1984, in addition, the right hand felt as if acid or a hot iron was placed against it and the skin was being peeled off (Figure 7.4). On 16 February 1984, percutaneous stimulation of the right C5 root identified radiologically, visualizing the clips of the previous rhizotomy, produced contractions in the right deltoid muscle but no reproducible sensory effect. A small lesion away from the ventral root had no significant effect. Subsequent stimulation of the C4 root produced paresthesias in the right C5 dermatome (epaulet region) with contraction of the right biceps. A radiofrequency lesion made at this site produced anesthesia in the epaulet region and eliminated the allodynia and hyperpathia but did not relieve the patient's sense of deep intermittent spontaneous pain in the same area. This deep pain was most severe in the morning, but it would be absent for hours at a time. The additional rhizotomy resulted in the loss of position sense at the right elbow (Figure 7.5). The patient was unchanged when last reviewed in July 1988, 4 years postoperatively.

Comment

A case of evoked pain in radicular distribution associated with cord injury, relieved by distal percutaneous radiofrequency rhizotomy.

Patient No. 4

This woman, born in 1948, developed multiple sclerosis in 1967 and by October 1987 was confined to bed, cachectic, unable to move either leg, with weakness (4/5) of the left upper extremity, normal sensation on the right side of the body, but ill-defined hypesthesia to all modalities on the left side of the body below the neck. She was totally incapacitated by constant knife-like pain in both hips, associated with constant hypertonicity of the trunk and both lower limbs and by excruciatingly painful violent muscle spasms in the same area spreading into the abdomen. She suffered from severe flexion contractures of the lower extremities and recurrent dislocation of the left hip (Figure 7.6). There was a low-level constant burning of both lower limbs, which was not a significant problem. In addition, there were excruciating electric shock sensations, once to twice daily, lasting hours at a time, in

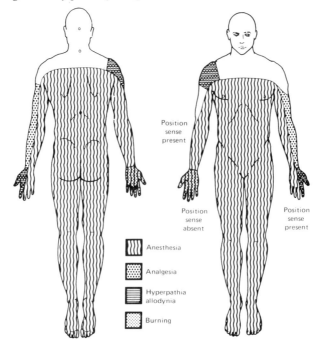

Figure 7.4 Type and location of pain in Patient 3 before operation

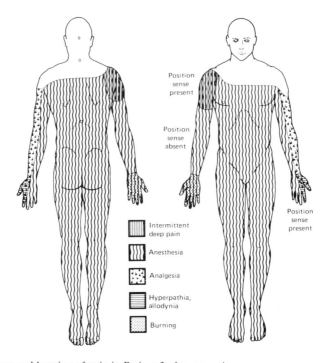

Figure 7.5 Type and location of pain in Patient 3 after operation

the trunk. She used an in-dwelling catheter and controlled evacuation with enemas. She had had bilateral iliopsoas tenotomy, fasciotomy of the tensor fasciae latae, adductor tenotomy of the hip, hamstring release and obturator neurectomies in July 1987, with some benefit to her motor problems. A Bischof myelotomy from T6 to T12 with bilateral open cordotomy at T5 were carried out on 18 January 1988, giving her total relief of pain and spasms up until the time of latest follow-up in July 1988. The fixed contractures persisted but she was now able to use her wheelchair and help in the management of her store. Unfortunately because of her paraplegia and cachectic state, she developed multiple pressure sores.

Comment

A patient with nociceptive pain not caused by cancer, relieved by bilateral cordotomy. In retrospect, Sindou's dorsal root entry zone operation might have been preferable, producing less sensory loss and possibly avoiding the pressure sores.

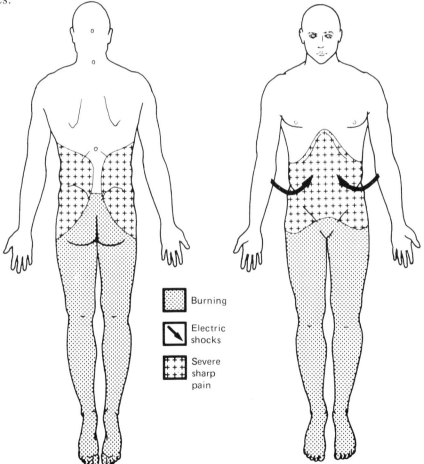

Figure 7.6 Type and location of pain in Patient 4 before operation

Patient No. 5

This man, born in 1932, suffered a fracture dislocation of C3–4 in a motor vehicle accident in 1979, rendering him totally quadriplegic at C3. He was treated conservatively and first noted pain 8 months after the injury, steadily increasing in severity and spreading to more of his body as time passed. The pain was sharp and steady with unexplained exacerbations, shooting into the testicles and up the trunk (Figure 7.7). This led to extensive negative psychological, genitourinary and gastrointestinal investigation, to herniorrhaphy, cholecystectomy, transurethral resection of the prostate and sphincterotomy. He also suffered from aching pain in both shoulders, aggravated by their passive movement. He could spend only one

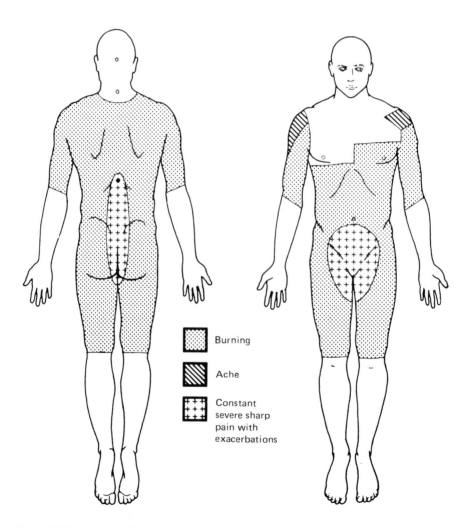

Figure 7.7 Type and location of pain in Patient 5

hour at a time in a chair and suffered from mild spasticity and spasms. On 1 and 8 November 1984, two-stage ventriculography and stereotactic mapping of the thalamus was carried out bilaterally, using microelectrode recording and micro-stimulation. Sites in both ventrobasal complexes were located where stimulation produced paresthesias in the trunk and legs. Stimulation of PVG produced no response. Following exploration, his pain disappeared until February 1985. After correction of an intercurrent penile implant infection, chronic stimulating elec-trodes were stereotactically inserted into both thalamic sensory nuclei on 28 February 1985, with revision of their position on 4 and 7 March 1985 and attachment to a radiofrequency-coupled dual channel receiver on 13 March 1985. Stimulation produced a tolerable burning tingling feeling in both legs and the trunk, associated with significant relief of pain. He continued to stimulate until September 1985 when a number of problems unrelated to the stimulator distracted him. A superficial scalp infection delayed re-exploration of his electrode until 20 January, 6 February and 13 February 1986, for apparent migration of the right thalamic electrode and technical difficulties with the left. At this time stereotactic thalamic exploration was repeated, the ventrobasal complex remapped, electrodes re-introduced and again attached to a dual channel stimulator. Following this, he continued to use his stimulator (2 h on and 2 h off at 60 Hz, 0.125 ms, 0.25 min off, 30 s on) producing burning paresthesia in the trunk and legs and suppressing his pain. At last follow-up, on 19 August 1988, he was spending 6 h/day in a chair, still requiring analgesia for his bilateral aching shoulder pain but not complaining of pain below his level of sensory loss $3\frac{1}{2}$ years after initial institution of chronic brain stimulation.

Comment

A patient with steady central pain of cord origin mimicking visceral disease, relieved by chronic brain stimulation. Coexistent nociceptive pain in the shoulder was not relieved.

Patient No. 6

This woman, born in 1927, suffered a coma producing subarachnoid hemorrhage in 1977 with delayed clipping of a left middle cerebral artery aneurysm complicated by postoperative spasm and massive infarction of the left cerebral hemisphere, sparing the thalamus. She recovered partly from her initial aphasia and right hemiplegia, becoming able to walk and attend to self-care. A few months after her subarach-noid hemorrhage, she began to notice pain which steadily worsened, becoming a serious problem after 1981. Various conservative means of treatment were tried including large doses of intramuscular morphine, demerol and other analgesics. By 10 April 1987 (Figure 7.8) she had constant burning in her right upper extremity and face and the feeling that it was immersed in ice-water. There were occasional intermittent spontaneous jabs of pain and severe hyperpathia and allodynia in the right half of the body, worst in the upper extremity, next worst in the face, least in the leg. She complained intermittently of mid-frontal headache and required Dilantin (diphenylhydantoin) and Tegretol (carbamazepine) to prevent epileptic seizures. She spoke in single sentences with little spontaneous speech and had a

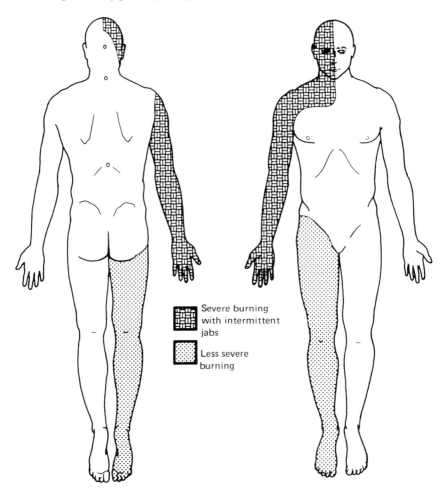

Figure 7.8 Type and location of pain in Patient 6

spastic right hemiparesis with dystonic posturing of the right upper extremity. Hyperpathia and allodynia were induced by pinprick, touch, hot and cold, vibration and movement of the entire right half of the body. On 14 December 1987, stereotactic CT-guided exploration of the left thalamus was carried out, mapping ventrobasal complex and PVG with microelectrodes. Stimulation of ventrobasal complex always aggravated her pain in the right upper extremity and was abandoned. Stimulation of right PVG, however, suppressed her hyperpathia after 15 min stimulation, an effect not reversed by 0.8 mg naloxone given intravenously. On 8 December 1987, an electrode was implanted in the left PVG and attached to a radiofrequency-coupled stimulator. This consistently suppressed her hyperpathia and her spontaneous pain from 10 out of 10 to 1–2 out of 10 when last seen on April 11, 1989.

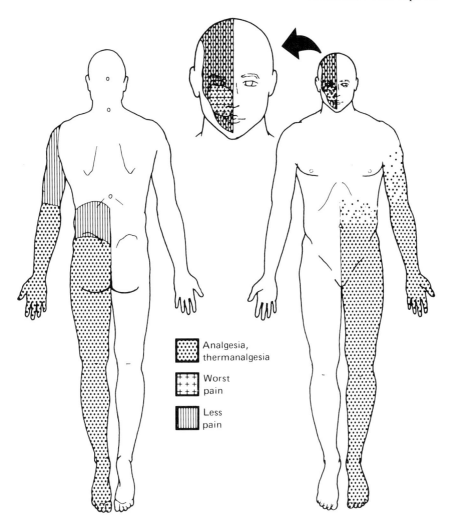

Figure 7.9 Type and location of pain in Patient 7

Comment

A patient with central pain of brain origin with dual spontaneous steady and intermittent pain associated with evoked pain. Presence of evoked pain has been noted to correlate with failure of stimulation of the ventrobasal complex to alleviate spontaneous pain, as it did in this patient. However, the pain was reduced by PVG stimulation.

Patient No. 7

This hypertensive and diabetic (Lente insulin 20 units/day) man, born in 1922, suddenly developed pain in the right eye, vomiting, dysphagia and right facial numbness in March 1981. He was noted to have vertigo, reduced hearing, hoarseness, reduced right-sided sweating, difficulty in looking to the right, minimal gait ataxia, right Horner's syndrome, horizontal and rotatory nystagmus (especially on looking to the right but also to the left), analgesia and thermanalgesia in the right trigeminal territory and in the left upper and lower extremities (see Figure 7.9). A few months after the stroke, he began to notice constant hot stinging pain, chiefly in the right V2 distribution, fading off into the adjacent V1 and V3 territory and associated with slight hyperpathia in the right cheek; he tended to pick at his right eye, forehead and scalp, to a degree sufficient to produce ulcers. The left leg felt constantly cold, the left upper extremity constantly numb. Although he could sleep well, he was unable to work or enjoy avocations; his pain was increased by activity but reduced by rest, so that he usually did not rise until noon. TENS and Tegretol (carbamazepine) induced temporary partial relief of pain; stellate block had no effect; application of cold to the cheek was beneficial. He was treated with aspirin and diazepam.

On 13 September 1982, 150 mg thiopental sodium intravenously reduced his pain from 8 to 4 out of 10, and a trial of percutaneous stimulation of the trigeminal nerve through the foramen ovale, producing paresthesias in his right cheek, abolished his pain. On 15 September 1982, two percutaneous dorsal cord stimulating electrodes were sutured to the dura of Meckel's cave, positioned to produce bipolar stimulation of the second division. After testing, they were attached to a radiofrequency-coupled receiver on 20 September 1982 and the patient followed closely from then until July 1988. Stimulation frequency varied over time from 20 to 120 Hz at 0.5 ms pulse width, producing paresthesias over the right cheek and reducing his pain from 8–10 out of 10 to 4–5 out of 10. Soon after rising in the morning he would begin stimulation and continue constantly throughout the day. Pain would subside within 15 min and recur within 15 min of turning off the stimulator. In March 1984 he developed keratitis in the right eye, requiring tarsorrhaphy. Over his follow-up period the degree of excoriation of the forehead and eye varied with time, periods of total healing being followed by recurrence of lesions, the whole process paralleling his degree of comfort. By 17 August 1984, he noticed that his pain seldom rose above a 5 out of 10 level and by 26 May 1986 his pain had become even less. At this time he reduced his dose of diazepam and aspirin and his facial excoriations healed permanently. When last seen in July 1988, 6 years after insertion of his stimulator, he stated that his pain was now so mild that he had ceased using the stimulator at all, although it still functioned technically.

Comment

A case of central pain associated with lateral medullary syndrome typically in the area of the trigeminal rather than the spinothalamic sensory loss, relieved by peripheral stimulation of the 5th nerve until the severity of the pain diminished spontaneously.

SUMMARY AND CONCLUSIONS

The roles of surgical procedures in the treatment of the various components of specific pain syndromes have been reviewed, developing a suggested protocol (summarized in Table 7.3) for the surgical treatment of intractable pain. This inevitably reflects the author's biases and will require continual revision as more objective clinical and laboratory data are amassed.

Table 7.3 Suggested protocol for surgical treatment of intractable pain

Type	Procedure of choice	Contraindications	Alternatives
Nociceptive	High cervical lateral percutaneous cordotomy	Respiratory, Pain above C5 / Bilateral or midline truncal pain	III ventricular morphine, stereotactic mesencephalic tractotomy, medial thalamotomy / Spinal morphine instillation
Central or deafferentation			
Major causalgia	Sympathectomy		As for other deafferentation pain
Brachial or lumbar plexus avulsion	DREZ	Infirmity	
V herpes zoster	?Trigeminal DREZ	Infirmity	
Other deafferentation			
Sympathetic hyperfunction	Sympathectomy		
Hyperpathia/allodynia	Percutaneous radiofrequency neurectomy, rhizotomy, ?cordotomy	Loss of essential function	
Spontaneous intermittent lancinating pain			
Spontaneous steady burning pain	Dorsal cord stimulation		Stimulation of ventrobasal complex
Cord central pain			
Spontaneous intermittent lancinating pain	Cordotomy, cordectomy, DREZ		
Spontaneous steady burning pain	Stimulation of ventrobasal complex		Stereotactic mesencephalic tractotomy or medial thalamotomy
Brain central pain			
Spontaneous intermittent lancinating pain	?PVG stimulation		?Stereotactic mesencephalic tractotomy or medial thalamotomy
Hyperpathia/allodynia			
Spontaneous steady burning pain	Stimulation of ventrobasal complex		Stereotactic mesencephalic tractotomy or medial thalamotomy

References

1. Ochoa, J. L., Torebjork, E., Marchettini, P. and Swak, M. Mechanisms of neuropathic pain: cumulative observations, new experiments, and further speculation. In *Advances in Pain Research and Therapy, Vol. 9* (ed. H. L. Fields, R. Dubner and F. Cervero), Raven, New York, pp. 431–450 (1985)
2. Tasker, R. R. and Lougheed, W. M. Neurosurgical techniques of sympathetic interruption. In *Pain and the Sympathetic Nervous System* (ed. M. Stanton-Hicks), Kluwer Norwell MA, 1989
3. Livingston, W. K. *Pain Mechanisms: a Physiological Interpretation of Causalgia and its Related States*, Macmillan, New York (1943)
4. Bowsher, D. The problem of central pain. *Verhandlungen der Deutschen Gesellschaft für innere Medizin*, **86**, 1525–1527 (1980)
5. Cassinari, V. and Pagni, C. A. *Central Pain: a Neurosurgical Survey*, Harvard, Cambridge (1969)
6. Levitt, M. Dysesthesias and self-mutilation in humans and subhumans: a review of clinical and experimental studies. *Brain Research Reviews*, **10**, 247–290 (1985)
7. Levitt, M. and Levitt, J. H. The deafferentation syndrome in monkeys: dysesthesias of spinal origin. *Pain*, **10**, 129–147 (1981)
8. Loeser, J. D., Ward, A. A. and White, L. E. Chronic deafferentation of human spinal cord neurons. *Journal of Neurosurgery*, **29**, 48–50 (1968)
9. Loh, L. and Nathan, P. W. Painful peripheral states and sympathetic blocks. *Journal of Neurology, Neurosurgery and Psychiatry*, **41**, 664–671 (1978)
10. Loh, L., Nathan, P. W. and Schott, G. D. Pain due to lesions of central nervous system removed by sympathetic block. *British Medical Journal*, **282**, 1026–1028 (1981)
11. Lombard, M. C. and Larabi, Y. Electrophysiological study of cervical dorsal horn cells in partially deafferented rats. In *Advances in Pain Research and Therapy, Vol. 5*, (ed. J. J. Bonica, U. Lindblom and A. Iggo), Raven Press, New York, pp. 147–154 (1983)
12. Lombard, M. C., Nashold, B. S., Albe-Fessard, D., Salman, N. and Sakr, C. Deafferentation hypersensitivity in the rat after dorsal rhizotomy: a possible animal model of chronic pain. *Pain*, **6**, 163–174 (1979)
13. Lombard, M. C., Nashold, B.S., Jr. and Pelissier, T. Thalamic recordings in rats with hyperalgesia. In *Advances in Pain Research and Therapy, Vol. 3* (ed. J. J. Bonica, J. C. Liebeskind and D. G. Albe-Fessard), Raven Press, New York, pp. 767–772 (1979)
14. Nashold, B. S., Jr. Central pain: its origins and treatment. *Clinical Neurosurgery*, **20**, 311–322 (1974)
15. Nathan, P. W. On the pathogenesis of causalgia in peripheral nerve lesions. *Brain*, **70**, 145–170 (1947)
16. Noordenbos, W. *Pain*, Elsevier, Amsterdam (1959)
17. Pagni, C. A. Place of stereotactic technique in surgery for pain. In *Advances in Neurology, Vol. 4* (ed. J. J. Bonica), Raven, New York, pp. 669–706 (1974)
18. Pagni, C. A. Central pain and painful anesthesia. In *Progress in Neurological Surgery, Vol. 8* (ed. H. Krayenbühl, P. E. Maspes and W. J. Sweet), pp. 132–257 (1977)
19. Pagni, C. A. Central pain due to spinal cord and brain stem damage. In *Textbook of Pain* (ed. P. D. Wall and R. Melzack), Churchill Livingstone, Edinburgh, pp. 481–495 (1984)
20. Roberts, W. J. A hypothesis on the physiological basis for causalgia and related pains. *Pain*, **24**, 297–311 (1986)
21. Sunderland, S. Pain mechanisms in causalgia. *Journal of Neurology, Neurosurgery and Psychiatry*, **39**, 471–480 (1976)
22. Wall, P. D. Signs of plasticity and reconnection in spinal cord damage. In *Ciba Foundation Symposium 34, Outcome of Severe Damage to the Central Nervous System*, Elsevier-Excerpta Medica-North-Holland, Amsterdam, p. 35 (1975)
23. Wall, P. D. On the origin of pain associated with amputation. In *Phantom and Stump Pain* (ed. J. Siegfried and M. Zimmerman), Springer-Verlag, Berlin, pp. 2–44 (1981)
24. Zimmermann, M. Peripheral and central nervous mechanisms of nociception pain, and pain therapy: facts and hypotheses. In *Advances in Pain Research and Therapy, Vol. 3* (ed. J. J. Bonica, J. C. Liebeskind and D. G. Albe-Fessard), Raven, New York, p. 3–32 (1979)
25. Tasker, R. R. Percutaneous cordotomy. *Comprehensive Therapy*, **1**, 51–56 (1975)
26. Tasker, R. R., Organ, L. W. and Hawrylyshyn, P. Deafferentation and causalgia. In *Pain* (ed. J. J. Bonica), Raven, New York, pp. 305–309 (1980)
27. Tasker, R. R., Organ, L. W. and Hawrylyshyn, P. The Thalamus and Midbrain of Man. A Physiological Atlas Using Electrical Stimulation. Wilkins R. H. (ed) Thomas, Springfield, Illinois, pp. (1982)

28. Tasker, R. R. Identification of pain processing systems by electrical stimulation of the brain. *Human Neurobiology*, **1**, 261–272 (1982)
29. Tasker, R. R. Percutaneous cordotomy – the lateral high cervical technique. In *Operative Neurosurgical Techniques, Indications, Methods, and Results* (ed. H. H. Schmidek and W. H. Sweet), Grune and Stratton, New York, pp. 1137–1153 (1982)
30. Tasker, R. R. Thalamic stereotaxic procedures. In *Stereotaxy of the Human Brain* (ed. G. Schaltenbrand and A. E. Walker), Stuttgart, Thieme, pp. 484–497 (1982)
31. Tasker, R. R., Tsuda, T. and Hawrylyshyn, P. Clinical investigation of deafferentation pain. In *Advances in Pain Research and Therapy, Vol. 5* (ed. J. J. Bonica, U. Lindblom and A. Iggo), Raven, New York, pp. 713–738 (1983)
32. Tasker, R. R. Deafferentation. In *Textbook of Pain* (ed. P. D. Wall and R. Melzack), Churchill Livingstone, Edinburgh, pp. 119–132 (1984)
33. Tasker, R. R. Stereotaxic surgery. In *Textbook of Pain* (ed. P. D. Wall and R. Melzack), Churchill Livingstone, Edinburgh, pp. 639–655 (1984)
34. Tasker, R. R. Surgical approaches to the primary afferent and the spinal cord. In *Advances in Pain Research and Therapy, Vol. 9* (ed. H. L. Fields, R. Dubner and F. Cervero), Raven, New York, pp. 299–324 (1985)
35. Tasker, R. R. Pain resulting from central nervous system pathology (central pain). In *Management of Pain in Clinical Practice* (ed. J. J. Bonica), Lea and Febiger, Philadelphia, pp. 262–282 (1988)
36. Tasker, R. R. The problem of deafferentation pain in the management of the patient with cancer. *Journal of Palliative Care*, **2**, 8–12 (1987)
37. Tasker, R. R. Percutaneous cordotomy: the lateral high cervical technique. In *Operative Neurosurgical Techniques, Indications, Methods and Results*, 2nd edn (ed. H. H. Schmidek and W. H. Sweet), Grune and Stratton, New York, pp. 1191–1205 (1988)
38. Tasker, R. R. Neurostimulation and percutaneous neural destructive techniques. In *Neural Blockade in Clinical Anesthesia and Management of Pain*, 2nd edn (ed. M. J. Cousins and P. O. Bridenbaugh), Lippincott, Philadelphia, pp. 1085–1117 (1988)
39. Tasker, R. R. and Dostrovsky, J. O. Deafferentation and central pain. In *Textbook of Pain*, 2nd edn, (ed. P. D. Wall and R. Melzack), Churchill Livingstone, Edinburgh, pp. 154–180 (1988)
40. Lindblom, U. Assessment of abnormal evoked pain in neurological pain patients and its relation to spontaneous pain: a descriptive and conceptual model with some analytical results. In *Advances in Pain Research and Therapy, Vol. 9* (ed. H. L. Fields, R. Dubner and F. Cervero), pp. 402–423 (1985)
41. Tasker, R. R. Effets sensitifs et moteurs de la stimulation thalamique chez l'homme. Applications cliniques. *Revue Neurologique* (*Paris*), **142**, 316–320 (1986)
42. Dostrovsky, J. O., Tasker, R. R., Yamashiro, K. *et al.* Sensations evoked by microstimulation in human ventral thalamus in relation to neuronal receptive fields. *Society for Neurosciences Abstracts*, **12**, 329 (1986)
43. Albe-Fessard, D., Tasker, R. R., Yamashiro, K. and Dostrovsky, J. Effects of stimulation of the primary thalamic somatic relay for the relief of central pain. *Pain Clinic*, **11**, 207–213 (1987)
44. Tasker, R. R., Gorecki, J., Lenz, F. A. *et al.* Thalamic microelectrode recording and neurostimulation in central and deafferentation pain. *Applied Neurophysiology*, **50**, 414–417 (1987)
45. Tasker, R. R., Lenz, F., Yamashiro, K. *et al.* Microelectrode techniques in localization of stereotactic targets. *Neurological Reviews*, **9**, 105–112 (1987)
46. Lenz, F. A., Dostrovsky, J. O., Kwan, H. C. *et al.* Methods for microstimulation and recording of single neurons and evoked potentials in the human central nervous system. *Journal of Neurosurgery*, **68**, 630–634 (1988)
47. Lenz, F. A., Dostrovsky, J. O., Tasker, R. R. *et al.* Single-unit analysis of the human ventral thalamic nuclear group: somatosensory responses. *Journal of Neurophysiology*, **59**, 299–316 (1988)
48. Lenz, F. A., Tasker, R. R., Dostrovsky, J. O. *et al.* Abnormal single-unit activity and responses to stimulation in the presumed ventrocaudal nucleus of patients with central pain. In *Proceedings of the Vth World Congress on Pain, Pain Research and Clinical Management, Vol. 3* (ed. R. Dubner, G. F. Gebhard and M. R. Bond), Elsevier, Amsterdam, pp. 157–164 (1988)
49. Lenz, F. A., Tasker, R. R., Dostrovsky, J. O. *et al.* Abnormal single-unit activity recorded in the somatosensory thalamus of the quadriplegic patient with central pain. *Pain*, **31**, 225–236 (1987)
50. Gorecki, J., Hirayama, T., Dostrovsky, J. O. *et al.* Thalamic stimulation and recording in patients with deafferentation and central pain. *Stereotactic and Functional Neurosurgery*, **52**, 219–226 (1989)
51. Hirayama, T., Dostrovsky, J. O., Gorecki, J. *et al.* Recordings of abnormal activity in patients with deafferentation and central pain. *Stereotactic and Functional Neurosurgery*, **52**, 120–126 (1989)

52. Davis, R. A. and Stokes, J. W. Neurosurgical attempts to relieve thalamic pain. *Surgery, Gynecology and Obstetrics*, **123**, 371–384 (1966)
53. Nashold, B. S., Jr. Brainstem stereotaxic procedures. In *Stereotaxy of the Human Brain: Anatomical, Physiological and Clinical Applications* (ed. G. Schaltenbrand and A. E. Walker), Georg Thieme, Stuttgart, pp. 475–483 (1982)
54. Rees, W. E. S. Multiple bilateral percutaneous rhizolysis in the treatment of the slipped disc syndrome. *Presented at the Annual Meeting of the AANS, St Louis* (1974)
55. Shealy, C. N. Percutaneous radiofrequency denervation of spinal facets. *Journal of Neurosurgery*, **43**, 448–451 (1975)
56. Fox, J. L. and Rizzoli, H. V. Identification of radiological coordinates for the posterior articular nerve of Luschka in the lumbar spine. *Surgical Neurology*, **1**, 343–346 (1973)
57. Pedersen, H. E., Blunck, C. F. J. and Gardner, E. The anatomy of lumbosacral posterior rami and meningeal branches of spinal nerves (sinu-vertebral nerves) with an experimental study of their functions. *Journal of Bone and Joint Surgery*, **38A**, 377 (1956)
58. Johnson, I. Radiofrequency percutaneous facet rhizotomy. *Journal of Neurosurgical Nursing*, **6**, 92–96 (1974)
59. Oudenhoven, R. C. Articular rhizotomy. *Surgical Neurology*, **2**, 275–278 (1974)
60. Burton, C. V. Percutaneous radiofrequency facet denervation. *Applied Neurophysiology*, **39**, 80–86 (1976)
61. McCulloch, J. A. Percutaneous radiofrequency lumbar rhizolysis (rhizotomy). *Applied Neurophysiology*, **39**, 87–96 (1976)
62. Dunsker, S. B., Wood, M., Lotspeich, E. S. and Maysfield, E. H. Percutaneous electrocoagulation of lumbar articular nerves. In *Pain Management* (ed. J. F. Lee), Williams and Wilkins, Baltimore, pp. 123–127 (1977)
63. Blume, H. G. Radiofrequency denervation in occipital pain: a new approach in 114 cases. In *Advances in Pain Research and Therapy, Vol 1* (ed. J. J. Bonica and D. Albe-Fessard), Raven, New York, pp. 691–698 (1976)
64. Blume, H. and Fromm, S. Radiofrequency denaturation in occipital pain: a new approach. In *Sixth International Congress of Neurological Surgery*, Excerpta Medica, Amsterdam, pp. 221–222 (1977)
65. Uematsu, S. Percutaneous electrothermocoagulation of spinal nerve trunk, ganglion, and rootlets. In *Operative Neurosurgical Techniques, Indications, Methods and Results* (ed. H. H. Schmidek and W. H. Sweet), Grune and Stratton, New York, pp. 1177–1198 (1982)
66. Kirschner, M. Elektrokoagulation des Ganglion Gasseri. *Zentralblatt für Chirurgie*, **47**, 2841–2843 (1932)
67. Härtel, F. Die Leitungsanästhesie und Injections-behandlung des Ganglion Gasseri und der Trigeminustäme. *Archiv für Klinische Chirurgie*, **100**, 193 (1912)
68. Sweet, W. H. and Wepsic, S. G. Controlled thermocoagulation of trigeminal ganglion and results for differential destruction of pain fibers. *Journal of Neurosurgery*, **29**, 143–156 (1974)
69. Nugent, G. R. and Berry, B. Trigeminal neuralgia treated by differential percutaneous radiofrequency coagulation of the gasserian ganglion. *Journal of Neurosurgery*, **40**, 517–523
70. Tew, J. M., Jr and Tobler, W. D. Percutaneous rhizotomy in the treatment of intractable facial pain (trigeminal, glossopharyngeal, and vagal nerves). In *Operative Neurosurgical Techniques, Indications, Methods and Results*, (ed. H. H. Schmidek and W. H. Sweet), Grune and Stratton, New York, pp. 1083–1100 (1982)
71. Latchaw, J. P., Jr, Hardy, R. W., Jr, Forsythe, S. B. and Cook, A. F. Trigeminal neuralgia treated by radiofrequency coagulation. *Journal of Neurosurgery*, **59**, 479–484 (1983)
72. Siegfried, J. and Broggi, G. Percutaneous thermocoagulation of the gasserian ganglion in the treatment of pain in advanced cancer. In *Advances in Pain Research and Therapy, Vol. 2* (ed. J. J. Bonica and V. Ventafridda), Raven, New York, pp. 463–468 (1979)
73. Maxwell, R. F. Surgical control of chronic migrainous neuralgia by trigeminal ganglio-rhizolysis. *Journal of Neurosurgery*, **57**, 459–466 (1982)
74. Watson, C. P., Morley, T. P., Richardson, J. C. et al. The surgical treatment of chronic cluster headache. *Headache*, **23**, 289–295 (1983)
75. Onofrio, B. M. and Campbell, J. K. Surgical treatment of chronic cluster headache. *Mayo Clinic Proceedings*, **61**, 537–544 (1986)
76. Tew, J. M. Jr, Keller, J. T. and Williams, D. S. Functional surgery of the trigeminal nerve. In *Treatment of Trigeminal Neuralgia. Functional Neurosurgery* (ed. T. Rasmussen and R. Marino), Raven, New York, p. 129 (1979)
77. Broggi, G. C. Surgical treatment of glossopharyngeal neuralgia and pain from cancer of the nasopharynx. *Journal of Neurosurgery*, **61**, 952–955 (1984)
78. Broggi, G. and Siegfried, J. Percutaneous differential radiofrequency rhizotomy of glosso-

pharyngeal nerve in facial pain due to cancer. In *Advances in Pain Research and Therapy, Vol. 2*, (ed. J. J. Bonica and V. Ventafridda), Raven, New York, pp. 469–473 (1979)

79. Isamat, F., Ferran, E. and Acebes, J. J. Selective percutaneous thermocoagulation rhizotomy in essential glossopharyngeal neuralgia. *Journal of Neurosurgery*, **55**, 575–580 (1981)

80. Lazorthes, Y. and Verdie, J. C. Radiofrequency coagulation of the petrous ganglion in glossopharyngeal neuralgia. *Neurosurgery*, **4**, 512 (1979)

81. Pagura, J. R., Schnapp, M. and Passarelli, P. Percutaneous radiofrequency glossopharyngeal rhizolysis for cancer pain. *Applied Neurophysiology*, **46**, 154–159 (1983)

82. Salar, G., Ori, C., Baratto, V. *et al.* Selective percutaneous thermolesions of the ninth cranial nerve by lateral cervical approach: Report of eight cases. *Surgical Neurology*, **20**, 276.

83. Giorgi, C. and Broggi, G. Surgical treatment of glossopharyngeal neuralgia and pain from cancer of the nasopharynx: a 20-year experience. *Journal of Neurosurgery*, **61**, 952–955 (1984)

84. Håkansson, S. Trigeminal neuralgia treated by the injection of glycerol into the trigeminal cistern. *Neurosurgery*, **9**, 638 (1981)

85. Taarnhoj, P. Decompression of the trigeminal root and the posterior part of the ganglion as treatment in trigeminal neuralgia. Preliminary communication. *Journal of Neurosurgery*, **9**, 288–290 (1952)

86. Sheldon, C. H. Depolarization in the treatment of trigeminal neuralgia: Evaluation of compression and electrical methods; clinical concept of neurophysiological mechanisms. In *Pain* (ed. R. S. Knighton and P. R. Dumke), Little Brown, Boston, pp. 373–386 (1966)

87. Mullan, S. and Lichtor, T. Percutaneous microcompression of the trigeminal ganglion for trigeminal neuralgia. *Journal of Neurosurgery*, **59**, 1007–1012 (1983)

88. Jannetta, P. J. Arterial compression of the trigeminal nerve at the pons in patients with trigeminal neuralgia. *Journal of Neurosurgery*, **26**, 159–162 (1967)

89. Uematsu, S., Udbarhelyi, G. B., Benson, D. W. and Siebens, A. A. Percutaneous radiofrequency rhizotomy. *Surgical Neurology*, **2**, 319–325 (1974)

90. McLaurin, R. L. Neurosurgical approaches to pain in cancer. In *Pain Management* (ed. J. F. Lee), Williams & Wilkins, Baltimore, pp. 186–194 (1977)

91. Loeser, J. D. Dorsal rhizotomy: indications and results. In *Advances in Neurology, Vol. 4* (ed. J. J. Bonica), Raven, New York, pp. 615–619 (1974)

92. Onofrio, B. M. Rhizotomy: What is its place in the treatment of pain. In *Advances in Neurology, Vol. 4* (ed. J. J. Bonica), Raven, New York, pp. 621–623 (1974)

93. Saris, S. C., Silver, J. M., Vieira, J. F. S. and Nashold, B. S. Jr., Sacrococcygeal rhizotomy for perineal pain. *Neurosurgery*, **19**, 789–793 (1986)

94. Sindou, M., Fischer, G. and Mansuy, L. Posterior spinal rhizotomy and selective posterior rhizidiotomy. *Progress in Neurological Surgery*, **7**, 201–250 (1976)

95. Smith, F. P. Trans-spinal ganglionectomy for relief of intercostal pain. *Journal of Neurosurgery*, **32**, 574–577 (1970)

96. Pagura, J. R. Percutaneous radiofrequency spinal rhizotomy. *Applied Neurophysiology*, **46**, 138–146 (1983)

97. Katz, J. Current role of neurolytic agents. In *Advances in Neurology, Vol. 4* (ed. J. J. Bonica), Raven, New York, pp. 471–476 (1974)

98. Meyerson, B. A., Arner, S. and Linderoth, B. Pros and cons of different approaches to the management of pelvic cancer pain. *Acta Neurochirurgica, Suppl.*, **33**, 407–419 (1984)

99. Moore, D. C. Role of nerve block with neurolytic solutions for pelvic visceral cancer pain. In *Advances in Pain Research and Therapy, Vol. 2* (ed. J. J. Bonica and V. Ventafridda), Raven, New York, pp. 593–596 (1979)

100. Ventafridda, V. and Martino, G. Clinical evaluation of subarachnoid neurolytic blocks in intractable cancer pain. In *Advances in Pain Research and Therapy, Vol. 1* (ed. J. J. Bonica and D. Albe-Fessard), Raven, New York, pp. 699–703 (1975)

101. Papo, I. and Visca, A. Phenol subarachnoid rhizotomy for the treatment of cancer pain. A personal account on 290 cases. In *Advances in Pain Research and Therapy, Vol 2* (ed. J. J. Bonica and V. Ventafridda), Raven, New York, pp. 339–346 (1979)

102. Swerdlow, M. Subarachnoid and extradural neurolytic blocks. In *Advances in Pain Research and Therapy, Vol. 2* (ed. J. J. Bonica and V. Ventafridda), Raven, New York, pp. 325–327 (1979)

103. Ventafridda, V., Fochi, C., Sganzerla, E. P. and Tamburini, M. Neurolytic blocks in perineal pain. In *Advances in Pain Research and Therapy, Vol. 2* (ed. J. J. Bonica and V. Ventafridda), Raven, New York, pp. 597–605 (1979)

104. Ventafridda, V. and Spreafico, R. Subarachnoid saline perfusion. In *Advances in Neurology, Vol. 4* (ed. J. J. Bonica), Raven, New York, pp. 477–484 (1974)

105. Spiller, W. G. and Martin, E. The treatment of persistent pain of organic origin in the lower part of

the body by division of the anterolateral column of the spinal cord. *Journal of the American Medical Association*, **58**, 1489–1490 (1912)
106. Mullan, S., Harper, P. V., Hekmatpanah, J. *et al*. Percutaneous interruption of spinal pain tracts by means of a strontium 90 needle. *Journal of Neurosurgery*, **20**, 931–939 (1963)
107. Rosomoff, H. L., Carroll, F., Brown, J. *et al*. Percutaneous radiofrequency cervical cordotomy: technique. *Journal of Neurosurgery*, **23**, 639–644
108. Piscol, K. Die 'offenen' spinalen Schmerzoperationen (anterolaterale Chordotomie und kommissurale Myelotomie) in der modernen Schmerzbekämpfung. *Langenbecks Archiv für Chirurgie*, **342**, 91–99 (1976)
109. Rosomoff, H. L. Percutaneous radiofrequency cervical cordotomy for intractable pain. *Sixth International Congress of Neurological Surgery: International Congress Series 148*, Excerpta Medica, Amsterdam, pp. 110–111 (1977)
110. Lipton, S. Percutaneous cordotomy. In *Textbook of Pain* (ed. P. D. Walls and R. Melzack), Churchill Livingstone, Edinburgh, pp. 632–638 (1984)
111. Meglio, M. and Cioni, B. The role of percutaneous cordotomy in the treatment of chronic cancer pain. *Acta Neurochirurgica*, **59**, 111–121 (1981)
112. Lahuerta, T., Lipton, S. and Wells, J. C. D. Percutaneous cervical cordotomy; results and complications in a recent series of 100 patients. *Annals of the Royal College of Surgeons of England*, **67**, 41–44 (1985)
113. Kühner, A. La cordotomie percutanée. Sa place actuelle dans la chirurgie de la douleur. *Anesthésie, Analgésie, Réanimation (Paris)*, **38**, 357–359 (1981)
114. Siegfried, J., Kühner, A. and Sturm, V. Neurosurgical treatment of cancer pain. Recent results. *Cancer Research*, **89**, 148–155 (1984)
115. Lorenz, R. Methods of percutaneous spinothalamic tract section. In *Advances and Technical Standards in Neurosurgery, Vol. 3* (ed. H. Krayenbühl), Springer Verlag, Vienna, pp. 123–145 (1976)
116. Ischia, S., Luzzani, A., Ischia, A. *et al*. Bilateral percutaneous cervical cordotomy: immediate and long-term results in 36 patients with neoplastic disease. *Journal of Neurology, Neurosurgery and Psychiatry*, **47**, 141–147 (1984)
117. Ischia, S., Luzzani, A., Ischia, A. *et al*. Subarachnoid neurolytic block (L5 S1) and unilateral percutaneous cervical cordotomy in the treatment of pain secondary to pelvic malignant disease. *Pain*, **20**, 139–149 (1984)
118. Ischia, S., Luzzani, A., Ischia, A. *et al*. Role of percutaneous cervical cordotomy in the treatment of neoplastic vertebral pain. *Pain*, **19**, 123–131 (1984)
119. Ischia, S., Ischia, A., Luzzani, A. *et al*. Results up to death in the treatment of persistent cervicothoracic (Pancoast) and thoracic malignant pain by unilateral percutaneous cervical cordotomy. *Pain*, **21**, 339–355 (1985)
120. Armour, D. Surgery of the spinal cord and its membranes. *Lancet*, ii, 691–697 (1927)
121. Cook, A. W., Nathan, P. W. and Smith, M. C. Sensory consequences of commissural myelotomy. A challenge to traditional anatomical concepts. *Brain*, **107**, 547–568 (1984)
122. Wertheimer, P. and Lecuire, J. La myelotomie commissurale postérieure. *Acta Chirugica Belgica*, **52**, 568–574 (1953)
123. Payne, N. S. Dorsal longitudinal myelotomy for the control of perineal and lower body pain. *Pain*, Suppl. 2, S320
124. Adams, J. E., Lippert, R. and Hosobuchi, Y. Commissural myelotomy. In *Operative Neurosurgical Techniques, Indications, Methods and Results* (ed. H. H. Schmidek and W. H. Sweet), Grune and Stratton, New York, pp. 1155–1161 (1982)
125. Broager, B. Commissural myelotomy. *Surgical Neurology*, **2**, 71–74 (1974)
126. Sourek, K. Mediolongitudinal myelotomy. In *Progress in Neurological Surgery, Vol. 8* (ed. H. Krayenbühl, P. E. Maspes and W. H. Sweet), Karger, Basel, pp. 15–34 (1977)
127. Hitchcock, E. R. Stereotactic cervical myelotomy. *Journal of Neurology, Neurosurgery and Psychiatry*, **33**, 224–230 (1970)
128. Eiras, J., Garcia, J., Gomez, J. *et al*. First results with extralemniscal myelotomy. *Acta Neurochirurgica*, Suppl. 30, 377–381 (1980)
129. Schvarcz, J. R. Stereotactic high cervical extralemniscal myelotomy for pelvic cancer pain. *Acta Neurochirurgica*, Suppl. 33, 431–435 (1984)
130. Papo, I. Spinal posterior rhizotomy and commissural myelotomy in the treatment of cancer pain. In *Advances in Pain Research and Therapy, Vol. 2* (ed. J. J. Bonica and V. Ventafridda), Raven, New York, pp. 439–447 (1979)
131. Crue, B. L., Jr, Todd, E. M., Carregal, E. J. A. and Kilham, O. Percutaneous trigeminal tractotomy. Case report utilizing stereotactic radiofrequency lesion. *Bulletin of the Los Angeles Neurological Society*, **32**, 86–92 (1967)

132. Crue, B. L., Todd, E. M. and Carregal, E. J. Percutaneous radiofrequency stereotactic trigeminal tractotomy. In *Pain and Suffering* (ed. B. L. Crue), Thomas, Springfield, pp. 69–79 (1970)
133. Fox, J. L. Delineation of the obex by contrast radiography during percutaneous trigeminal tractotomy. Technical note. *Journal of Neurosurgery*, **36**, 107–112 (1972)
134. Fox, J. L. Percutaneous trigeminal tractotomy. Variations in delineation of the obex using emulsified pantopaque. *Confins de la Neurologie*, **36**, 97–100 (1974)
135. Hitchcock, E. R. Stereotactic trigeminal tractotomy. *Annals of Clinical Research*, **2**, 131–135 (1970)
136. Hitchcock, E. R. and Schvarcz, J. R. Stereotaxic trigeminal tractotomy for post-herpetic facial pain. *Journal of Neurosurgery*, **37**, 412–417 (1972)
137. Schvarcz, J. R. Spinal cord stereotactic techniques re trigeminal nucleotomy and extralemniscal myelotomy. *Applied Neurophysiology*, **41**, 99–112 (1978)
138. Schvarcz, J. R. Stereotactic spinal trigeminal nucleotomy for dysesthetic facial pain. In *Advances in Pain Research and Therapy, Vol. 3* (ed. J. J. Bonica, J. C. Liebeskind and D. G. Albe-Fessard), Raven, New York, pp. 331–336 (1979)
139. Todd, E. M., Crue, B. L. and Carregal, E. J. A. Posterior percutaneous tractotomy and cordotomy. *Confins de la Neurologie*, **31**, 106–115 (1969)
140. Hyndman, O. R. Lissauer's tract section. A contribution to chordotomy for the relief of pain. (Preliminary report). *Journal of the International College of Surgeons*, **5**, 394–400 (1942)
141. Sindou, M. *Etude de la Jonction Radicellomédullaire Postérieure. La Radicellotomie Postérieure Sélective dans la Chirurgie de la Douleur.* Medical thesis, Lyon (1972)
142. Sindou, M. and Lapras, C. Neurosurgical treatment of pain in the Pancoast-Tobias syndrome: sélective posterior rhizotomy and open anterolateral C2-cordotomy. In *Advances in Pain Research and Therapy, Vol. 4* (ed. J. J. Bonica), Raven, New York, pp. 199–206 (1982)
143. Sindou, M., Fischer, G., Goutelle, A. and Mansuy, L. La radicellotomie postérieure sélective. Premiers résultats dans la chirurgie de la douleur. *Neurochirurgie*, **20**, 391–408 (1974)
144. Sindou, M., Mifsud, J. J., Boisson, D. and Goutelle, A. Selective posterior rhizotomy in the dorsal root entry zone for treatment of hyperspasticity and pain in the hemiplegic upper limb. *Neurosurgery*, **18**, 587–595 (1986)
145. Hitchcock, E. R. Stereotaxic pontine spinothalamic tractotomy. *Journal of Neurosurgery*, **39**, 746–752 (1973)
146. Hitchcock, E., Sotelo, M. G. and Kim, M. C. Analgesic levels and technical method in stereotactic pontine spinothalamic tractotomy. *Acta Neurochirurgica*, **77**, 29–36 (1985)
147. Hitchcock, E. R., Kim, M. C. and Jotelo, M. Further experience in stereotactic pontine tractotomy. *Applied Neurophysiology*, **48**, 242–246
148. Barbéra, J., Barcia-Salorio, J. L. and Broseta, J. Stereotaxic pontine spinothalamic tractotomy. *Surgical Neurology*, **11**, 111–114 (1979)
149. Spiegel, E. A. and Wycis, H. T. *Stereoencephalotomy. II. Clinical and Physiological Applications.* Grune and Stratton, New York (1962)
150. Wycis, H. T. and Spiegel, E. A. Long-range results in the treatment of intractable pain by stereotaxic midbrain surgery. *Journal of Neurosurgery*, **19**, 101–107 (1962)
151. Mazars, G., Pansini, A. Chiarelli, J. Coagulation du faisceau spino-thalamique et du faisceau quinto-thalamique par stéréotaxie. Indications – résultats. *Acta Neurochirurgica*, **8**, 324–326
152. Mazars, G., Roge, R. and Pansini, A. Stereotactic coagulation of the spinothalamic tract for intractable trigeminal pain. *Journal of Neurology, Neurosurgery and Psychiatry*, **23**, 352 (abstract) (1960)
153. Turnbull, I. M. Bilateral cingulumotomy combined with thalamotomy or mesencephalic tractotomy for pain. *Surgery, Gynecology and Obstetrics*, **134**, 958–962 (1972)
154. Nashold, B. S., Jr and Wilson, W. P. Central pain. Observations in man with chronic implanted electrodes in the midbrain tegmentum. *Confins de la Neurologie*, **27**, 30–44 (1966)
155. Nashold, B. S., Jr, Wilson, W. P. and Slaughter, D. G. Sensations evoked by stimulation in the midbrain of man. *Journal of Neurosurgery*, **30**, 14–24 (1969)
156. Nashold, B. S., Wilson, W. P. and Slaughter, D. G. Stereotaxic midbrain lesions for central dysesthesia and phantom pain. *Journal of Neurosurgery*, **30**, 116–126 (1969)
157. Nashold, B. S., Jr, Wilson, W. P. and Slaughter, D. G. The midbrain and pain. In *Advances in Neurology, Vol. 4* (ed. J. J. Bonica), Raven, New York, pp. 191–196 (1974)
158. Nashold, B. S., Slaughter, D. G., Wilson, W. P. and Zorub, D. Stereotactic mesencephalotomy. In *Progress in Neurological Surgery, Vol. 8* (ed. H. Krayenbühl, P. E. Maspes and W. H. Sweet), Karger, Basel, pp. 35–49 (1977)
159. Spiegel, E. A., Kletzkin, M., Szekely, E. G. and Wycis, H. T. Pain reactions upon stimulation of the tectum mesencephali. *Journal of Neuropathology and Experimental Neurology*, **13**, 212–220 (1954)

160. Walker, A. E. Somatotopic localization of spinothalamic and secondary trigeminal tract in mesencephalon. *Archives of Neurology and Psychiatry*, **48**, 884–889 (1942)
161. Amano, K., Tanikawa, T., Iseki, H. *et al*. Single neuron analysis of the human midbrain tegmentum. *Applied Neurophysiology*, **41**, 66–78 (1978)
162. Amano, K., Iseki, H., Notani, M. *et al*. Rostral mesencephalic reticulotomy for pain relief with reference to electrode trajectory and clinical results. *Applied Neurophysiology*, **42**, 316 (1979)
163. Amano, K., Kawamura, H., Tanikawa, T. *et al*. Long-term followup study of rostral mesencephalic reticulotomy for pain relief – report of 34 cases. *Applied Neurophysiology*, **49**, 105–111 (1986)
164. Frank, F., Tognetti, F., Gaist, G. *et al*. Stereotaxic rostral mesencephalotomy in treatment of malignant faciothoracobrachial pain syndromes. *Journal of Neurosurgery*, **56**, 807–811 (1982)
165. Frank, F., Fabrizi, A. P., Gaist, G. *et al*. Stereotactic lesions in the treatment of chronic cancer pain syndromes: mesencephalotomy versus multiple thalamotomies in the treatment of chronic cancer pain syndromes. *Applied Neurophysiology*, **50**, 314–318 (1987)
166. Gioia, D. F., Wallace, P. B., Fuste, F. J. and Greene, M. A stereotaxic method of surgery for the relief of intractable pain. *International Surgery*, **48**, 409–416 (1967)
167. Helfant, M. H., Leksell, L. and Strang, R. R. Experience with intractable pain treated by stereotaxic mesencephalotomy. *Acta chirurgica scandinavica*, **129**, 573–580 (1965)
168. de Montreuil, C. B., Lajat, Y., Resche, F. *et al*. Apport de la neuro-chirurgie stéréotaxique dans le traitement des algies des cancers cervico-faciaux. *Annals d'Oto-Laryngologie et de Chirurgie Cervico-faciale (Paris)* **100**, 181–186 (1983)
169. Torvik, A. Sensory motor and reflex changes in two cases of intractable pain after stereotactic mesencephalic tractotomy. *Journal of Neurology, Neurosurgery and Psychiatry*, **22**, 299–305 (1959)
170. Voris, H. C. and Whisler, W. W. Results of stereotaxic surgery for intractable pain. *Confins de la Neurologie*, **37**, 86–96 (1975)
171. Whisler, W. W. and Voris, H. C. Mesencephalotomy for intractable pain due to malignant disease. *Applied Neurophysiology*, **47**, 52–56 (1978)
172. Monnier, M. and Fischer, R. Localisation, stimulation et coagulation du thalamus chez l'homme. *Journal de Physiologie*, **43**, 818 (1951)
173. Ervin, F. R. and Mark, V. H. Stereotactic thalamotomy in the human. II. Physiologic observations on the human thalamus. *Archives of Neurology*, **3**, 368–380 (1960)
174. Mark, V. H., Ervin, F. R. and Yakovlev, P. I. Correlation of pain relief, sensory loss, and anatomical lesion sites in pain patients treated by stereotactic thalamotomy. *Transactions of the American Neurological Association*, **86**, 86–90 (1961)
175. Mark, V. H., Ervin, F. R. and Yakovlev, P. Stereotactic thalamotomy. III. The verification of anatomical lesion sites in the human thalamus. *Archives of Neurology*, **8**, 78–88 (1963)
176. Mark, V. H. and Ervin, F. R. Role of thalamotomy in treatment of chronic severe pain. *Postgraduate Medicine*, **35**, 563–571 (1965)
177. Mark, V. H. and Tsutsumi, H. The suppression of pain by intrathalamic lidocaine. In *Advances in Neurology, Vol. 4* (ed. J. J. Bonica), Raven, New York, pp. 715–721 (1974)
178. Mark, V. H., Ervin, F. R. and Hackett, T. P. Clinical aspects of stereotactic thalamotomy in the human. I. The treatment of chronic severe pain. *Archives of Neurology*, **3**, 351–367 (1960)
179. Hassler, R. The division of pain conduction into systems of pain sensation and pain awareness. In *Pain: Basic Principles – Pharmacology – Therapy* (ed. R. Janzen, W. D. Keidel, A. Herz and C. Steichele), Georg Thieme, Stuttgart, pp. 98–112 (1972)
180. Halliday, A. M. and Logue, V. Painful sensations evoked by electrical stimulation in the thalamus. In *Neurophysiology Studied in Man* (ed. G. G. Somjen), Excerpta Medica, Amsterdam, pp. 221–230 (1972)
181. Hitchcock, E. R. and Teixeira, M. J. A comparison of results from center-median and basal thalamotomies for pain. *Surgical Neurology*, **15**, 341–351 (1981)
182. Talairach, J., Tournoux, P. and Bancaud, J. Chirurgie pariétale de la douleur. *Acta Neurochirurgica*, **8**, 153–250 (1960)
183. Willis, W. D. The origin and destination of pathways involved in pain transmission. In *Textbook of Pain* (ed. P. D. Wall and R. Melzack), Churchill Livingstone, Edinburgh, pp. 88–99 (1984)
184. Sano, K. Intralaminar thalamotomy (thalamolaminotomy) and posterior hypothalamotomy in the treatment of intractable pain. In *Progress in Neurological Surgery, Vol. 8* (ed. J. Krayenbühl, P. E. Maspes and W. H. Sweet), Karger, Basel, pp. 50–103 (1977)
185. Sano, K. Stereotaxic thalamolaminotomy and posteromedial hypothalamotomy for the relief of intractable pain. In *Advances in Pain Research and Therapy, Vol. 2* (ed. J. J. Bonica and V. Ventafridda), Raven, New York, pp. 475–485 (1979)
186. Sano, K., Yoshioka, M., Ogashiwa, M. *et al*. Thalamolaminotomy: a new operation for relief of intractable pain. *Confins de la Neurologie*, **27**, 63–66 (1966)

187. Sano, K., Yoshioka, M., Sekino, H. *et al.* Functional organization of the internal medullary lamina in man. *Confins de la Neurologie*, **32**, 374–380 (1970)
188. Hécaen, H., Talairach, J., David, M. and Dell, M. B. Coagulations limitées du thalamus dans les algies du syndrome thalamique. *Revue Neurologique, Paris*, **81**, 917–931 (1949)
189. Bettag, W. and Yoshida, T. Uber stereotaktische Schmerzoperationen. *Acta Neurochirurgica*, **8**, 299–317 (1960)
190. Richardson, D. E. Recent advances in the neurosurgical control of pain. *Southern Medical Journal*, **60**, 1082–1086 (1967)
191. Uematsu, S., Konigsmark, B. and Walker, A. E. Thalamotomy for alleviation of intractable pain. *Confins de la Neurologie*, **36**, 88–96 (1974)
192. Adams, J. E. and Rutkin, B. B. Lesions of the centrum medianum in the treatment of movement disorders. *Confins de la Neurologie*, **26**, 231–236 (1965)
193. Askenasy, H. M. and Levinger, M. Stereoencephalotomy for relief of pain. *Harefuah*, **74**, 85–89 (1968)
194. Bulacio, E. N., Pozzetti, A. and Barros, M. Dolor crónico Effedos de lesiones en núcleos centro-medianus y parafasciculares. *Buenos Aires Medicine*, **32**, 363–372 (1972)
195. Cooper, I. S. Clinical and physiologic implications of thalamic surgery for disorders of sensory communication. Thalamic surgery for intractable pain. *Journal of Neurological Sciences*, **2**, 493–519 (1965)
196. Forster, D. M. C., Leksell, L., Meyerson, B. A. and Steiner, L. Gamma thalamotomy in intractable pain. In *Pain: Basic Principles – Pharmacology – Therapy* (ed. R. Janzen, W. D. Keidel, A. Herz and C. Steichele), Thieme, Stuttgart, pp. 194–198 (1972)
197. Hassler, R. and Riechert, T. Klinische und anatomische Befunde bei stereotaktischen Schmerzoperationen im Thalamus. *Archiv für Psychiatrie und Nervenkrankheiten*, **200**, 93–122 (1959)
198. Kudo, T., Yoshii, N. and Shimizu, S. Stereotaxic surgery for pain relief. *Journal of Experimental Medicine*, **96**, 219–234 (1968)
199. Leksell, L., Meyerson, B. A. and Forster, D. M. C. Radiosurgical thalamotomy for intractable pain. *Confins de la Neurologie*, **34**, 264 (1972)
200. Mundinger, F. Stereotaktische Operationen gegen anderweitig unbehandelbar schwere Schmerzzustände. *Zeitschrift für Allgemeinmedizin*, **50**, 860–864 (1974)
201. Niizuma, H., Kwak, R., Saso, S. *et al.* Follow-up results of center median thalamotomy for central pain. *Applied Neurophysiology*, **43**, 336 (1980)
202. von Orthner, H. Weitere klinische und anatomische Erfahrungen mit zerebralen Schmerzoperationen. *Confins de la Neurologie*, **27**, 71–74 (1966)
203. von Orthner, H. and Roeder, F. Further clinical and anatomical experience with stereotactic operations for relief of pain. *Confins de la Neurologie*, **27**, 418–430 (1966)
204. Richardson, D. E. Thalamotomy for control of chronic pain. *Acta Neurochirurgica*, Suppl. 21, 77–88 (1974)
205. Steiner, L., Forster, D., Leksell, L. *et al.* Gammathalamotomy in intractable pain. *Acta Neurochirurgica*, **52**, 173–184 (1980)
206. Sugita, K., Musuga, N., Takaoka, Y. and Doi, T. Results of stereotaxic thalamotomy for pain. *Confins de la Neurologie*, **34**, 265–274 (1972)
207. Tsubokawa, T. and Moriyasu, N. Follow-up results of centre median thalamotomy for relief of intractable pain. *Confins de la Neurologie*, **37**, 280–284 (1975)
208. Urabe, M. and Tsubokawa, T. Stereotaxic thalamotomy for the relief of intractable pain. *Tohoku Journal of Experimental Medicine*, **85**, 286–300 (1965)
209. Yoshimasu, N., Ishijima, B. and Sano, K. Pain and the internal medullary lamina. *Applied Neurophysiology*, **45**, 498–499 (1982)
210. Fairman, D. Unilateral thalamic tractotomy for the relief of bilateral pain in malignant tumours. *Confins de la Neurologie*, **29**, 146–158 (1967)
211. Fairman, D. Hypothalamotomy as a new perspective for alleviation of intractable pain and regression of metastatic malignant tumours. In *Present Limits of Neurosurgery* (ed. I. Fusek and Z. Kune), Avicenum, Prague, pp. 525–528 (1972)
212. Fairman, D. and Llavallol, M. A. Thalamic tractotomy for the alleviation of intractable pain in cancer. *Cancer*, **31**, 700–707 (1973)
213. Pilon, R. N. and Baker, A. R. Control of chronic pain by means of an epidural catheter. *Cancer*, **37**, 903–905 (1976)
214. Yaksh, T. L. Spinal opiate analgesia: characteristics and principles of action. *Pain*, **11**, 293–341 (1981)
215. Wang, J. K., Nauss, L. A. and Thomas, J. E. Intrathecally applied morphine in man. *Anesthesiology*, **50**, 149–151 (1975)

216. Ventafridda, V., Figliuzzi, M., Tamburini, M. *et al.* Clinical observation on analgesia elicited by intrathecal morphine in cancer patients. In *Advances in Pain Research and Therapy, Vol. 3* (ed. J. J. Bonica, J. C. Leibeskind and D. Albe-Fessard), Raven, New York, pp. 559–565 (1979)
217. D'Annunzio, V., Denaro, F. and Meglio, M. Personal experience with intrathecal morphine in the management of pain from pelvic cancer. *Acta Neurochirurgica*, Suppl. 33, 421–425 (1984)
218. Meyerson, B. A., Arner, S. and Linderoth, B. Pros and cons of different approaches to the management of pelvic cancer pain. *Acta Neurochirurgica*, Suppl. 33, 407 (1984)
219. Onofrio, B. M., Yaksh, T. L. and Arnold, P. G. Continuous low-dose intrathecal morphine administration in the treatment of chronic pain of malignant origin. *Mayo Clinic Proceedings*, **56**, 516–520 (1981)
220. Penn, R. D., Paice, J. A., Gottschalk, W. and Ivankovich, A. D. Cancer pain relief using chronic morphine infusion. *Journal of Neurosurgery*, **61**, 302–306 (1984)
221. Penn, R. D. and Paice, J. A. Chronic intrathecal morphine for intractable pain. *Journal of Neurosurgery*, **67**, 182–186 (1987)
222. Poletti, C., Cohen, A. M., Todd, D. P. *et al.* Cancer pain relieved by long-term epidural morphine with permanent indwelling systems for self-administration. *Journal of Neurosurgery*, **55**, 581–584 (1981)
223. Poletti, C. E., Schmidek, H. H., Sweet, W. H. and Pilon, R. N. Intraspinal and intraventricular implantable systems and agents for long-term relief of cancer pain. In *Operative Neurosurgical Techniques, Indications, Methods and Results* (ed. H. H. Schmidek and W. H. Sweet), Grune and Stratton, New York, pp. 1145–1153 (1988)
224. Sheller, A. G., Hadley, M. N. and Wilkinson, E. Administration of intraspinal morphine sulphate for the treatment of intractable cancer pain. *Neurosurgery*, **18**, 740–747 (1986)
225. Yaksh, T. L. and Onofrio, B. M. Retrospective consideration of the doses of morphine given intrathecally by chronic infusion in 163 patients by 19 physicians. *Pain*, **31**, 211–223 (1987)
226. Obbens, E. A. M. T., Hill, C. S., Leavens, M. E. *et al.* Intraventricular morphine administration for control of chronic cancer pain. *Pain*, **28**, 61–68 (1987)
227. Lenz, A., Galli, G. and Marini, G. Intraventricular morphine in the treatment of pain secondary to cancer. In *Operative Neurosurgical Techniques, Indications, Methods and Results* (ed. H. H. Schmidek and W. H. Sweet), Grune and Stratton, New York, pp. 1077–1088 (1988)
228. Luft, R. and Olivecroma, H. Experiences with hypophysectomy in man. *Journal of Neurosurgery*, **10**, 301–316 (1953)
229. Perrault, M., LeBeau, J., Klotz, B. *et al.* L'hypophysectomie totale dans le traitement du cancer du sein; premier cas français; avenir de la méthode. *Therapie*, **7**, 290–300
230. Shimken, H. R., Ortega, P. and Naffziger, H. C. Effects of surgical hypophysectomy in a man with malignant melanoma. *Journal of Clinical Endocrinology and Metabolism*, **12**, 439–453 (1952)
231. Tindall, G. T., Christy, J. H., Nixon, D. W. *et al.* Trans-sphenoidal hypophysectomy for pain of disseminated carcinoma of the breast and prostate gland. In *Pain Management* (ed. J. F. Lee), Williams and Wilkins, Baltimore, pp. 172–185 (1977)
232. Morricca, G. Chemical hypophysectomy for cancer pain. In *Advances in Neurology, Vol. 4* (ed. J. J. Bonica), Raven, New York, pp. 707–714 (1974)
233. Lipton, S. Percutaneous cervical cordotomy and the injection of the pituitary with alcohol. *Anaesthesia*, **33**, 953–957 (1978)
234. Lipton, S., Miles, J., Williams, N. and Bark-Jones, N. Pituitary injection of alcohol for widespread cancer pain. *Pain*, **5**, 73–82 (1978)
235. Madrid, J. L. Chemical hypophysectomy. In *Advances in Pain Research and Therapy, Vol. 2* (ed. J. J. Bonica and V. Ventafridda), Raven, New York, pp. 381–391 (1979)
236. Morricca, G. Neuroadenolysis for diffuse intractable cancer pain. In *Advances in Pain Research and Therapy, Vol. 1* (ed. J. J. Bonica and D. Albe-Fessard), Raven, New York, pp. 863–869 (1976)
237. Miles, J. Chemical hypophysectomy. In *Advances in Pain Research and Therapy, Vol. 2* (ed. J. J. Bonica and V. Ventafridda), Raven, New York, pp. 373–380 (1979)
238. Miles, J. Neurological advances in the relief of pain. *British Journal of Hospital Medicine*, **30**, 348–353 (1983)
239. Miles, J. Pituitary destruction. In *Textbook of Pain* (ed. P. D. Wall and R. Melzack), Churchill Livingstone, Edinburgh, pp. 656–665 (1984)
240. Yanagida, H., Corssen, G., Trouwborst, A. and Erdmann, W. Relief of cancer pain in man: alcohol-induced neuroadenolysis vs electrical stimulation of the pituitary gland. *Pain*, **19**, 133–141 (1984)
241. Capper, S. J., Conlon, J. M., Lahuerta, J. *et al.* Peptide concentrations in the CSF following injection of alcohol into the pituitary gland. *Pain*, Suppl 2, S316 (1984)

242. Takeda, F., Fujii, T., Uki, J. *et al.* Cancer pain relief and tumor regression by means of pituitary neuroadenolysis and surgical hypophysectomy. *Neurologia Medico-Chirugica (Tokyo)*, **23**, 41–49 (1983)

243. Takeda, F., Uki, J., Fujii, T. *et al.* Pituitary neuroadenolysis to relieve cancer pain: Observations of spread of ethanol installed into the sella turcica and subsequent changes of the hypothalamo-pituitary axis at autopsy. *Neurologia Medico-Chirugica (Tokyo)*, **23**, 50–54 (1983)

244. Reynolds, D. V. Surgery in the rat during electrical analgesia induced by frontal brain stimulation. *Science*, **164**, 444–445 (1969)

245. Richardson, D. E. and Akil, H. Pain reduction by electrical brain stimulation in man. I. Acute administration in periaqueductal and periventricular sites. *Journal of Neurosurgery*, **47**, 178–183 (1977)

246. Richardson, D. E. and Akil, H. Pain reduction by electrical brain stimulation in man. Part 2. Chronic self-administration in the periventricular gray matter. *Journal of Neurosurgery*, **47**, 184–194 (1977)

247. Richardson, D. E. Analgesia produced by stimulation of various sites in the human beta-endorphin system. *Applied Neurophysiology*, **45**, 116–122 (1982)

248. Boivie, J. and Meyerson, B. A. A correlative anatomic and clinical study of pain suppression by deep brain stimulation. *Pain*, **13**, 113–126 (1982)

249. Meyerson, B. A., Boethius, J. and Carlsson, A. M. Percutaneous central gray stimulation for cancer pain. *Applied Neurophysiology*, **41**, 57–65 (1978)

250. Meyerson, B. A. Aspects on the present state of intracerebral stimulation for pain. In *Brain Stimulation and Neuronal Plasticity* (ed. T. Tsubokawa), Neuron, Tokyo, pp. 33–54 (1985)

251. Ray, C. D. and Burton, C. V. Deep brain stimulation for severe chronic pain. *Acta Neurochirurgica*, Suppl. 30, 289–293 (1980)

252. Richardson, D. E. and Akil, H. Long term results of periventricular gray self-stimulation. *Neurosurgery*, **1**, 200–202 (1977)

253. Richardson, D. E. Long-term follow-up of deep brain stimulation for relief of chronic pain in the human. In *Modern Neurology* (ed. M. Brock), Springer-Verlag, Berlin, pp. 449–453 (1982)

254. Tsubokawa, T., Katayama, Y., Yamamoto, T. and Hirayama, T. Deafferentation pain and stimulation of the thalamic sensory relay nucleus: clinical and experimental study. *Applied Neurophysiology*, **48**, 166–171 (1985)

255. Tsubokawa, T., Hirayama, T., Yamamoto, T. *et al.* Differential effects between thalamic sensory relay nucleus and periaqueductal gray stimulation on neural activity within the normal and deafferented trigeminal medullary dorsal horn. In *Brain Stimulation and Neuronal Plasticity* (ed. T. Tsubokawa), Neuron, Tokyo, pp. 65–76 (1985)

256. Tasker, R. R. Safety and efficacy of chronic neural stimulators. Contract with Canada Department of Health and Welfare (in preparation)

257. Hosobuchi, Y. Analgesia induced by brain stimulation with chronically implanted electrodes. In *Operative Neurosurgical Techniques, Indications, Methods and Results*, 2nd edn (ed. H. H. Schmidek and W. H. Sweet), Grune and Stratton, New York, pp.1089–1095 (1988)

258. Levy, R. M., Lamb, S. and Adams, J. E. Treatment of chronic pain by deep brain stimulation: long-term follow-up and review of the literature. *Neurosurgery*, **21**, 885–893 (1987)

259. Young, R. F. and Brechner, T. Electrical stimulation of the brain for relief of intractable pain due to cancer. *Cancer*, **57**, 1266–1272 (1986)

260. Young, R. F. and Chambi, V. I. Pain relief by electrical stimulation of the periaqueductal and periventricular gray matter. *Journal of Neurosurgery*, **66**, 364–371 (1987)

261. Condouris, G. A. Local anesthetics as modulators of neural information. In *Advances in Pain Research and Therapy, Vol. 1* (ed. J. J. Bonica and D. Albe-Fessard), Raven, New York, pp. 663–667 (1976)

262. Arminio, J. A. A new concept for the treatment of hyperpathia after nerve trauma. *Delaware Medical Journal*, **47**, 363–369 (1975)

263. Battista, A. F. Pain of peripheral nerve origin: fascicle ligation for the prevention of painful neuroma. In *Advances in Pain Research and Therapy, Vol. 3* (ed. J. J. Bonica, J. C. Lebeskind and D. G. Albe-Fessard), Raven, New York, pp. 167–172 (1979)

264. Baumgartner, C. Surgical stump revision as a treatment of stump and phantom pains. In *Phantom and Stump Pain* (ed. J. Siegfried and M. Zimmermann), Springer-Verlag, Berlin, pp. 118–122 (1981)

265. Narakas, A. O. The effects on pain of reconstructive neurosurgery in 160 patients with traction and/or crush injury to the brachial plexus. In *Phantom and Stump Pain* (ed. J. Siegfried and M. Zimmermann), Springer-Verlag, Berlin, pp. 126–147 (1981)

266. Noordenbos, W. and Wall, P. Implications of the failure of nerve resection and graft to cure chronic pain produced by nerve lesions. *Journal of Neurology, Neurosurgery and Psychiatry*, **44**, 1068–1073 (1981)
267. Coggeshall, R. E. Afferent fibers in the ventral root. *Neurosurgery*, **4**, 443–448 (1979)
268. Coggeshall, R. E., Applebaum, M. L., Fazen, M. *et al*. Unmyelinated axons in human ventral roots, a possible explanation for the failure of dorsal rhizotomy to relieve pain. *Brain*, **98**, 157–166 (1975)
269. Osgood, C. P., Dujovmy, M., Faille, R. and Atrassy, M. Microsurgical lumbosacral ganglionectomy, anatomic rationale, and surgical results. *Acta Neurochirurgica*, **35**, 197–204 (1976)
270. Fink, R. A. Neurosurgical treatment of nonmalignant intractable rectal pain: microsurgical commissural myelotomy with carbon dioxide laser. *Neurosurgery*, **14**, 64–65 (1984)
271. von Roeder, F. and Orthner, H. Erfabrungen mit stereotaktishen Eingriffen. III. Mitteilung. *Confins de la Neurologie*, **21**, 51–97 (1961)
272. Orthner, H. and Roeder, F. Further clinical and anatomical experiences with stereotactic operations for relief of pain. *Confins de la Neurologie*, **27**, 418–430 (1966)
273. Shieff, C. and Nashold, B. S. Jr. Stereotactic mesencephalic tractotomy in thalamic pain. *British Journal of Neurosurgery*, **1**, 305–310 (1987)
274. Albe-Fessard, D., Dondey, M., Nicolaidis, S. and LeBeau, J. Remarks concerning the effect of diencephalic lesions on pain and sensitivity with special reference to lemniscally mediated control of noxious afferences. *Confins de la Neurologie*, **32**, 174–184 (1970)
275. Siegfried, J. and Krayenbühl, H. Clinical experience in the treatment of intractable pain. In *Pain: Basic Principles – Pharmacology – Therapy* (ed. R. Janzen, W. D. Keidel, A. Herz and C. Steichele), Georg Thieme, Stuttgart, pp. 202–204 (1972)
276. Portenoy, R. K. and Foley, K. M. Chronic use of opioid analgesics in nonmalignant pain: report of 38 cases. *Pain*, **25**, 171–186 (1986)
277. Levin, A. B., Ramirez, L. F. and Katz, J. The use of stereotactic chemical hypophysectomy in the treatment of thalamic pain syndrome. *Journal of Neurosurgery*, **59**, 1002–1006 (1983)
278. Gybels, J. Electrical stimulation of the brain for pain control in humans. *Verhandlungen der Deutschen Gesellschaaft für innere Medizin*, **86**, 1553–1559 (1980)
279. Hosobuchi, Y., Adams, J. E. and Linchitz, R. Pain relief by electrical stimulation of the central gray matter in humans and its reversal by naloxone, *Science*, **179**, 181–186 (1977)
280. Schvarcz, J. R. Chronic self-stimulation of the medial posterior inferior thalamus for the alleviation of deafferentation pain. *Acta Neurochirurgica*, Suppl. 20, 295–301 (1980)
281. Carstens, E., Guinan, M. J. and MacKinnon, J. D. Naloxone does not consistently affect inhibition of spinal nociceptive transmission produced by medial diencephalic stimulation in the cat. *Neuroscience Letters*, **42**, 71–76 (1983)
282. Mayer, D. J. and Price, D. P. Central nervous system mechanisms of analgesia. *Pain*, **2**, 379–404 (1976)
283. Melzack, R. and Wall, P. Pain mechanisms; a new theory. *Science*, **150**, 971–979 (1965)
284. Wall, P. D. and Sweet, W. H. Temporary abolition of pain in man. *Science*, **155**, 108–109 (1967)
285. Campbell, J. N. and Long, D. M. Peripheral nerve stimulation in the treatment of intractable pain. *Journal of Neurosurgery*, **45**, 692, 699 (1976)
286. Picaza, J. A. Peripheral nerve stimulation for pain control. *Journal of the Florida Medical Association*, **63**, 903–905 (1976)
287. Picaza, J. A., Cannon, B. W., Hunter, S. E. *et al*. Pain suppression by peripheral nerve stimulation. Part III. Observations with implanted devices, *Surgical Neurology*, **4**, 115–126 (1975)
288. Picaza, J. A., Hunter, J. E. and Cannon, B. W. Session in peripheral nerve and neuromuscular stimulation. Pain suppression: chronic effects. *Neurology*, **1**, 226–227 (1977)
289. Picaza, J. A., Hunter, S. E. and Cannon, B. W. Pain suppression by peripheral nerve stimulation. Chronic effects of implanted devices. *Applied Neurophysiology*, **40**, 223–234 (1977–8)
290. Sheldon, C. H. Depolarization in the treatment of trigeminal neuralgia: evaluation of compression and electrical methods: clinical concept of neurophysiological mechanism. In *Pain* (ed. R. S. Knighton and P. R. Dumke), Little, Brown, Boston, pp. 373–386 (1966)
291. Atkinson, J. R. Clinical monopolar stimulation implant on gasserian ganglion for anesthesia dolorosa. *Presented at 32nd Annual Meeting, American Association of Neurological Surgeons, Mexico* (1970)
292. Meyerson, B. A. and Håkansson, S. Alleviation of atypical trigeminal pain by stimulation of the gasserian ganglion via an implanted electrode. *Acta Neurochirurgica*, Suppl. 30, 303–330 (1980)
293. Meyerson, B. A. and Håkansson, S. Longterm results of stimulation via an implanted gasserian electrode for atypical facial pain. *Acta Neurochirurgica*, Suppl. 33, 479–480 (1984)
294. Steude, V. Radiofrequency electrical stimulation of the gasserian ganglion in patients with atypical

trigeminal pain. Methods of percutaneous temporary test-stimulation and permanent implantation of stimulation devices. *Acta Neurochirurgica*, Suppl. 33, 481–486 (1984)

295. Meyerson, B. A. and Håkansson, S. Suppression of pain in trigeminal neuropathy by electric stimulation of the gasserian ganglion. *Neurosurgery*, **18**, 59–66 (1986)

296. Gorecki, J. P., Tasker, R. R. and Hirayama, T. Chronic gasserian ganglion stimulation in the management of central and deafferentation pain. *Transplantation and Implantation Today*, **4**, 42–48 (1987)

297. Shealy, C. N., Mortimer, J. T. and Hagfors, N. R. Dorsal column electroanalgesia. *Journal of Neurosurgery*, **32**, 560–564 (1970)

298. Burton, C. V. Session on spinal cord stimulation. Summary of proceedings. *Surgical Neurology*, **1**, 285–289 (1977)

299. Fox, J. L. Dorsal column stimulation for relief of intractable pain: problems encountered. *Surgical Neurology*, **2**, 59–64 (1974)

300. Lazorthes, Y. and Verdie, J. C. Indications et techniques de stimulation analgésique médullaire et périphérique. *Annales de L'Anesthésiologie Française*, **19**, 439–444 (1978)

301. Long, D. M. and Erickson, D. E. Stimulation of the posterior columns of the spinal cord for the relief of intractable pain. *Surgical Neurology*, **4**, 134–141 (1975)

302. Nashold, B. S., Jr, Somjen, G. and Friedman, H. The effects of stimulating the dorsal columns of man. *Medical Progress through Technology*, **1**, 89–91 (1972)

303. Sweet, W. H. and Wepsic, J. G. Stimulation of the posterior columns of the spinal cord for pain control: indications, technique, and results. *Clinical Neurosurgery*, **2**, 278–310 (1974)

304. Dooley, D. M. A technique for the epidural percutaneous stimulation of the spinal cord in man. *Presented at the Annual Meeting of American Association of Neurological Surgeons, 1975, Miami Beach* (1975)

305. Erickson, D. L. Percutaneous trial of stimulation for patient selection for implantable stimulating electrodes. *Journal of Neurosurgery*, **43**, 440–444 (1975)

306. Hoppenstein, R. Percutaneous implantation of chronic spinal cord electrode for control of intractable pain. Preliminary report. *Surgical Neurology*, **4**, 195–198 (1975)

307. Lazorthes, Y., Verdie, J. C. and Arbus, L. Stimulation analgésique medullaire antérieure et postérieur par technique d'implantation percutanée. *Acta Neurochirurgica*, **40**, 253–276 (1978)

308. Martinez, S. N. Experience with spinal epidural stimulation in pain. In *Recent Advances in Treatment of Pain*, Montreal Neurological Institute, Montreal (1983)

309. North, R. B., Fischell, T. A. and Long, D. M. Chronic dorsal column stimulation via percutaneously inserted epidural electrodes. *Neurosurgery*, **1**, 215–280 (1977)

310. Richardson, R. R., Sigueira, E. B. and Cerullo, L. J. Spinal epidural neurostimulation for treatment of acute and chronic intractable pain: initial and long-term results. *Neurosurgery*, **5**, 344–348 (1979)

311. Urban, B. J. and Nashold, B. S., Jr. Percutaneous epidural stimulation of the spinal cord for relief of pain. Long-term results. *Journal of Neurosurgery*, **48**, 323–328 (1978)

312. Jacobs, M. J. H. M., Jörning, P. J. G., Soures, R. J. et al. Epidural spinal cord electrical stimulation improves microvascular blood flow in severe limb ischemia. *Annals of Surgery*, **207**, 179–183 (1988)

313. Murphy, D. F. and Giles, K. E. Dorsal column stimulation for pain relief from intractable angina pectoris. *Pain*, **28**, 365–368 (1987)

314. Mazars, G. J. Intermittent stimulation of nucleus ventralis posterolateralis for intractable pain. *Surgical Neurology*, **4**, 93–95 (1975)

315. Adams, J. E., Hosobuchi, Y. and Fields, H. L. Stimulation of internal capsule for relief of chronic pain. *Journal of Neurosurgery*, **41**, 740–744 (1974)

316. Adams, J. E. and Hosobuchi, Y. Session on deep brain stimulation. Technique and technical problems. *Neurosurgery*, **1**, 196–199 (1977)

317. Adams, J. E. Technique and technical problems associated with implantation of neuroaugmentative devices. *Applied Neurophysiology*, **40**, 111–123 (1977–8)

318. Hosobuchi, Y., Adams, J. E. and Fields, H. L. Chronic thalamic and internal capsule stimulation for the control of facial anesthesia dolorosa and the dysesthesia of thalamic syndrome. In *Advances in Neurology, Vol. 4* (ed. J. J. Bonica), Raven, New York, pp. 783–787 (1974)

319. Hosobuchi, Y., Adams, J. E. and Rutkin, B. Chronic thalamic and internal capsule stimulation for the control of central pain. *Surgical Neurology*, **4**, 91–92 (1975)

320. Hosobuchi, Y. The current status of analgesic brain stimulation. *Acta Neurochirurgica*, Suppl. 30, 219–227 (1980)

321. Mazars, G. J., Merienne, L. and Cioloca, C. Emploi des stimulateurs thalamiques dans le traitement de certains types de douleurs. *Annales de Médecine Interne*, **12b**, 869–871 (1975)

322. Mazars, G. J., Merienne, L. and Cioloca, C. Comparative study of electrical stimulation of posterior thalamic nuclei, periaqueductal gray, and other midline mesencephalic structures in man. In *Advances in Pain Research and Therapy, Vol. 3* (ed. J. J. Bonica), Raven, New York, pp. 541–546 (1979)
323. Mundinger, F. and Salamao, J. F. Deep brain stimulation in mesencephalic lemniscus medialis for chronic pain. *Acta Neurochirurgica,* Suppl. 30, 245–258 (1980)
324. Turnbull, I. M., Shulman, R. and Woodhurst, W. B. Thalamic stimulation for neuropathic pain. *Journal of Neurosurgery*, 52, 486–493 (1980)
325. Weir Mitchell, S. *Injuries of Nerves and their Consequences*. Dover, New York (reproduction of 1st edition by J. B. Lippincott, Philadelphia, 1872) (1965)
326. Bonica, J. J. Causalgia and other reflex sympathetic dystrophies. In *Advances in Pain Research and Therapy, Vol. 3* (ed. J. J. Bonica, J. C. Liebeskind and D. G. Albe-Fessard), Raven, New York, pp. 141–166 (1979)
326a Homans, J.Minor causalgia: a hyperesthetic neurovascular syndrome. *New England Journal of Medicine*, 222, 870–874 (1940)
327. Payne, R. Neuropathic pain syndromes, with special reference to causalgia and reflex sympathetic dystrophy. *Clinical Journal of Pain*, 2, 59–73 (1986)
328. Rowlingson, J. C. The sympathetic dystrophies. *International Anesthesiology Clinics*, 321, 117–129 (1983)
329. Shumaker, H. B. Jr. A personal view of causalgia and other reflex dystrophies. *Annals of Surgery*, 201, 278–289 (1985)
330. Tahmoush, A. J. Causalgia: redefinition as a clinical pain syndrome. *Pain*, 10, 187–197 (1981)
331. Saris, S. C., Vieira, J. F. S. and Nashold, B. S., Jr. Dorsal root entry zone coagulation for intractable sciatica. *Applied Neurophysiology*, 51, 206–211 (1988)
332. Bernard, E. J., Jr, Nashold, B. S., Jr and Caputi, F. Clinical review of nucleus caudalis dorsal root entry zone lesions for facial pain. *Applied Neurophysiology*, 51, 218–224 (1988)
333. Carlsson, C. A., Persson, K. and Pelletieri, L. Painful scars after thoracic and abdominal surgery. *Acta chirurgica scandinavica*, 151, 309–311 (1985)
334. Conacher, I. D. Percutaneous cryotherapy for post-thoracotomy neuralgia. *Pain*, 25, 227–228 (1986)
335. Smith, E. P. Trans-spinal ganglionectomy for relief of intercostal pain. *Journal of Neurosurgery*, 32, 574–577 (1970)
336. Carlen, P. L., Wall, P. D., Nodvorna, H. and Steinbach, T. Phantom limbs and related phenomena in recent traumatic amputations. *Neurology*, 288, 211–217 (1978)
337. Siegfried, J. and Cetinalp, E. Neurosurgical treatment of phantom limb pain: a survey of methods. In *Phantom and Stump Pain* (ed. J. Siegfried and M. Zimmermann), Springer Verlag, Berlin, pp. 148–155 (1981)
338. Jansen, T. S. and Rasmussen, P. Amputation. In *Textbook of Pain* (ed. P. D. Wall and R. Melzack), Churchill Livingstone, Edinburgh, pp. 402–412 (1984)
339. Sherman, R. A., Sherman, C. J. and Parker, L. Chronic phantom and stump pain among American veterans: results of a survey. *Pain*, 18, 83–95 (1984)
340. Iaocono, R. P., Linford, J. and Sandyk, R. Pain management after lower extremity amputation. *Neurosurgery*, 20, 496–500 (1987)
341. Saris, S. C., Iacono, R. P. and Nashold, B. S., Jr. Dorsal root entry zone lesions for post-amputation pain. *Journal of Neurosurgery*, 62, 72–76 (1985)
342. Saris, S. C., Iacono, R. P. and Nashold, B. S., Jr. Successful treatment of phantom pain with dorsal root entry zone coagulation. *Applied Neurophysiology*, 51, 1188–1197 (1988)
343. Krainick, J. U. and Thoden, U. Spinal cord stimulation in post-amputation pain. In *Phantom and Stump Pain* (ed. J. Siegfried and M. Zimmermann), Springer-Verlag, Berlin, pp. 163–166 (1981)
344. Krainick, J. U., Thoden, U. and Riechert, R. Pain reduction in amputees by long-term spinal cord stimulation. *Journal of Neurosurgery*, 52, 346–350 (1980)
345. De la Porte, C. and Siegfried, J. Lumbosacral spinal fibrosis (spinal arachnoiditis). Its diagnosis and treatment by spinal cord stimulation. *Spine*, 8, 593–603 (1983)
346. Loeser, J. D. Herpes zoster and postherpetic neuralgia. *Pain*, 25, 149–164 (1986)
347. Milligan, N. S. and Nash, T. P. Treatment of post-herpetic neuralgia. A review of 27 consecutive cases. *Pain*, 23, 381–386 (1985)
348. Demierre, B. and Siegfried, J. Traitement neurochirurgical de la névralgie postherpétiforme. *Médecine et Hygiène*, 41, 1960–1965 (1983)
349. Friedman, A. H., Nashold, B. S., Jr and Ovelinen-Levitt, J. Dorsal root entry zone lesions for the treatment of post-herpetic neuralgia. *Journal of Neurosurgery*, 60, 1258–1262 (1984)
350. Nashold, B. S., Jr, Ostdahl, R. H., Bullitt, E. *et al.* Dorsal root entry zone lesions: a new

neurosurgical therapy for deafferentation pain. In *Advances in Pain Research and Therapy, Vol. 5* (ed. J. J. Bonica, U. Lindblom, and A. Iggo), Raven, New York, pp. 739–750 (1983)

351. Friedman, A. H. and Bullitt, E. Dorsal root entry zone lesions in the treatment of pain following brachial plexus avulsion, spinal cord injury and herpes zoster. *Applied Neurophysiology*, **51**, 164–169 (1988)

352. Nashold, B. S., Jr, Lopes, H., Chodakiewitz, J. and Bronec, P. Trigeminal DREZ for craniofacial pain. In *Surgery in and around the Brain Stem and the Third Ventricle* (ed. M. Samii), Springer-Verlag, Berlin, pp. 54–59 (1986)

353. Wynn Parry, C. B. Management of pain in avulsion lesions of the brachial plexus. In *Advances in Pain Research and Therapy, Vol. 5* (ed. J. J. Bonica, U. Lindblom and A. Iggo), Raven, New York, pp. 751–761 (1983)

354. Demierre, B. and Siegfried, J. Douleurs apres irradiation thérapeutique. Discussion des mécanismes et proposition de traitement. *Médecine et Hygiène*, **42**, 1777–1782 (1984)

355. Nashold, B. S., Jr and Ostdahl, R. H. Dorsal root entry zone lesions for pain relief. *Journal of Neurosurgery*, **51**, 59–69 (1979)

356. Thomas, D. G. T. and Sheehy, J. P. R. Dorsal root entry zone lesions (Nashold's procedure) for pain relief following brachial plexus avulsion. *Journal of Neurology, Neurosurgery and Psychiatry*, **46**, 924–928 (1983)

357. Friedman, A. H. and Bullitt, E. Dorsal root entry zone lesions in the treatment of pain following brachial plexus avulsion, spinal cord injury and herpes zoster. *Applied Neurophysiology*, **51**, 164–169 (1988)

358. Campbell, J. N., Solomon, C. T. and James, C. S. The Hopkins experience with lesions of the dorsal horn (Nashold's operation) for pain from avulsion of the brachial plexus. *Applied Neurophysiology*, **51**, 170–174 (1988)

359. Ishijima, B., Shimoji, K., Shimizu, H. *et al*. Lesions of spinal and trigeminal dorsal root entry zone for deafferentation pain. *Applied Neurophysiology*, **51**, 175–187 (1988)

360. Moossy, J. J. and Nashold, B. S., Jr. Dorsal root entry zone lesions for conus medullaris root avulsions. *Applied Neurophysiology*, **51**, 198–205 (1988)

361. Botterell, E. H., Callaghan, J. C. and Joussse, A. T. Pain in paraplegia: clinical management and surgical treatment. *Proceedings of the Royal Society of Medicine*, **47**, 17–24 (1953)

362. White, J. C. Anterospinal chordotomy – its effectiveness in relieving pain of non-malignant disease. *Neurochirurgia*, **6**, 83–102 (1963)

363. White, J. C. and Sweet, W. H. *Pain and the Neurosurgeon: A Forty Year Experience*, Thomas, Springfield, Illinois, pp. 435–447 (1969)

364. Druckman, R. and Lende, R. Central pain of spinal origin: pathogenesis and surgical relief in one patient. *Neurology*, **15**, 518–522 (1965)

365. Melzack, R. and Loeser, J. D. Phantom body pain in paraplegics: evidence for a central 'pattern-generating mechanism' for pain. *Pain*, **4**, 195–210 (1978)

366. Durward, Q. J., Rice, G. P., Ball, M. J. *et al*. Selective spinal cordectomy: clinicopathological correlation, *Journal of Neurosurgery*, **56**, 359–367 (1982)

367. Jefferson, A. Cordectomy for intractable pain. In *Persistent Pain, Vol. 4* (ed. S. Lipton and J. Miles), Grune and Stratton, New York, pp. 115–132 (1983)

368. Nashold, B. S., Jr and Bullitt, E. Dorsal root entry zone lesions to control central pain in paraplegics. *Journal of Neurosurgery*, **55**, 414–419 (1981)

369. Nashold, B. S., Jr, Ostdahl, R. H., Bullitt, E. *et al*. Dorsal root entry zone lesions: a new neurosurgical therapy for deafferentation pain. In *Advances in Pain Research and Therapy, Vol. 5* (ed. J. J. Bonica, U. Lindblom and A. Iggo), Raven, New York, pp. 739–750 (1983)

370. Richter, H. P. and Seitz, K. Dorsal root entry zone lesions for the control of deafferentation pain: experience in ten patients. *Neurosurgery*, **15**, 956–959 (1984)

371. Sweet, W. H. and Poletti, C. E. Operations in the brain stem and spinal canal, with an appendix on open cordotomy. In *Textbook of Pain* (ed. P. D. Wall and R. Melzack), Churchill Livingstone, Edinburgh, pp. 615–631 (1984)

372. Friedman, A. H. and Nashold, B. S., Jr. DREZ lesions for relief of pain related to spinal cord injury. *Journal of Neurosurgery*, **65**, 465–469 (1986)

373. Richardson, R. R., Meyer, P. R. and Cerullo, L. J. Neurostimulation in the modulation of intractable paraplegic and traumatic neuroma pains. *Pain*, **8**, 76–84 (1980)

374. Gildenberg, R. Stereotactic treatment of head and neck pain. *Research and Clinical Studies in Headache*, **5**, 102–121 (1978)

375. Namba, S., Nakao, Y., Matsumoto, Y. *et al*. Electrical stimulation of the posterior limb of the internal capsule for treatment of thalamic pain. *Applied Neurophysiology*, **47**, 137–148 (1984)

376. Niizuma, H., Kwak, R., Ikeda, S. *et al* Follow-up results of centromedian thalamotomy for central

pain. *Applied Neurophysiology*, **45**, 324–325 (1982)
377. Mazars, G. J., Merienne, L. and Cioloca, C. Traitment de certaines types de douleurs par les stimulateurs thalamiques implantables. *Neurochirugie*, **20**, 117–124 (1974)
378. Levy, R. M., Lam, S. and Adams, J. E. Deep brain stimulation for chronic pain: long-term follow-up in 145 patients, 1972–1984. *Pain*, Suppl. 2, S115 (1984)
379. Demierre, B. and Siegfried, J. Le syndrome douloureux thalamique. Corrélations radiologico-cliniques et traitement par la stimulation intermittente des noyaux sensitifs du thalamus. *Neurochirurgie*, **31**, 281–285 (1985)
380. Mundinger, F. and Neumueller, H. Programmed stimulation for control of chronic pain and motor disease. *Applied Neurophysiology*, **45**, 102–111 (1982)
381. Siegfried, J. and Demierre, B. Thalamic electrostimulation in the treatment of thalamic pain syndrome. *Pain*, Suppl. 2, S116 (1984)
382. Siegfried, J. and Pamir, M. N. Electrical stimulation in humans of the sensory thalamic nuclei and effects on dyskinesias and spasticity. In *Clinical Aspects of Sensory Motor Integration* (ed. A. Struppler and A. Weindl), Springer-Verlag, Berlin, pp. 283–288 (1985)
383. Fields, H. L. and Adams, J. E. Pain after cortical injury relieved by electrical stimulation of the internal capsule. *Brain*, **97**, 169–178 (1974)

8
Deafferentation syndromes and dorsal root entry zone lesions

Kim J. Burchiel

INTRODUCTION

The principle of a chronic pain state which results from loss of primary afferent input to the central nervous system, so-called 'deafferentation pain', has been dealt with in the preceding chapter. Patients with these disorders represent one of the most challenging, and often intractable, problems confronting health care professionals who deal with chronic pain management. Until recently, there has been relatively little to offer these patients. Non-surgical treatment has been limited to sedative, antidepressant or anticonvulsant medication, or psychologic counseling and support. In most cases these regimens were palliative, at best. On the other hand, surgical therapy often employed ineffective and ill-advised neurodestructive procedures.

Beginning in 1972, Sindou and his colleagues at Lyons began to consider the dorsal root entry zone (DREZ) as a possible target for pain surgery. His group undertook anatomic studies and some preliminary surgical trials in humans in order to determine whether a destructive procedure at this level was effective for pain control [1–4]. They proposed that the DREZ was constituted by (1) the central portion of the dorsal roots, (2) Lissauer's tract, and (3) laminae I–V of the dorsal horn. Their detailed anatomic studies have been reviewed recently [5]. The essence of their argument is that as the dorsal roots fuse with the DREZ, the fibers destined for the lemniscal pathway, i.e. large myelinated axons (A-α/β), become segregated into the medial-most part of the root. Conversely, the pain-signalling axons (A-δ and C fibers), which enter Lissauer's tract and the superficial dorsal horn, are found more laterally in the root (Figure 8.1). Their principle was that section of the lateral root and Lissauer's tract down to the level of the gray matter of the dorsal horn would selectively interrupt nociceptive input to the spinal cord, without complete sacrifice of remaining lemniscal fibers. This principle has been successfully applied in the 'selective posterior rhizotomy' operation since that time and represents one of the two major techniques of DREZ surgery for pain control.

In 1975, Nashold and his associates at Duke University performed for the first time a procedure in a patient with brachial plexus avulsion and deafferentation pain of that extremity [7]. The operation involved destruction of the superficial dorsal root entry zone (DREZ) of the spinal cord over the segments of previous nerve

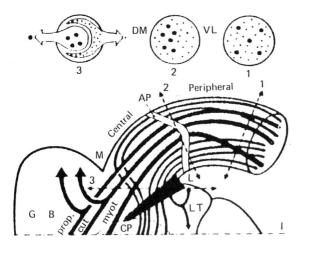

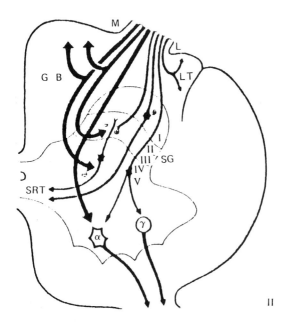

Figure 8.1 Fiber organization of the dorsal root at its entry zone into spinal cord. Top, organization of fibers at the dorsal root/spinal cord junction in man. Each rootlet has both a peripheral and central component. The junction between the two constitutes the pial ring (AP). Peripherally the fibers have no organization, as shown in the cross-section of the rootlet (1). Near the pial ring, the small fibers are situated on the rootlet surface, predominantly on its lateral side (2). In its central component these small fibers group laterally (3) to enter Lissauer's tract (LT) and the posterior horn (CP). The large fibers are situated centrally for the myotactic fibers and medially (2,3) for the lemniscal (proprioceptive and cutaneous) ones. Selective posterior rhizotomy affects the black triangle. Bottom, posterior rootlet projections to the spinal cord. The small fibers terminate on the spinoreticulothalamic (SRT) cells which they activate, and by polysynaptic arcs on the γ and α motoneurons of the anterior horn. The short collaterals of the large fibers (of cutaneous or proprioceptive origin) terminate on and inhibit the SRT cells. From Sindou, M. and Goutelle, A. Surgical posterior rhizotomies for the treatment of pain. In *Advances and Technical Standards in Neurosurgery* (ed. H. Krayenbuhl), Springer-Verlag, Wien, pp. 147–185 (1983) with permission

root avulsion. The rationale for the procedure was their belief that when neurons in the dorsal horn which are normally involved in the signalling of pain are deprived of their normal afferent input they behave in a pathologic way. According to this reasoning, this abnormal neuronal behavior is experienced by the patient as pain. Thus, the destruction of those neurons generating abnormal activity would relieve the discomfort. This initial DREZ procedure was successful in relieving the patient's pain, and since that time Nashold and his colleagues, as well as a number of other groups, have had very gratifying results with the use of DREZ lesions for brachial plexus avulsion pain, as well as a host of other deafferentation pain syndromes.

Both Sindou's selective posterior rhizotomy and Nashold's DREZ lesion procedure have produced convincing and long-lasting pain relief in patients afflicted with deafferentation pain. These surgical procedures represent the neurosurgical 'state-of-the-art' in controlling these difficult disorders. In this chapter, we briefly review the anatomy and physiology of the dorsal horn as well as the pathophysiologic correlates of the injured or deafferented dorsal horn. The rest of this section dwells on the indications, technique and outcome from surgery in the region of the DREZ.

ANATOMY AND PHYSIOLOGY OF THE DORSAL HORN

Chapter 1 reviewed our current understanding of the anatomy and physiology of the dorsal horn. The reader is directed there for a more complete discussion of these issues. Below we reiterate some of that background information that is germane to the discussion of deafferentation pain.

Several investigators have recently questioned whether all nociceptive fibers enter the spinal cord via the dorsal root [8,9]. Anatomic data indicated that up to 30% of axons entering through the ventral root were unmyelinated C-fiber afferents. It was postulated that these primary afferents originated in the dorsal root ganglion, but that their centrally projecting processes looped back into ventral root and entered spinal cord via the ventral root. However, this challenge to the law of Bell and Magendie has been mitigated by the finding that the majority of these ventral root unmyelinated afferents do not enter the cord through the ventral root, but simply loop deeply into the ventral root before re-entering the dorsal root to reach the dorsal horn eventually [10].

Capping the dorsal horn is a short intersegmental pathway, Lissauer's tract (LT). This area plays an important part in the intersegmental modulation of the nociceptive afferents [11]. The deeper and more lateral portion of the LT mediates interconnections of the inhibitory substantia gelatinosa (*see below*), while the more medial and superficial LT contains the collateral fibers of the primary nociceptive afferents which run rostral and caudal one or two segments from the point of entry of the dorsal root (Figure 8.2).

Beneath this tract, the dorsal horn can be divided cytoarchitectonically into five laminae as originally described by Rexed: I (marginal layer), II–III (substantia gelatinosa), IV–V (nucleus proprius) (*see* Figure 1.3, Chapter 1). Large myelinated non-nociceptive axons (A-α/β) enter the spinal cord in the medial dorsal root, while nociceptive axons (A-δ and C fibers) enter laterally (Figure 8.1). The medial axons (tactile, proprioceptive) bifurcate, sending one axon into the ipsilateral dorsal column and one into the dorsal horn. Lateral axons enter the spinal cord

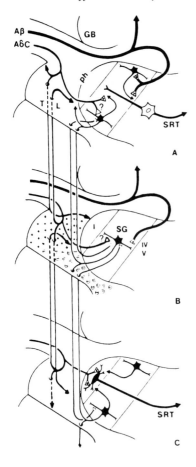

Figure 8.2 Modulation of nociceptive radicular afferents in the DREZ. On entering the spinal cord, the nociceptive A-δ and C fibers are lateral in the posterior rootlet to penetrate into Lissauer's tract (TL) and reach the posterior horn (ph), either directly or through a two-segment ascending or descending trajectory. There they relay on to the apical dendrites of the spinoreticulothalamic (SRT) cells of lamina I marginal cells (part C) and lamina IV and V nucleus proprius neurons (part A), whereas the lemniscal A-β fibers are medial in the posterior rootlet. They form long axons ascending in the dorsal column and short recurrent collaterals ending in the substantia gelatinosa (SG) where they relay on to the apical dendrites of the nucleus proprius neurons. These collaterals also activate the small cells constituting the SG, which is an inhibitory structure according to the gate control theory (part B). Thus, the lemniscal fibers prevent nociceptive A-δ and C afferents from entering the SRT pathway. This constitutes a local segmental modulating system. On entering the cord, the afferents also undergo modulation from the neighboring roots through the TL associative fibers (part B). Its internal region (site of the ascending and descending collaterals of the nociceptive fibers) transmits the excitatory effects of the adjacent roots. In contrast, its external part (site of the SG longitudinal interconnecting axons called fasciculus proprius) presumably conveys the inhibitory influences of the neighboring segments. From Sindou, M. and Daher, A. Spinal cord ablation procedures for pain. In *Proceedings of the Vth World Congress on Pain* (ed. R. Dubner, G. F. Gebhart and M. R. Bond), Elsevier, Amsterdam, pp. 477–495 (1988) with permission

where they ascend and descend 1–2 segments in Lissauer's tract, entering laminae I and II from the lateral side. After one or more synapses, the final output cells, the spinothalamic tract neurons from lamina I and lamina V, send their axons across the midline to enter the contralateral ascending anterolateral system. Although our understanding of the spinal somatosensory system continues to evolve rapidly, a simplified schematic depiction of the anatomic segmental and intersegmental relationships within the dorsal horn is given in Figure 8.2.

Laminae II–III contain small enkephalinergic interneurons which have synaptic input from both large and small primary afferent fibers as well as from fibers which descend from the brain stem in the dorsolateral fasciculus (DLF). These interneurons project to both laminae I and IV–V where they make presynaptic contact on spinothalamic projection neurons that possess opioid receptors. There is evidence that release of opioid neurotransmitter (enkephalin) at these presynaptic sites by either stimulation of the interneuron from the DLF, primary afferent stimulation, or direct injection of opioid substances into the region of the dorsal horn, inhibits the activity of both nociceptive specific (marginal) and wide-dynamic-range neurons in response to a nociceptive stimulus [12–14]. Thus, these enkephalinergic interneurons are thought to inhibit the transmission of nociceptive input at the level of the dorsal horn.

There is evidence that nociceptive primary afferents use the peptide neurotransmitter substance P as their neurotransmitter at the primary synapse. However, it is likely that substance P is not the only nociceptive neurotransmitter. A large variety of other neuropeptides probably also have a role in both the signalling and inhibition of nociception. In particular, somatostatin appears to have an inhibitory function in the nociceptive pathway. In addition, there is evidence that some excitatory amino-acid transmitters are involved. The neurochemistry of the dorsal horn is extraordinarily complex, and the interested reader is directed to recent reviews of the subject [15–17].

PATHOPHYSIOLOGY OF THE DEAFFFERENTED DORSAL HORN

Several theories have been put forth to explain the pathophysiology of the seemingly paradoxical clinical circumstance of severe, unremitting, distressing pain in a hypesthetic or anesthetic body region (*see* Table 1.3, Chapter 1).

The first, and often incorrectly implied as proven, hypothesis is that deafferentation of dorsal horn nociceptive transmission neurons produces a kind of 'denervation hypersensitivity' of the cell. The analogy has been to the case of skeletal muscle, where denervation produces hypersensitivity to acetylcholine, and spontaneous myofibrillar activity (fibrillations and fasciculations). This state of deafferentation hyperactivity has also been compared to an 'epileptic-like' phenomenon [18]. There are conflicting data about whether this type of denervation supersensitivity occurs after *neuronal* deafferentation. Different studies of the dorsal horn in experimental animals after dorsal rhizotomy and other deafferenting lesions have both shown hyperactivity and spontaneous discharges [19,21], and no hyperactivity [22,23].

Another view is that, after deafferentation, the dorsal horn nociceptive neurons are released from 'powerful central inhibitory systems'. Some experimental evidence does seem to indicate that descending inhibition is diminished after dorsal horn deafferentation [24,25]. It has also been shown that receptive fields for dorsal horn neurons remaining after injury manifest dramatic shifts in their receptive fields and response characteristics [21,26]. This may imply either a change in descending control, plasticity or even sprouting at the segmental level. How these observations might relate to the genesis of a clinical pain syndrome is not clear.

Lastly, it has been stated that deafferentation leads to a fundamental change in the neurochemical milieu of the dorsal horn. In experimental preparations there is gliosis in Lissauer's tract and the substantia gelatinosa, as well as loss of substantia gelatinosa interneurons and somatostatin terminals. It appears that, after injury, levels of enkephalin, substance P and somatostatin all decrease. The possibility is that there is either a denervation supersensitivity to substance P, or an 'imbalance' of somatostatin/enkephalin [15].

Suffice it to say that the mechanism of deafferentation pain is not at all understood. However, it is instructive to keep in mind that, empirically, ablative lesions of the DREZ have been reported to be effective in controlling these pains. James Watt observed that the science of thermodynamics owed more to the steam engine than the reverse. Perhaps, in the same vein, the search for an explanation of the mechanism of deafferentation pain will be largely directed by the careful analysis of patient outcome, satisfactory and unsatisfactory, after DREZ surgery.

NON-SURGICAL MANAGEMENT OF DEAFFERENTATION PAIN

Deafferentation pain is typically intractable to conventional therapy. There is a consensus that deafferentation pain is relatively refractory to opiates, possibly because, in many cases, the neural substrate that would normally possess opioid receptors has been damaged or destroyed by the deafferenting process. Non-opioid analgesics and non-steroidal anti-inflammatory agents have little or no effect on this type of pain.

Available pharmacologic options can be broadly categorized in two groups: (1) anticonvulsants, such as phenytoin or carbamazepine, and (2) antidepressants, such as amitriptyline or doxepin. A general rule is that pains that are described as fleeting, lancinating, radiating, or electric in quality will best respond to anticonvulsant therapy, particularly to carbamazepine [27]; pains that are constant or burning in character will be better treated by the antidepressants. Because of the distressing quality of deafferentation pain, and the general tendency of 'central pains' to increase with stress, anxiolytic agents may also be useful. The use of these anxiolytic or other major psychotropic drugs must be approached with great caution, as they may produce behavioral and cognitive impairment, psychologic dependence and profound withdrawal effects.

Transcutaneous neurostimulation is rarely effective in these cases because the analgesic potential of this technique is dependent on intact sensation in the area of pain. This is, of course, not the situation in patients with deafferentation. Psychologic counseling, relaxation techniques, biofeedback or a formal 'pain clinic program' in the outpatient or inpatient setting may be of some palliative benefit.

Overall, the best non-surgical therapy for deafferentation pain has been only marginally effective [28,29]. This fact must be considered when we judge the indications and results of DREZ lesions and other surgery for these conditions.

TECHNIQUES FOR DREZ SURGERY

The procedure of selective posterior rhizotomy (SPR), as envisaged by Sindou [1], involves destruction of the lateral dorsal root and the medial portion of LT. It consists of microsurgical incision and bipolar coagulation performed ventrolaterally at the entrance of the rootlets into the dorsolateral sulcus, along the spinal cord segments elected to be operated on. The lesion, which penetrates the lateral part of the DREZ and the medial part of LT, extends down to the apex of the dorsal horn, recognized by its brown-gray color. The lesions are 2 mm deep and made at a 45 degree angle (Figure 8.3). Although autopsy confirmation is lacking, these lesions are presumed, first to destroy preferentially the pain pathway, i.e. the lateral dorsal root which contains nociceptive A-δ and C fibers, the medial part of LT that contains the excitatory nociceptive primary afferent collateral fibers, and possibly the superficial laminae of the dorsal horn; and, secondly, to preserve, at least partially, the inhibitory structures of the DREZ, namely the lemniscal fibers reaching the dorsal column, as well as their recurrent collaterals to the dorsal horn and the inhibitory intersegmental fibers of the lateral LT [5].

Selective surgical destruction of the superficial laminae of the dorsal horn for treating pain was first described by Nashold [7]. Early on, the technique involved the use of an RF electrode without temperature control. Thermocoupled temperature monitoring electrodes have become available for the DREZ operation only in

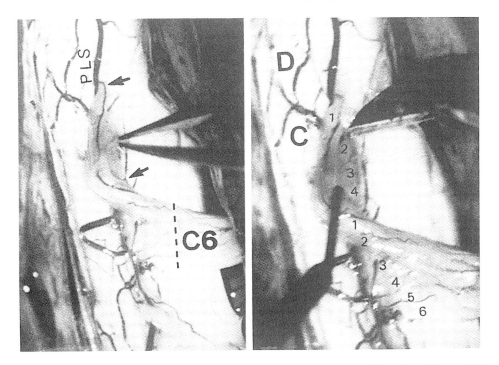

Figure 8.3 Technique of selective posterior rhizotomy at the cervical level. Through a right cervical hemilaminectomy with conservation of the spinous processes and after opening the dura and arachnoid membranes the posterolateral aspect of the spinal cord is approached under the microscope (at the level of the 6th posterior root). a, The right C6 root (which has six rootlets) has been retracted toward the inside to make the ventrolateral region of the spinal cord rootlet junction accessible (arrows). The ventrolateral region is the site of small pial vessels which are coagulated by means of a bipolar forceps. b, The ventrolateral selective incision is made along the six rootlets in the lateral sulcus of the posterolateral sulcus (PLS) using a small piece of a razor blade. The incision is 1 mm deep in the Lissauer tract and makes a 45 degree angle. From Sindou, M. and Goutelle, A. Surgical posterior rhizotomies for the treatment of pain. In *Advances and Technical Standards in Neurosurgery* (ed. H. Krayenbuhl), Springer-Verlag, Wien, pp. 147–185 (1983), with permission

the past few years. Early experience with RF DREZ lesions without temperature monitoring reflected a relatively high rate of postoperative neurologic complications related to damage to the dorsal columns or corticospinal tract. In comparison, since utilization of the temperature-controlled electrodes has become routine, results have shown a significant decrease in the postoperative neurologic morbidity [30]. Recent reports of DREZ lesions made by CO_2 laser have also indicated that the damage to tracts in proximity to the DREZ can be largely avoided by a discrete laser lesion [31,32].

Nashold's current technique involves performing the DREZ lesion with the patient under general anesthesia in the prone position. A laminectomy or hemilaminectomy is performed over the involved segments of the cervical spinal cord, usually C5–T1. The dura is opened, exposing the cord. This operation is commonly performed for patients with avulsion of the brachial plexus. In these patients the area of root avulsion is devoid of dorsal roots, and often shows some distortion of the normal surface anatomy of the cord (Figure 8.4). Often comparison with the normal side is helpful in localizing the area of the DREZ on the injured side.

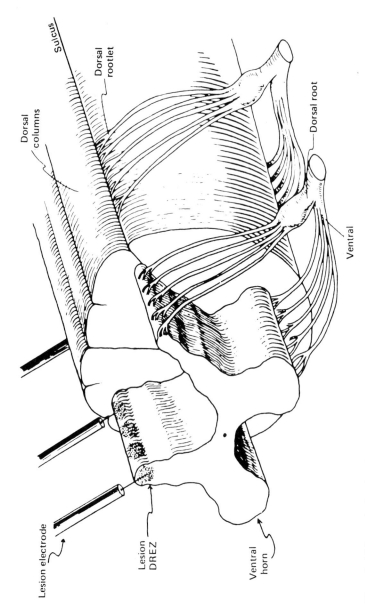

Figure 8.4 Schematic drawing showing the dorsal root entry zone and the region for DREZ lesions. From Nashold, B. S., Jr and Ostdahl, R. H. Dorsal root entry zone lesions for pain relief. *Journal of Neurosurgery*, **51**, 59–69 (1979), with permission

Usually, in the cervical spinal cord, electrophysiologic techniques are not necessary or practical, because the levels of root avulsion are readily identifiable, the root levels can be localized by direct inspection, and the upper extremity is often completely deafferented. For other deafferentation pain states, evoked potential monitoring is important for localization of the proper cord segment for DREZ lesion [34,35] (Figure 8.5).

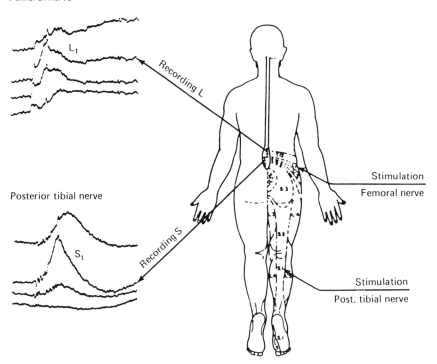

Figure 8.5 Electrophysiologic localization of the dorsal root entry zones on the conus medullaris. From Nashold, B. S., Jr, Higgins, A. C. and Blumenkopf, B. Dorsal root entry zone lesions for pain relief. In *Pain* (ed. P. D. Wall and R. Melzack), Churchill Livingstone, Edinburgh, pp. 2433–2437 (1984), with permission

The DREZ can be identified adjacent to the intermediolateral sulcus which delineates the lateral edge of the dorsal columns. It is not clear which laminae of the dorsal horn need to be destroyed to alleviate the pain maximally. Available autopsy data [36,37] indicate that the deeper layers (IV–VI) were coagulated by DREZ lesion. Nevertheless, the intent of the operation was to disrupt at least the first five layers of Rexed (2 mm depth) [18].

Once satisfactory anatomic localization of the DREZ is accomplished, the DREZ lesion is carried out either by RF electrode or by CO_2 laser (Figure 8.6). In the first case, thermal coagulative lesions can be created with an insulated steel wire 0.018 mm in diameter, with a 2 mm uninsulated tip. Early on in Nashold's series, a radiofrequency generator was set to deliver 30–35 mA for 15 s. In later patients, a 0.25 mm thermistor electrode with a 2 mm tip was used. The electrode was

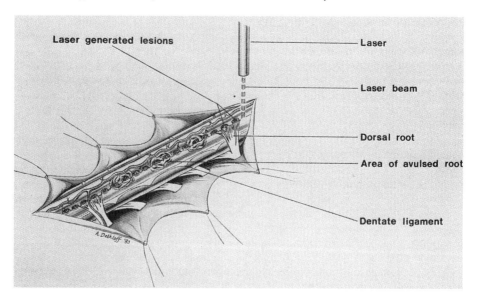

Figure 8.6 Diagram showing the method for producing DREZ lesions using a laser. From Levy, W. J., Nutkiewicz, A., Ditmore, Q. M. *et al.* Laser-induced dorsal root entry zone lesions for pain control. *Journal of Neurosurgery*, **59**, 884–886 (1983), with permission

introduced 2 mm into the cord parenchyma at an angle of about 25 degrees to the vertical plane, though the intermediolateral sulcus. This electrode was heated to 75–80°C for 15 s for each lesion. In either instance, the lesions were made by inserting the coagulator tip along the entrance of the dorsal nerve root to a depth of 2 mm. The operating microscope was employed to determine the exact position at which the rootlets entered the cord. The lesions were placed 0.5–1 mm apart so that approximately 25 lesions were made per spinal segment. Lesions were made from half a spinal segment above to half a segment below the area of pain. The overall length and number of DREZ lesions depends on the number of involved segments [18].

Laser lesions of the DREZ are made using the CO_2 laser operating at 5 W for 1 s at a focal spot size of 300–400 μm, or with an argon laser at a power output of 6–7 W, for 1 s at a spot size of 150 μm. The surgical wound limits the angle of attack of the laser, so the denticulate ligaments are divided and a traction suture placed in the ligament to allow rotation of the cord the requisite 25–30 degrees. This allows a vertically orientated laser beam to enter the dorsal horn at the appropriate angle to minimize damage to the adjacent tracts [32]. Before DREZ lesion by this method, the vasculature overlying the DREZ is coagulated either with the defocused laser or bipolar coagulation. A sequence of laser lesions is then carried out during brief periods of respiratory arrest to eliminate respiratory movement and to ensure complete immobility while the lesions are being made. A series of 5–10 contiguous lesions are made during approximately 30 s of respiratory arrest, and then the patient is ventilated for several minutes before the next series of lesions. This sequence is repeated until the DREZ lesions have been made at all segments involved.

INDICATIONS FOR DREZ SURGERY

For much of the remainder of this chapter, we consider three conditions that fall under the rubric of deafferentation pain: brachial plexus avulsion, central pain of paraplegics, and postherpetic neuralgia. All these conditions share the feature of damage to afferent pathways and, to some extent, damage to the dorsal horn itself. It is for these three syndromes that we have most data for DREZ surgery, and in which DREZ lesions represent a major advance over other therapeutic modalities.

A second group of disorders are also briefly discussed: pains of 'peripheral origin'. This includes, for example, phantom pain, post-thoracotomy pain, or neuropathic pain. These syndromes likewise are manifestations of primary afferent injury, but in these instances the injury is limited to the peripheral nervous system. This subdivision of 'peripheral' and 'central' origin of pains may be more convenient than accurate, because increasing data indicate that many, if not all, peripheral injuries are associated with persistent central nervous system changes. Nevertheless, on a purely empirical basis, response to DREZ lesion surgery can be predicted by whether a patient falls into this (admittedly inexact) definition. Thus, it is retained here for the purposes of this discussion. Nashold [38] has recently reviewed much of the data concerning deafferentation pain as it relates to the DREZ operation.

Before serious contemplation of operative intervention in these patients, it is imperative for the treating physicians to proceed with a complete evaluation of the medical history, neurologic status, psychologic profile, drug usage history and social background of the patient. The psychologic evaluation and drug utilization review are particularly important. Psychologic inventory should include a detailed interview, personality (i.e. Minnesota Multiphasic Personality Inventory) assessment and in some cases formal psychometric and neuropsychologic testing. In most cases it is best to address issues of drug withdrawal and detoxification pre-operatively, if possible, as this will also often greatly clarify the nature of the pain problem, and the contribution of drug dependence to the syndrome.

Brachial plexus avulsion

This relatively common injury [39] typically occurs in the setting of a vehicular accident involving a helmeted motorcyclist. In this particular injury, the impact is usually borne by the head and shoulder striking the pavement or other surface. The helmeted head is driven contralaterally, and the ipsilateral shoulder is forcefully depressed. This creates stretching of the brachial plexus, more of the upper roots than lower roots because the more superior tethering of the upper roots places them under relatively more tension by the downward movement of the shoulder. The force generated by this stretching avulses both the dorsal and ventral roots, as well as radicular vessels at several levels, and often the victim is left with a totally deafferented arm. Often there is associated head, neck, shoulder and upper extremity injury. In a patient with a pelvic fracture, or direct penetrating trauma to the sacral plexus, an analogous injury to the sacral roots and spinal cord may occur.

The pain usually begins at an early stage after the injury, often within hours to days [40]. The pain is constant and severe and commonly refractory to even potent opiate analgesics. The patient may describe two pain components: the first is a constant pain described as 'burning', 'aching', or 'crushing'; the second is a sharp, lancinating pain often described as 'electrical' in quality. These latter pains usually occur in partially innervated regions, or at the transition zone between normal and anesthetic dermatomes, either on the arm or on the chest wall. They may be triggered by light tactile stimulation of the transition zone, and may cause the patient scrupulously to avoid contact of that zone with clothes, bed-coverings, or other individuals.

On neurologic examination the patient may exhibit a partial to complete deafferentation of the upper extremity, depending on the extent of the injury. Complete anesthesia of the entire upper extremity is not uncommon. If trigger areas occur in the arm, the patient may guard the extremity, to some extent reminiscent of a causalgic syndrome. Atrophy and flaccidity of the involved myotomes is readily apparent in chronic cases. A Horner's syndrome may be seen ipsilaterally when the T1 or T2 roots are involved.

A recurring request of these patients seems to be to have the arm 'taken off'. To the naive clinician this has a certain appeal, but this particular procedure would be rewarded with disastrous consequences, as the patient would be left with no extremity and all of the pain [41]! With the minor exception of other surgical options discussed below, virtually the only surgical procedure with any consistent effectiveness for brachial plexus avulsion pain is DREZ lesion.

Pre-operatively, a myelogram or intrathecally enhanced CT scan should be done to prove and delineate the root avulsion. The myelographic abnormality at the level of avulsion may be as little as some deformity of the root sleeve, but more commonly an obvious pseudomeningocele extending out of the neural foramen pointing to the plexus is seen at one or more levels. Not only does this make the diagnosis of avulsion certain, but also may serve as guide to the surgeon for what to expect upon direct visualization of the spinal cord at the time of surgery. However, the levels of avulsion may extend rostral and caudal to the myelographically proven pseudomeningoceles.

Central pain in paraplegics

Injury to the spinal cord is associated with an estimated risk of 5–25% of the development of an intractable pain syndrome [28,42–49]. In contradistinction to brachial plexus avulsion pain, the discomfort may arise months or even years after the injury [43]. In fact, particularly late-onset pain may herald the development of a post-traumatic syringomyelia at and above the injury site [18]. The pain is described much as is that which occurs after brachial plexus avulsion, and can usually be divided into two components. In the first type, patients may complain of exquisite sensitivity of the transitional zone of decreased perception at and just below the level of injury. Light tactile stimulation of this region may produce lancinating, burning or electrical sensations in the transitional zone or just below it for a segment or two. The second component, which may merge with the first, is radiating or non-radiating pain perceived in the buttock, lower extremities or diffusely below the level of injury.

Pre-operative evaluation of these patients is complicated by issues of spinal stability, as many patients will have had spinal stabilization procedures and instrumentation. Review of plain radiographs is essential to evaluate the status of bony fusion, if any. A persistently unstable spine may require re-fusion, particularly following the laminectomy required to perform the DREZ lesions. A pre-operative myelogram or intrathecally enhanced CT scan is helpful to assess the status of the spinal cord, to inspect for arachnoiditis, spinal cord tethering, blockage of CSF flow, spinal cord atrophy, or extradural fibrosis. Delayed CT scanning 6 h after instillation of intrathecal contrast may reveal syringomyelia [18,50]. In cases without metallic instrumentation, the MRI (magnetic resonance imaging) scan is the diagnostic procedure of choice.

Postherpetic neuralgia

The clinical features of postherpetic neuralgia (PHN) are described in detail in Chapter 9 [51–54].

As early as 1891, Barensprung described inflammation in the dorsal ganglion of patients with herpes zoster. Later studies have demonstrated that the inflammatory process spreads distally along the peripheral nerves, causing atrophy of the large myelinated fibers, and centrally along the roots and meninges [55]. Autopsy studies have demonstrated inflammatory changes in the dorsal and ventral horns of the spinal cord [56,57]. These neuropathologic findings indicate that the dorsal root ganglion cell is the primary target of the viral infection, and that the resultant pain is usually associated with some degree of deafferentation.

Patients typically complain of two types of pain. The first is a constant burning aching pain often associated with a region of allodynia. Pain is often triggered in this region by light tactile stimulation of the atrophic and scarred cutaneous areas of previous vesicular eruption. The second pain is a deep itching or formication ('crawling') feeling. As with the other deafferentation syndromes, pharmacologic management is usually only partially effective (*see* Chapter 10), and neurodestructive techniques have not provided lasting benefit. Several recent reviews have described the experience with both medical and surgical management of PHN in detail [51,53,54, and *see* Chapter 9].

Following their experience with brachial plexus avulsion and other deafferentation pain states, Nashold and his group applied DREZ lesion surgery to patients with intractable postherpetic pain. The surgical technique involved laminectomies two vertebral levels above the affected dermatomes. The DREZ to be coagulated was localized with the assistance of direct spinal cord evoked potentials produced by monopolar stimulation of the intercostal nerve root immediately adjacent to the area affected by the herpes. The intercostal nerve was stimulated at < 4 Hz, 0.05–0.5 ms pulse duration, and 0.5–5 V amplitude. Averaged evoked potential recordings were obtained from the DREZ. The DREZ of interest was identified as that having the maximal evoked potential (Figure 8.5).

RESULTS OF DREZ SURGERY

The reported results of SPR and DREZ lesion surgery are shown in Tables 8.1 and 8.2, respectively. Representative series of patients are discussed below.

Table 8.1 Results of selective posterior rhizotomy (SPR)

Etiologies	No. of cases	Results on spontaneous pain		Results on hyperalgesia		Follow-up range
		Good (> 50%) n	(< 50%) n	Good (> 50%) n	(< 50%) n	
Group I (pure neurogenic pain): 42 cases						
Post-amputation (stump 3, stump + phantom 1)	4	3	1	1	0	2–14 years
Peripheral nerve injury (trauma 2, post-surgical 2)	4	3	1	2	0	16m–4 years
Brachial plexus injury (avulsion)	8	3	5	2	1	15m–13 years
Brachial plexopathy (post-radiation Rx)	3	1	1	1	0	3–4 years
Herpes zoster	4	0	4	4	0	3–13 years
Cervical (1) or thoracic (6) cord lesions	7	5	2	2	0	
Conus medullaris lesions	8 }16*	8 }14	0 }2	1 }4	0 }0	6m–7 years
Cauda equina lesions *	1	1	0	1	0	
Total:	42	25	16	15	2	
Miscellaneous						
Idiopathic perineal pain	1	1	0	0	0	3 years
Reflex sympathetic dystrophy	1	0	1	0	1	13 years
Thalamic syndrome	1	0	1	1	0	4 years
Group II (pain associated with spasticity): 57 cases						
Lower limbs (bilateral 39, unilateral 3) (MS, trauma, . . .)	42	40	2	7	4	6m–14 years
Upper limb (unilateral)(trauma, stroke, . . .)	15	14	.	1	0	13m–13 years
Total:	57	54	3	8	4	
Overall results	99 cases	79	19	23	6	

From Sindou, M. and Daher, A. Spinal cord ablation procedures for pain. In *Proceedings of the Vth World Congress on Pain* (ed. R. Dubner, G. F. Gebhart and M. R. Bond), Elsevier, Amsterdam, pp. 477–495 (1988), with permission.

* Origin: trauma 11, gunshot 1, tumor 2, Pott 1, post-surgical 1.

Brachial plexus avulsion

Sindou and Daher [5] reported eight cases of pain associated with brachial plexus avulsion, with follow-up ranging from 15 months to 13 years, all subjected to SPR. Three of eight (37.5%) patients reported good (> 50%) relief of spontaneous pain. Of the three patients in this group with cutaneous hyperalgesia, two (66%) reported good postoperative pain relief. There were no reported complications in this group.

The most complete reporting of Nashold's results with RF DREZ lesions [58] for brachial plexus avulsion pain with follow-up of up to 10 years indicated that 45 of 57 (79%) patients had good results. Careful follow-up (14 months to 10 years) in 39 of these cases demonstrated lasting good results in 54%. Furthermore, multiple closely spaced lesions seemed to produce the best long-term results [61]. With recent refinements in the technique, minor neurological morbidity can be expected in approximately 5%.

Dr David Thomas at the National Hospital in London has likewise reported on the results of RF DREZ procedures performed in 41 patients, 34 of whom had brachial plexus avulsion pain, mainly resulting from motorcycle accidents [62]. He found that after a follow-up interval of 4–44 months, pain relief was good (> 75% pain relief) in 62%, fair (25–75% relief) in 24%, and poor (< 25% relief) in 14%. Of the 21 patients followed for at least 18 months, good pain relief persisted in 12 (57%), and fair relief persisted in six (29%). In 17 cases out of 34 there were no postoperative changes in sensorimotor function. However, there were minor motor changes in nine cases (27%), sensory changes in 4 cases (12%), and both motor and sensory changes in another 4 cases (12%).

Samii and Moringlane [63] have reported 22 patients with brachial plexus avulsion pain that underwent RF DREZ as long as four years before follow-up: 17 patients (77%) had very good pain relief (> 70%), three had good relief (14%) and in two cases (9%) there was a fair result (< 50%). Although 18 patients of his entire series of 35 cases (51%) with DREZ lesions for a variety of indications complained about slight ipsilateral leg weakness, sensory loss or paresthesias postoperatively, none of the patients suffered permanent deficit attributable to the surgical procedure.

Smaller series have been compiled by a number of other groups. Richter and Seitz [64] and Dieckmann and Veras [65] have reported good results with the RF DREZ lesion procedure in 75% and 78% of patients, respectively. Young *et al.* [66] compared the results of RF lesions using current monitoring or temperature monitoring with those after laser DREZ lesion. They found that RF lesions performed without and with temperature monitoring gave good results in four out of six (67%) and five out of seven (71%) cases, respectively, whereas CO_2 laser lesions produced good results in only two out of four (50%).

Moossy *et al.* [59] described the experience of Nashold's group with conus medullaris root avulsions. Pain secondary to these lesions was considered to have an etiology similar to that after brachial plexus avulsion. However, lumbosacral root avulsion pain responded even more favorably, with 83% showing good long-term pain relief after DREZ lesions to the conus.

Thus, RF DREZ lesions performed for pain associated with brachial plexus avulsion can be expected to produce favorable results in approximately 75% of cases. The role of laser DREZ lesions and SPR for this disorder cannot be evaluated fully, because of the relatively small number of cases performed. Nevertheless, DREZ surgery for this type of chronic pain appears to be by far the most efficacious treatment available.

Table 8.2 Documented results of DREZ surgery

Authors and follow-up	No. of cases	Technique*	Brachial plexus avulsion	Lumbosacral avulsion	Spinal cord injury	Cauda equina injury	Post-amputation	Post-herpetic	Miscellaneous[†]	Complications below the lesion[‡]
Nashold et al. 6m–10 years	158	RF	47/57[a] (80%)	5/6[b] (83%)	23/56[c] (50%)		8/22[d] (36%)	10/17[e] (59%)		RF (amp) M: 50% S: 71% RF (t°)
Samii et al. ≤ 4 years	33	RF	20/22 (90%)		4/5 (80%)		1/2 (50%)		MS 1/1; periph. nerve 2/2	51% (M,S)
Richter et al. 6–30 m	10	RF	6/8 (75%)		0/2 (0%)					44% (M,S)
Thomas et al. 4–44m	34	RF	20/34 (58%)							50% (M,S)
Dieckmann et al. 2–16m	18	RF	7/9 (78%)		0/2 (0%)		4/5 (80%)	0/1 (0%)	arachn. 0/1	22% (M,S)
Young et al. ≤ 5 years	21	RF (amp)	4/6 (67%)	1/2 (50%)	3/5 (60%)	2/2 (100%)	2/3 (67%)	2/3 (67%)		52% (M,S)
	26	RF (t°)	5/7 (71%)	2/2 (100%)	4/8 (50%)	2/2 (100%)	2/3 (67%)	3/4 (75%)		4% (M,S)
	20	CO$_2$L	2/4 (50%)	0/1 (0%)	3/6 (50%)	1/2 (50%)	1/2 (50%)	2/5 (40%)		15% (M,S)
Powers et al. 2–19m	21	Ar L	2/2 (100%)		6/7 (85%)		2/3 (67%)		arachn. 1/3; post-rhiz. 2/2; periph. nerve 0/3	10% (S)

	N	Lesion									
Levy *et al.*	3	CO_2 L	1/1 (100%)		0/1 (0%)					arachn.	0%
Malin and Winkelmuller 9m–2 years	4	RF	3/4 (75%)								?
Krause and Balakrishnan	7	RF (amp)	4/7 (57%)								43% (M,S)
Total	355		119/161 (74%)	8/11 (73%)	43/92 (47%)	5/6 (83%)	20/40 (50%)	17/30 (57%)		7/13 (54%)	RF (amp 50%; RF (t°) 5%; Laser 0–10%

Depicted as good results/total patients (N/N)

* RF, radiofrequency; amp, current-controlled RF lesions; t°, temperature-controlled RF lesions; CO_2 carbon dioxide; Ar, argon; L, laser

† multiple sclerosis; periph. nerve, peripheral nerve lesion; arachn., lumbar arachnoiditis; post. rhiz., posterior rhizotomy

‡ M, motor, S, sensory. Superscripts a, b, c, d, e, refer to references 58, 59, 43, 60 and 52, respectively.

Adapted from Sindou, M. and Daher, A. Spinal cord ablation procedures for pain. In *Proceedings of the Vth World Congress on Pain* (ed. R. Dubner, G. F. Gebhart and M. R. Bond). Elsevier, Amsterdam, pp. 477–495 (1988) with permission.

Central pain in paraplegics

The results of DREZ lesions for relief of pain related to spinal cord injury have most recently been reported by Friedman and Nashold [43]. Fifty-six patients with intractable pain following spinal cord injury were treated at Duke with RF DREZ lesions, and evaluated from 6 months to 6 years postoperatively. Patients with good results were defined as either pain free, or having minimal pain not requiring analgesics. The fair pain relief group included those patients using supplemental non-narcotic analgesia, and a poor result was a patient requiring narcotic analgesia postoperatively. By these criteria, 28 (50%) of patients had good pain relief following DREZ lesion, five (9%) were afforded fair pain relief, and 23 (41%) received poor pain relief. These statistics are comparable to those of Young *et al.* [66] using either RF or laser DREZ lesions.

In the spinal cord injury patients, the distribution of the pain seems to be of considerable prognostic significance. Unilateral pain seems to respond particularly well [43]. Pains that are described as beginning at the physiologic level of the spinal cord injury and extending caudally for a variable number of dermatomes respond well. In Nashold's series, good results were seen in this particular sub-group in 74% of patients. In contrast, pains that are characterized as diffusely involving the body caudal to the level of spinal cord injury, or predominantly midline perineosacral, respond very poorly, only 20% obtaining good relief of pain in Nashold's experience [43]. Powers *et al.* [32] and Young *et al.* [66] have made similar observations. This diffuse pain caudal to the spinal cord injury level, does not appear to be generated in the dorsal horn, as extending the lesions from the level of the injury down into the sacral dermatomes does not affect it. The author has had similar results with extensive DREZ lesions in patients with spinal cord injuries. These findings suggest that this nociceptive input may originate at suprasegmental levels.

Of Nashold's 56 patients, nine experienced CSF leak (16%) and two required further surgery to correct this. Three patients experienced new weakness (5%), and two patients complained of new dysesthesias (4%). Recurrence of pain in surgical failures was typically reported within 3 months (21/23 treatment failures).

Sindou and Daher [5] observed that patients with what they termed purely 'neurogenic' pain after spinal cord injury (trauma, gunshot, tumor, Pott's disease, or post-surgical) respond well to SPR at the involved levels. Fourteen of 16 patients (8%) with pain related to cord injury had a good result (> 50% relief) at follow-up of 6 months to 7 years. A mixed, but related group of 57 cases were those he described as having pain associated with spasticity of either the lower limbs (42 cases secondary to trauma, multiple sclerosis, etc.) or upper limbs (15 cases from trauma, stroke, etc.). These cases responded with good results 96% and 93% of the time, respectively. In this latter group of 57 there were two deaths (4%) related to respiratory failure in severely impaired MS patients, and one patient (2%) manifested a postoperative Brown-Séquard syndrome.

Postherpetic neuralgia

The latest follow-up from Nashold's series is a report of 17 cases that underwent DREZ lesion surgery, and were reviewed 6–25 months postoperatively [52]. Ten patients of this group reported good pain relief (59%), and one patient had partial relief (6%). In the initial four patients in this group, DREZ lesions were made without the benefit of a temperature-monitoring probe; all four of these patients experienced ipsilateral leg weakness postoperatively. However, at follow-up 6 weeks postoperatively, three of these patients had improved significantly and showed no obvious impairment of gait. Subsequent patients had DREZ lesions using a temperature-monitored electrode, and no patient in the later group showed more than a minor weakness of iliopsoas ipsilaterally. All of the patients had a change in touch sensation for a variable number of dermatomes below the level of the lesions. Many of the patients also noted pain in the region of the laminectomy. Thus, the risk of major morbidity from a temperature-controlled DREZ lesion for PHN in Nashold's hands appears to be in the range of 6%. Young *et al.* have reported a small series using both RF and laser DREZ techniques with good results, ranging from 75% for a temperature-monitored RF electrode to 40% for the CO_2 laser [66].

In a manner similar to the experience with central pain after spinal cord injury, the nature and distribution of the pain predicted the outcome from DREZ lesion surgery. In PHN, pain that is described by the sufferer as superficial with a burning quality, exacerbated by light stroking of the skin surrounding anesthetic scars, was routinely relieved after DREZ lesion [52]. Pain identified as deep cramping, or constricting, often occurring in untriggered paroxysms, did not respond as well [67].

OTHER INDICATIONS FOR DREZ SURGERY: PAINS OF PERIPHERAL ORIGIN

Post-amputation pain

DREZ lesions have a limited, but definite, role in the management of postamputation pain. Saris *et al.* [60] have reported a series of 22 cases with limb amputations of various causes, and either phantom pain, stump pain or both. Follow-up was 6 months to 4 years. Only eight patients had pain relief, no patient with stump pain alone had relief, and only two of seven patients with stump and phantom pain were improved. However, good results were obtained in six of nine (67%) patients with phantom pain alone, and five of six (83%) patients with traumatic amputations associated with root avulsion.

Using RF DREZ lesions, Young *et al.* [66] have similarly obtained good results in 67% of a group of postamputation pain patients. In a small series of patients, Dieckmann and Veras [65] have also found that phantom pain after amputation is reduced in 80% of cases after DREZ lesion. Sindou and Daher [5] found that SPR also relieved either stump or stump and phantom pain in three of four cases (75%) after follow-up of 2–14 years.

Thus, DREZ lesions may be used for postamputation pain, but at present it appears that they are most useful in cases in which phantom rather than stump pain, possibly due to neuromata, predominates.

Peripheral neuropathy

A few cases of pain associated with peripheral nerve lesions treated with DREZ surgery have been reported. Nashold *et al.* [18] treated five cases of median or ulnar painful traumatic neuropathy with RF DREZ lesions and four (80%) were improved at 6–12-month follow-up. Samii and Moringlane [63] had good results with RF DREZ in two patients with peripheral nerve lesions. In three out of four (75%) cases of peripheral nerve injury, Sindou and Daher [5] had good results with SPR. Therefore, despite the small numbers of reported operations, the results seem promising.

OTHER SURGICAL PROCEDURES FOR DEAFFERENTATION PAIN

Several other surgical procedures may also be considered for patients with deafferentation pain. Neurostimulation techniques may be worth consideration, and are non-destructive. Epidural spinal cord stimulation can be effective for the segmental pains of paraplegics that occur at the transition zone between normal and absent sensation, and in patients with postherpetic neuralgia. Peripheral nerve stimulation is usually quite effective for control of pain related to nerve injury [68]. Recently, deep brain stimulation (DBS) in the region of the periventricular or periaqueductal gray, or thalamus, has been shown to be effective for a number of types of deafferentation pains [69,70]. For further discussion of surgical treatments of pain *see* Chapter 7.

References

1. Sindou, M. *Etude de la Jonction Radiculo-medullaire Posterieure: la Radicellotomie Posterieure Selective dans la Chirurgie de la Douleur.* These Med., Lyon, p. 182 (1972)
2. Sindou, M., Fischer, G. and Baleydier, C. Fiber organization at the posterior spinal cord-rootlet junction in man. *Journal of Comparative Neurology*, **153**, 15–26 (1974)
3. Mansuy, L. and Sindou, M. Physiology of pain at spinal cord level: neurosurgical aspects. In *Neurological Surgery. International Congress Series, no. 433* (ed. R. Carrea), Excerpta Medica, Amsterdam, pp. 257–263 (1978)
4. Sindou, M., Mifsud, J. J., Boisson, D. and Goutelle, A. Selective posterior rhizotomy in the dorsal root entry zone for the treatment of hyperspasticity and pain in the hemiplegic upper limb. *Neurosurgery*, **18**, 587–595 (1986)
5. Sindou, M. and Daher, A. Spinal cord ablation procedures for pain. In *Proceedings of the Vth World Congress on Pain* (ed. R. Dubner, G. F. Gebhart and M. R. Bond), Elsevier, Amsterdam, pp.477–495 (1988)
6. Sindou, M. and Goutelle, A. Surgical posterior rhizotomies for the treatment of pain. In *Advances and Technical Standards in Neurosurgery* (ed. H. Krayenbuhl), Springer-Verlag, Wien, pp. 147–185 (1983)
7. Nashold, B. S., Jr, Urban, B. and Zorub, D. S. Phantom relief by focal destruction of substantia gelatinosa of Rolando. *Advances in Pain Research Therapy*, **1**, 959–963 (1976)
8. Coggeshall, R. E., Applebaum, M. L., Fazen, M. *et al.* Unmyelinated axons in human ventral roots, a possible explanation for the failure of dorsal rhizotomy to relieve pain. *Brain*, **98**, 157–166 (1975)
9. Coggeshall, R. E. and Ito, H. Sensory fibres in ventral roots L$_7$ and S$_1$ in the cat. *Journal of Physiology*, **267**, 215–235 (1977)
10. Willis, W. D. *The Pain System*, Karger, Basel, p. 346 (1985)
11. Denny-Brown, D., Kirk, E. J. and Yanagisawa, N. The tract of Lissauer in relation to sensory transmission in the dorsal horn of spinal cord in the macaque monkey. *Journal of Comparative Neurology*, **151**, 175–200 (1973)

12. LeBars, D., Guilbaud, G., Jurna, I. *et al.* Differential effects of morphine on responses of dorsal horn lamina V type cells elicited by A and C fiber stimulation in the spinal cat. *Brain Research*, **115**, 518–524 (1976)
13. Light, A. R. and Perl, E. R. Spinal termination of functionally identified primary afferent neurons with slowly conducting myelinated fibers. *Journal of Comparative Neurology*, **186**, 133–150 (1979)
14. Zieglgansberger, W. and Bayerl, H. The mechanisms of inhibition of neuronal activity by opiates in the spinal cord of the cat. *Brain Research*, **115**, 111–128 (1976)
15. Blumenkopf, B. Neuropharmacology of the dorsal root entry zone. *Neurosurgery*, **15**, 900–903 (1984)
16. Howe, J. R. and Zieglgansberger, W. Spinal peptidergic and catecholaminergic systems and nociception. *Neurosurgery*, **15**, 904–912 (1984)
17. Yaksh, T. L. and Stevens, C. W. Properties of the modulation of spinal nociceptive transmission by receptor-selective agents. In *Proceedings of the Vth World Congress on Pain*, (ed. R. Dubner, G. F. Gebhart and M. R. Bond), Elsevier, Amsterdam, pp. 417–435 (1988)
18. Nashold, B. S., Jr, Higgins, A. C. and Blumenkopf, B. Dorsal root entry zone lesions for pain relief. In *Pain* (ed. P. D. Wall and R. Melzack), Churchill Livingstone, Edinburgh, pp. 2433–2437 (1984)
19. Loeser, J. D. and Ward, A. A., Jr. Some effects of deafferentation on neurons of the cat spinal cord. *Archives of Neurology*, **17**, 629–636 (1967)
20. Kjerulf, T. D. and Loeser, J. D. Neuronal hyperactivity following deafferentation of the lateral cuneate nucleus. *Experimental Neurology*, **39**, 70–85 (1973)
21. Basbaum, A. I. and Wall, P. D. Chronic changes in the response of cells in adult cat dorsal horn following partial deafferentation: The appearance of responding cells in a previously non-responsive region. *Brain Research*, **116**, 181–204 (1976)
22. Brinkhus, H. B. and Zimmermann, M. Characteristics of spinal dorsal horn neurons after partial chronic deafferentation by dorsal root transection. *Pain*, **15**, 221–236 (1983)
23. Pubols, L. M. and Goldberger, M. E. Recovery of function in dorsal horn following partial deafferentation. *Journal of Neurophysiology*, **43**, 102–118 (1980)
24. Teasdale, R. D. and Stravraky, G. W. Responses to deafferented spinal neurons to corticospinal impulses. *Journal of Neurophysiology*, **16**, 367–375 (1953)
25. Ovelmen-Levitt, J., Johnson, B., Bedenbaugh, P. and Nashold, B. S., Jr. Dorsal root rhizotomy and avulsion in the cat: A comparison of long-term effects on dorsal horn neuronal activity. *Neurosurgery*, **15**, 921–927 (1984)
26. Devor, M. and Wall, P. D. Reorganization of spinal cord sensory map after peripheral nerve injury. *Nature*, **276**, 75–76 (1978)
27. Swerdlow, M. The treatment of shooting pain. *Postgraduate Medical Journal*, **56**, 159–161 (1980)
28. Melzack, R. and Loeser, J. D. Phantom body pain in paraplegia: Evidence for a central 'pattern generating mechanism' for pain. *Pain*, **4**, 195–210 (1979)
29. Pagni, C. A. Central pain and painful anesthesia: Pathophysiology and treatment of sensory deprivation syndromes due to central and peripheral nervous system lesions. *Progress in Neurological Surgery*, **8**, 132–257 (1976)
30. Sweet, W. H. and Poletti, C. E. Operations in the brain stem and spinal cord, with an appendix on open cordotomy. In *Pain*, (ed. P. D. Wall and R. Melzack), Churchill Livingstone, Edinburgh, pp. 615–631 (1984)
31. Levy, W. J., Nutkiewicz, A., Ditmore, Q. M. *et al.* Laser-induced dorsal root entry zone lesions for pain control. *Journal of Neurosurgery*, **59**, 884–886 (1983)
32. Powers, S. K., Adams, J. E., Edwards, S. B. *et al.* Pain relief from dorsal root enry zone lesions made with argon and carbon dioxide microsurgical lasers. *Journal of Neurosurgery*, **61**, 841–847 (1984)
33. Nashold, B. S., Jr and Ostdahl, R. H. Dorsal root entry zone lesions for pain relief. *Journal of Neurosurgery*, **51**, 59–69 (1979)
34. Campbell, J. A. and Miles, J. Evoked potentials as an aid to lesion making in the dorsal root entry zone. *Neurosurgery*, **15**, 951–952 (1984)
35. Nashold, B. S., Jr, Ovelmen-Levitt, J., Sharpe, R. *et al.* Intraoperative evoked potentials recorded in man directly from dorsal roots and spinal cord. *Journal of Neurosurgery*, **62**, 680–693 (1985)
36. Richter, H-P and Schachenmayr, W. Is the substantia gelatinosa the target in dorsal root entry zone lesions? An autopsy report. *Neurosurgery*, **15**, 913–916 (1984)
37. Iacono, R. P., Aguirre, M. L. and Nashold, B. S., Jr. Anatomic examination of human DREZ lesions. *Applied Neurophysiology*, **51**, 225–229 (1988)
38. Nashold, B. S., Jr. Deafferentation pain in man and animals as it relates to the DREZ operation. *Canadian Journal of Neurological Sciences*, **15**, 5–9 (1988)
39. Parry, C. B. W. Pain in avulsion of the brachial plexus. *Neurosurgery*, **15**, 960–965 (1984)

40. Malin, J-P and Winkelmuller, W. Phantom phenomenon (phantom arm) following cervical root avulsion. Effect of dorsal root entry zone thermocoagulation. *European Archives of Psychiatry and Neurological Science*, **235**, 53–56 (1985)
41. Krause, B. L. and Balakrishnan, V. Dorsal root entry zone radiofrequency lesion for pain relief in brachial plexus avulsion. *New Zealand Medical Journal*, **99**, 851–853 (1986)
42. Nashold, B. S., Jr and Bullitt, E. Dorsal root entry zone lesions to control central pain in paraplegics. *Journal of Neurosurgery*, **55**, 414–419 (1981)
43. Friedman, A. H. and Nashold, B. S., Jr. DREZ lesions for relief of pain related to spinal cord injury. *Journal of Neurosurgery*, **65**, 465–469 (1986)
44. Botterell, E. H., Callaghan, J. C. and Jousse, A. T. Pain in paraplegia. Clinical management and surgical treatment. *Proceedings of the Royal Society of Medicine*, **47**, 281–288 (1954)
45. Davis, L. and Martin, J. Studies upon spinal cord injuries. II. The nature and treatment of pain. *Journal of Neurosurgery*, **4**, 483–491 (1947)
46. Kuhn, W. G., Jr. The care and rehabilitation of patients with injuries of the spinal cord and cauda equina. A preliminary report on 113 cases. *Journal of Neurosurgery*, **4**, 40–68 (1947)
47. Munro, D. Two-year end-results in the total rehabilitation of veterans with spinal-cord and cauda-equina injuries. *New England Journal of Medicine*, **242**, 1–16 (1950)
48. Nepomuceno, C., Gowens, H., Stover, S. L. *et al.* Pain in the spinal cord injured. *Archives of Physical Medicine*, **58**, 532–533 (1977)
49. White, J. C. and Sweet, W. H. *Pain and the Neurosurgeon: A Forty Year Experience*, Charles C. Thomas, Springfield, Illinois (1969)
50. Osborne, D. R. S., Vavoulis, G., Nashold, B. S., Jr *et al.* Late sequelae of spinal-cord trauma: myelographic and surgical correlation. *Journal of Neurosurgery*, **57**, 18–23 (1982)
51. Watson, P. N. and Evans, R. J. Postherpetic neuralgia. *Archives of Neurology*, **43**, 836–840 (1986)
52. Friedman, A. H. and Nashold, B. S. Jr. Dorsal root entry zone lesions for the treatment of postherpetic neuralgia. *Neurosurgery*, **15**, 969–970 (1984)
53. Portenoy, R. K., Duma, C. and Foley, K. M. Acute herpetic and postherpetic neuralgia: Clinical review and current management. *Annals of Neurology*, **20**, 651–664 (1986)
54. Loeser, J. D. Herpes zoster and postherpetic neuralgia. *Pain*, **25**, 149–164 (1986)
55. Denny-Brown, D., Adams, R. D. and Fitzgerald, P. J. Pathologic features of herpes zoster: a note on 'geniculate' herpes. *Archives of Neurology and Psychiatry*, **51**, 215–231 (1944)
56. Smith, F. P. Pathological studies of spinal nerve ganglia in relation to intractable intercostal pain. *Surgical Neurology*, **10**, 50–53 (1978)
57. Watson, C. P. N., Morshead, C., Van der Kooy, D. *et al.* Postherpetic neuralgia: Postmortem analysis of a case. *Pain*, **54**, 123–158 (1988)
58. Nashold, B. S., Jr. Current status of the DREZ operation: 1984. *Neurosurgery*, **15**, 942–944 (1984)
59. Moossy, J. J., Nashold, B. S., Jr, Osborne, D. and Friedman, A. H. Conus medullaris nerve root avulsions. *Journal of Neurosurgery*, **66**, 835–841 (1987)
60. Saris, S. C., Iacono, R. P. and Nashold, B. S., Jr. Dorsal root entry zone lesions for post-amputation pain. *Journal of Neurosurgery*, **62**, 72–76 (1985)
61. Friedman, A. H., Nashold, B. S. Jr and Bronec, P. R. Dorsal root entry zone lesions for the treatment of brachial plexus avulsion injuries: A follow-up study. *Neurosurgery*, **22**, 369–373 (1988)
62. Thomas, D. G. T. and Jones, S. J. Dorsal root entry zone lesions (Nashold's procedure) in brachial plexus avulsion. *Neurosurgery*, **15**, 966–968 (1984)
63. Samii, M. and Moringlane, J. R. Thermocoagulation of the dorsal root entry zone for the treatment of intractable pain. *Neurosurgery*, **15**, 953–955 (1984)
64. Richter, H-P. and Seitz, K. Dorsal root entry zone lesions for the control of deafferentation pain: Experiences in ten patients. *Neurosurgery*, **15**, 956–959 (1984)
65. Dieckmann, G. and Veras, G. High-frequency coagulation of dorsal root entry zone in patients with deafferentation pain. *Acta Neurochirurgica*, Suppl. 33, 445–450 (1984)
66. Young, R. F., Foley, K., Israel, Chambi V. *et al.* Dorsal root entry zone lesions: Part I: a comparison of radiofrequency and laser techniques; Part II: clinical experience in 67 patients over five years. *Journal of Neurosurgery*, 1989, in press
67. Friedman, A. H., Nashold, B. S., Jr. and Ovelmen-Levitt, J. Dorsal root entry zone lesions for the treatment of post-herpetic neuralgia. *Journal of Neurosurgery*, **60**, 1258–1262 (1984)
68. Waisbrod, H., Panhans, C., Hansen, D. *et al.* Direct nerve stimulation for painful peripheral neuropathies. *Journal of Bone and Joint Surgery*, **67**, 470–472 (1985)
69. Young, R. F., Kroening, R., Fulton, W. *et al.* Electrical stimulation of the brain in treatment of chronic pain. Experience over 5 years. *Journal of Neurosurgery*, **62**, 389–396 (1985)
70. Hosobuchi, Y. Subcortical electrical stimulation for control of intractable pain in humans. Report of 122 cases (1970–1984). *Journal of Neurosurgery*, **64**, 543–553 (1986)

9
Postherpetic neuralgia: clinical features and treatment

C. P. N. Watson

INTRODUCTION

Postherpetic neuralgia (PHN) is a common cause of neuropathic pain which can be quite difficult to manage. The natural history, clinical and pathologic features are becoming clearer and a concept of the pathogenesis of the pain can be formulated. There has been a confusing variety of published therapeutic approaches over the years, mainly because of a lack of controls and failure to understand the importance of the natural history of the condition. Despite the fact that there is no panacea for all patients, the pain is ameliorated by treatment in many patients as well as improving with time. This chapter gives an overview of the clinical features of PHN and emphasizes guidelines for management based on the literature and on the author's experience.

ORIGIN

PHN is a consequence of herpes zoster (HZ) which is caused by re-activation of the varicella zoster virus (VZV) usually contracted in childhood. On initial exposure, VZV causes varicella in which the virus disseminates hematogenously from the nasopharynx to the skin and mucous membranes. Later in the course of the illness it is presumed to enter sensory nerve fibres and to be transported to the trigeminal, geniculate and dorsal root ganglia where it comes to be dormant for many years. It is thought that with declining immune surveillance accompanying advancing age, or because of an immunocompromised state, the virus re-erupts in the sensory ganglion to cause a hemorrhagic inflammatory reaction and to re-infect segmental skin and mucous membrane areas and occasionally the spinal cord and meninges in the manifestation referred to as herpes zoster. This disorder is often very painful, either before the rash for up to two weeks, during or after the rash appears. Usually this pain subsides but if it persists or recurs with healing it is referred to as PHN.

DEFINITION OF PHN

In the broadest sense PHN is pain occurring in the dermatomal distribution affected by herpes zoster. It is important to be more precise than this because the management of pain occurring immediately in association with the rash probably differs in most cases from that of pain persisting after the rash has healed. Certainly the pathologic features of HZ and PHN are quite dissimilar. Interpretation of published therapies depends on this discrimination also because of the pain's natural history. A reasonable definition of PHN is pain persisting after 1 month, the time it usually takes the rash to heal.

NATURAL HISTORY AND EFFECT OF AGE

The incidence of PHN (as previously defined as pain persisting for > 1 month) has been variously estimated at 9% [1], 9.7% [2] and 14.3% [3]. Of these cases 35% [4] to 55% [1] still had pain at 3 months and in 22% [1] to 33% [4] severe pain persisted for at least 1 year. Thus of 100 patients, at 3 months as few as five and at one year only three patients continued to suffer severe pain. These data emphasize that any study of the treatment of this disorder should concentrate on patients with severe pain at 1 or even 3 or 6 months to ensure a fairly stable, chronic status. Thirty-three of our 63 patients with severe PHN of duration > 1 year became pain free on no therapy at follow-up assessment. Thus, some longstanding cases may also subside with time.

Despite this overall low incidence and marked tendency for PHN to improve with time, Demoragas and Kierland [4] found that the incidence and the severity (as measured by duration) were directly related to age. Their study revealed that 50% at age 60 years and nearly 75% at age 70 years with herpes zoster developed PHN 1 month or more after the rash.

SEX INCIDENCE AND DERMATOMAL DISTRIBUTION

Hope-Simpson [3], in his study of 46 cases, found that 65% of his cases of PHN occurred in female patients. No sex difference, interestingly, has been found for herpes zoster [1–4].

A study of 208 of our patients revealed that the dermatomal distribution of PHN reflected that of herpes zoster [1,2,5], there being a predilection for thoracic dermatomes, especially T5 and T6, and for the ophthalmic division of the trigeminal nerve (Figure 9.1). This is also demonstrated by Table 9.1 which shows the usual proportion of all dermatomes occupied by trigeminal and thoracic segments in comparison to those affected in PHN.

NATURE OF THE PAIN AND AFFECTED SKIN

Noordenbos [6] described both steady and paroxysmal, brief aspects to the pain experienced. We administered the McGill Pain Questionnaire to 50 patients with severe PHN and found that the most frequent words chosen corroborated these qualities. 'Nagging', 'burning' and 'gnawing' reflected a constant quality. 'Flicker-

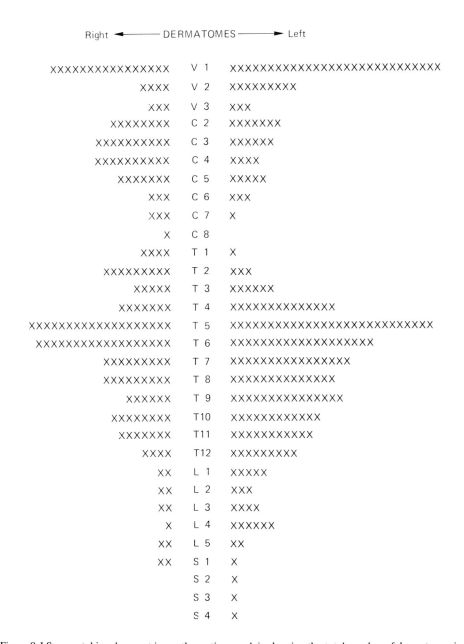

Figure 9.1 Segmental involvement in postherpetic neuralgia showing the total number of dermatomes in 208 patients

Table 9.1 Dermatomal distribution* in 208 cases of postherpetic neuralgia

Dermatomes	Number of patients and dermatomal area affected in each	Patients and dermatomal areas affected (%)	Usual skin area represented by the group of dermatomes (%)
Trigeminal	47	22.59	3.45
Cervical	24	11.55	24.14
Thoracic	115	55.28	41.37
Lumbar	19	9.14	17.25
Sacral	3	1.44	13.79

* Each group of segments expressed as a percentage of all dermatomes affected compared with the usual percentage that each group of segments represents of the dermatomes of the normal skin surface.

ing', 'sharp', 'shooting' and 'stabbing' described a brief component. The descriptor 'tender' was often chosen, referring to aggravation by contact with even the lightest of clothing. Unbearable itch or formication may also be encountered. Physical activity, ambient temperature change and emotional upset were all frequently mentioned by our patients as factors exacerbating their misery.

Shortly after the acute phase has healed, the skin exhibits a reddish, purple or brownish hue. As this fades, silvery or white scarring remains, sometimes with a pigmented border or background. Most of our subjects (Table 9.2) had scarring with reduced or absent appreciation of touch and pinprick. In 40% this sensory reduction extended outside the scarring for a dermatome or more into normal-appearing skin. The exaggerated sensations of hyperesthesia, dysesthesia or allodynia (pain from a non-painful stimulus) were also frequently encountered. A true hyperpathic response was less common and present in 25% of cases.

Table 9.2 Clinical features of affected skin in 158 patients with postherpetic neuralgia

Clinical features	Present (%)	Absent (%)	Uncertain (%)
Scarring	95	5	0
Analgesia or hypalgesia to pinprick	92	5	3
Anesthesia or hypesthesia to light touch	90	8	2
Hyperesthesia, dysesthesia or allodynia to light stroking	65	28	7

PATHOLOGY AND PATHOGENESIS

The pathologic changes occurring in the nervous system with HZ are well known. A hemorrhagic inflammation involves the dorsal aspect of the dorsal root ganglion, peripheral nerve, nerve root and sometimes the leptomeninges and spinal cord [7]. In the months following the acute infection, fibrosis occurs in the dorsal root ganglion [7], peripheral nerve [8] and nerve root [7]. Degeneration occurs in the ipsilateral posterior column by as early as the ninth day after the eruption and disappears by between 5 and 9 months after the onset of the illness [7]. The presence of pain is not stated in most of these longstanding cases. Case 7 of Head and Campbell [7] suffered severe pain at 2 months and died at 3 months after the onset. They found 'sclerosis' in part of the ganglion and peripheral nerve and nerve root. 'Small round cells' were seen around the ganglion and 'degeneration' was seen in the nerve, nerve root and ipsilateral posterior column. Zacks *et al.* [8] looked at nerves peripherally near scarred skin in four subjects. Two of these had pain, 2 and 14 months after the rash. The authors found that an early phase of Wallerian degeneration went on to proliferation of collagen, transforming the nerve into a nearly solid mass of fibrous tissue containing rare, small, myelinated fibers. Noordenbos [6] noted a decrease in the number of large myelinated fibers and an increase in small unmyelinated fibers.

Watson *et al.*, in a detailed study of a case of PHN of 4 years' duration [9], found atrophy of the dorsal horn of the affected side over four segments despite fibrosis of only one ganglion. The presence of at least some unmyelinated dorsal root axons was inferred because there was no reduction in substance P staining in the dorsal horn. This neurotransmitter is utilized by small-diameter nociceptive afferents and contributes significantly to the substance P found in this area.

There is, then, evidence in PHN for an imbalance in fiber input (reduced large, inhibitory fibers and intact or increased small, excitatory fibers) to an abnormal dorsal horn which may contain hypersensitive, deafferented neurones. This would account for the fact that clinically both peripheral and central factors seem to be involved in the perceived pain. The pain is obviously influenced by the periphery because normally innocuous stimulation of the skin produces hyperesthesia, dysesthesia and allodynia. Hyperpathia, the failure of surgery involving further peripheral deafferentation and the limited success of dorsal root entry zone (DREZ) lesions suggest a central mechanism. It has been suggested that pain relief in PHN by antidepressants may act by replenishing or increasing a serotonin- or noradrenaline-mediated inhibition of pain transmission [10]

PREVENTION OF PHN

The various therapeutic approaches to preventing PHN are summarized in Table 9.3. A number of uncontrolled studies of small numbers of patients with acute herpes zoster treated with corticosteroids have claimed a reduction in PHN [11–14]. Two controlled studies have demonstrated a preventative effect [15,16]. Eaglstein *et al.* [15] randomly allocated 35 patients with acute herpes zoster in a double-blind fashion to either oral triamcinolone or placebo. Considering patients over 60 years of age, 11 (73%) of 15 of the control group developed PHN versus three (30%) of ten in the steroid-treated group. Merselis *et al.* [17] cautioned about the risk of generalized herpes zoster as a result of steroid therapy of the acute rash in their report of 17 such cases. Neither Eaglstein *et al.* nor Keczkes and Basheer encountered dissemination of the eruption, the latter investigators pointing out that the severely affected patients of Merselis and coworkers all had leukemia or other serious underlying disease and were probably immunosuppressed because of this or the treatment [16]. A recent randomized double-blind placebo-controlled trial compared prednisolone combined with oral acyclovir versus placebo together with acyclovir in HZ [18]. This study found no difference in the incidence of PHN at 6 months follow-up. The acyclovir was given to prevent dissemination of HZ; this trial needs to be substantiated. The bulk of the evidence to date provides

Table 9.3 Agents used to prevent postherpetic neuralgia

Agent	Source	Study population	Effective	No. of patients treated/total	Controlled trial	Randomized	Double-blind
Steroids							
Triamcinolone	Eaglstein et al., 1970 [15]	Herpes zoster	Yes	15/35	Yes	Yes	Yes
Prednisolone	Keczkes and Basheer, 1980 [16]	Herpes zoster	Yes	20/40	Yes	Yes	No
Prednisolone	Esmann et al., 1987 [18]	Herpes zoster	No	39/78	Yes	Yes	Yes
Sympathetic block (1% lidocaine hydrochloride with norepinephrine bitartrate)	Colding 1969 [19] Colding 1973 [20]	Herpes zoster Herpes zoster	Yes Yes	71/303 155/483	No No		
Amantadine hydrochloride	Galbraith 1983 [21]	Herpes zoster	Yes	33/67	Yes	Yes	Yes
Levodopa and benserazide	Kernbaum and Hauchecorne, 1981 [22]	Herpes zoster	Yes at 21 days; no at 60 days	25/47	Yes	Yes	Yes
Vidarabine	Whitley et al., 1976 [25]	Herpes zoster immunosuppressed	Reduced duration but not incidence	63/121	Yes	Yes	Yes
Interferon-α	Merigan et al., 1978 [24]	Herpes zoster, cancer	Reduced severity and duration	45/90	Yes	Yes	Yes

Acyclovir	Peterslund et al., 1981 [27]	Herpes zoster immunocompetent	No	Yes	Low dose, 27/56; High dose, 19/29	Yes	Yes	Yes
	Bean et al., 1982 [29]	Herpes zoster immunocompetent	No	Yes	19/29	Yes	Yes	Yes
	Balfour et al., 1983 [31]	Herpes zoster immunocompromised	No	Yes	94	Yes	Yes	Yes
Acyclovir vs vidarabine	Shepp et al., 1986 [32]	Herpes zoster immunocompromised	No difference	Yes	22	Yes	Yes	No
Adenosine monophosphate	Sklar et al., 1985 [33]	Herpes zoster	Yes	Yes	17/32	Yes	Yes	Yes

reasonable support for the use of moderate doses of an agent such as prednisone (60 mg daily) at the onset of HZ, with gradual reduction in dosage over 2 weeks in the non-immunosuppressed patient.

Colding [19,20] reported that sympathetic blockade with local anesthetic in acute herpes zoster markedly reduced the incidence of PHN. Although he treated a large number of patients in this fashion, his work was uncontrolled, the median age of the group followed was not stated, and a substantial number of patients were unavailable for follow-up.

Galbraith [21] reported a double-blind, placebo-controlled trial of amantadine hydrochloride for the acute illness in a population with a mean age of 70 years. He found a reduction by half in the time taken to achieve total pain relief with this agent. A double-blind placebo-controlled study of levodopa and benserazide [22] claimed a reduction in PHN in patients aged $\geq$ 65 years. Although a difference was detected at 21 days, no such effect was present at 60 days after the onset of the rash. Intramuscular interferon-α reduced both the severity and duration of PHN in patients with malignant neoplasms in two randomized placebo-controlled double-blind studies [23,24]. Intravenous vidarabine reduced the duration but not the incidence of PHN in a double-blind placebo-controlled study of herpes zoster in immunosuppressed patients [25]. The authors concluded that because of its potential toxicity the drug should be reserved for immunocompromised patients. Well-controlled studies [26–30] have shown that acyclovir did not reduce the incidence or severity of PHN in immunocompetent [26–30] or immunocompromised adults [31], although intravenously it shortened the period of acute pain and accelerated cutaneous healing [26–29]. A randomized study that compared acyclovir with vidarabine in immunocompromised patients found no difference in the incidence of PHN at 28 days or more after the rash [32].

A randomized placebo-controlled double-blind trial of intramuscular adenosine monophosphate (AMP) has been reported to reduce PHN markedly [33]. However, the number of patients in this trial was small and concern has been expressed that the groups were not comparable as to severity of disease, and also about the toxicity of AMP in humans [34].

TREATMENT OF PHN

Over the past 50 years the medical literature has contained a bewildering array of medical and surgical approaches to the treatment of PHN (Table 9.4). This has demonstrated the difficulty in managing this disorder. Problems in interpreting some of these studies include a failure to discriminate the pain of acute herpes zoster from true PHN, a failure to appreciate the natural history of the pain, and the lack of adequate controls and follow-up. None the less, some useful practical information may be obtained.

Medical treatment

Antidepressants and neuroleptics

Farber and Burks [35] used high doses of chlorprothixene in patients with postherpetic pain of duration 2 days to 8 weeks. In an uncontrolled study of 30 subjects of unstated age, they found total relief of pain within 72 h in all save one. Nathan [36] attempted to duplicate this work in established PHN (median duration 1 year) by the same method and also by a lower-dose double-blind placebo-controlled study. He concluded that dosages < 100 mg/24 h were ineffective. The higher-dose regimen helped about one-third of patients but only in the short term and with a high incidence of side-effects. Woodforde *et al.* [37] were the first to recognize that amitriptyline hydrochloride could afford relief in truly chronic postherpetic pain problems. They thought that all 14 of their patients were depressed, and that formed their rationale for using the drug. They used an initial dose of 10 mg four times a day, achieving at least good relief in 11 patients for one to 11 months. Merskey and Hester [38] suggested that tricyclic antidepressants and phenothiazines might have an analgesic action, in their discussion of a variety of chronic pain problems, including a description of seven patients with PHN. Taub [39] reported treating five subjects with PHN of > 3 months duration with amitriptyline and a phenothiazine (perphenazine, fluphenazine, or thioridazine). In a later publication, Taub and Collins [40] used amitriptyline hydrochloride, 75 mg every night with fluphenazine, 1 mg three times a day, in 17 patients with pain of duration > 1 year. The subjects in both studies had good relief with some mild residual pain at 6 months to 3 years follow-up. Taub [39] commented on the ineffectiveness of amitriptyline alone, using it mainly to combat the depressive potential of the phenothiazine. Watson *et al.* [10] randomly allocated 24 patients with PHN to treatment with amitriptyline or placebo in a double-blind study, finding good results in 16 (67%) of the 24 patients. Most patients were not depressed, nor could an effect of the drug on depression be found in those who were. Doses of amitriptyline hydrochloride were lower than those used for depression (75 mg median). Follow-up was a median of 12 months, with good results maintained in 12 (55%) of 22. Significant side-effects were few. Of 19 assessable patients, ten maintained a good response at 5 years, with only four receiving amitriptyline and six no medication. A therapeutic window might exist for this drug in some patients, further emphasizing the need to start therapy with small doses (10–25 mg every night) [41].

Anticonvulsants

Studies utilizing the anticonvulsants carbamazepine, phenytoin and valproic acid for PHN have been either unimpressive [42] or difficult to interpret because of the concomitant use of antidepressants [42–45]. Although carbamazepine is a popular agent for the paroxysmal lancinating pain that commonly occurs, there is no conclusive evidence to justify its use in this fashion.

Topical capsaicin

Capsaicin (8-methyl-*N*-vanillyl-6-nonenamide) is the pungent principle of hot paprika or chili peppers. The chemical structure is similar to that of oil of cloves, an old remedy for toothache, which produces a long-lasting trigeminal anesthesia. Capsaicin selectively stimulates and then blocks unmyelinated sensory afferents from skin and mucous membranes [46–50]. Many of these contain substance P, an excitatory peptide neurotransmitter and other neurotransmitters such as calcitonin gene-related peptide and somatostatin. It is thought that capsaicin initially releases

Table 9.4 Treatment of postherpetic neuralgia (PHN)

Treatment mode	Source	Agent	PHN (>1 month)	Effective	Number of subjects	Controlled trial	Crossover	Randomized	Double-blind
Anti-depressants	Farber and Burks, 1974 [35]	Chlorprothixene	Some	Yes	30	No			
	Nathan, 1978 [36]	Chlorprothixene	Yes	No No	(A) 13 (B) 19	Yes No	Yes	Yes	Yes
	Woodforde et al., 1965 [37]	Amitriptyline	Yes	Yes	14	No			
	Taub, 1973 [39]	Amitriptyline and perphenazine or fluphenazine or thioridazine	Yes	Yes	5	No			
	Taub and Collins, 1974 [40]	Amitriptyline plus fluphenazine	Yes	Yes	17	No			
	Watson et al., 1982 [10]	Amitriptyline	Yes	Yes	24	Yes	Yes	Yes	Yes
Anti-convulsants	Killian and Fromm, 1968 [42]	Carbamazepine	Longstanding	No	6	Yes	No	Yes	Yes
	Hatangdi et al., 1976 [43]	Carbamazepine or phenytoin plus nortriptyline	Yes	Yes	34	No			
	Gerson et al., 1977 [44]	Carbamazepine plus clomipramine	Yes	Yes	16	Yes (TENS)	Yes	Yes	
	Raftery, 1969 [45]	Valproic acid plus amitriptyline	Yes	Yes	10	No	Yes	Yes	No

Treatment	Reference	Method	?		n				
Local anesthetic spray and/or vibration	Russell et al., 1957 [53]	Vibration	?	Yes	100	No			
	Taverner, 1960 [54]	Ethyl chloride	Yes	Yes	16	No			
	Todd et al., 1965 [55]	Ethyl chloride and vibration	Yes	Yes	86	No			
Sympathetic block	Colding, 1969 [19]	1% Lidocaine with noradrenaline	Yes	No	34	No			
	Colding, 1973 [20]	1% Lidocaine with noradrenaline	Yes	No	67	No			
Transcutaneous nerve stimulation (TENS)	Nathan, 1974 [36]	Continuous TENS	Yes	Yes	30	No			
	Gerson et al., 1977 [44]	Intermittent TENS	Yes	No	17	No			
	Haas, 1977 [59]	TENS	Yes	Yes	11	No			
Acupuncture	Lewith et al., 1983 [60]	Acupuncture	Yes	No	30/62	Yes (vs mock TENS)	No	Yes	No
Epidural steroids	Forrest, 1980 [56]	Methyl-prednisolone	Yes	Yes	37	No			
Topical capsaicin	Bernstein et al., 1987 [51]	Capsaicin	Yes	Yes	12	No			
	Watson et al., 1988 [52]	Capsaicin	Yes	Yes	33	No			

and then depletes substance P and that it relieves pain in this fashion. Two open-label studies support an analgesic action of capsaicin ointment in PHN. One of these involved 12 patients and found that 9 (75%) experienced 'substantial relief of pain' [51]; it was not clear how many actually had a good or satisfactory response. We have carried out an open-label trial of 33 patients and found a good response in 56% with some significant change in 79% [52]. Burning after application was a significant problem. Preliminary results from a randomized double-blind parallel trial support these findings. We would suggest the following guidelines for the use of capsaicin:

1. It must be used 4–5 times daily (if used less, it may not effectively deplete substance P).
2. It should be used for 4 weeks. (Patients may not get relief for 2 or 3 weeks.)
3. Patients should be seen regularly to encourage persistence and deal with capsaicin-induced burning.
4. If burning occurs it may be ameliorated by the previous application of 5% lidocaine ointment, by covering a small area of skin initially, and by regular analgesics.
5. Hands should be washed after use to avoid eye exposure by inadvertent contact and the ointment should be kept above the eyebrow and away from the eye if used for ophthalmic nerve involvement.

Miscellaneous therapies

Russell *et al.* [53] advocated repeated nerve blocks, interspinal ligament injection of hypertonic saline solution, or skin infiltration with procaine hydrochloride for relief of hyperesthesia and spontaneous pain in PHN. They also discussed the use of a hand vibrator over the injured skin. Of 100 patients they provided details for only five. No duration of antecedent pain was stated. Taverner [54] reported 16 cases treated with ethyl chloride spray to the scarred area. Symptoms for 12 of these were relieved for 3–21 months, with their pain duration being 10 months to 13 years. The spray was applied daily to twice a week. The author commented on the failure of vibration in his experience, cautioning about the risk of skin injury. Todd *et al.* [55] reported on 86 patients with PHN of at least 3 months: 58 (67%) obtained relief with a combination of ethyl chloride spray followed by the application of a hand vibrator; follow-up was 6 months to 6 years. Colding [19,20] concluded that sympathetic blocks for established PHN were of no value. Forrest [56] treated 37 patients with postherpetic pain of > 6 months' duration with three epidural injections of methylprednisolone acetate at weekly intervals. At 1 year 89% of the patients were free of pain, with 'some patients' followed up for > 3 years. Forrest postulated that the steroid, local anesthetic used, or preservative might be the effective component. In view of the pathologic findings of fibrosis and lack of inflammation, it is difficult to explain how local steroids might be effective; a systemic effect would be one explanation. We have been unable to reproduce this study in an uncontrolled pilot study using the identical protocol, which to date includes 10 patients with PHN of > 3 months' duration and followed up for at least 2 months. Another study [57] of five patients with true PHN, treated with epidural bupivacaine hydrochloride and methylprednisolone, concluded that no patient had more than 50% relief at 1 and 5 months.

Nathan and Wall [58] used prolonged transcutaneous electrical nerve stimulation (TENS) and found good results in 11 of 30 patients with established PHN. Voltage, pulse width, frequency, site of application, and duration were all controlled by the patient. Generally, the subjective sensation of the input was non-painful and tingling. Pain relief often outlasted stimulation by hours. Follow-up duration was not clearly stated in all. Gerson *et al.* [44] found the intermittent use of TENS unsuccessful in 17 patients with chronic PHN. Haas [59] concluded that TENS was helpful in nine of 11 patients, with follow-up over 1–18 months. Lewith *et al.* [60] concluded that acupuncture was of little value in PHN when compared with placebo (mock TENS) in 62 patients. Claims have been made for a variety of other therapies, but these studies suffer from small numbers of patients, lack of controls, inadequate data about the patient population, and/or lack of adequate follow-up.

Surgical treatment

A number of surgical approaches to PHN have been described and discussed over the years. The early literature was reviewed by White and Sweet [61] in their book. Results at that time were generally unsatisfactory and the number of patients studied few. Hitchcock and Schvarcz [62] reported success with stereotaxic trigeminal tractotomy in three cases of ophthalmic PHN with follow-up of 4, 9 and 11 months. Nashold *et al.* [63] described 12 patients with PHN treated by dorsal root entry zone (DREZ) lesions with good results in six for up to 2 years. Friedman *et al.* [64] reported 12 postherpetic DREZ lesions with eight achieving good relief over 6–12 months. They found better relief with superficial burning pain and hyperesthesia than with deep aching pain. No significant postoperative deficits were noted, and they concluded that DREZ lesions were a satisfactory treatment for PHN in patients who failed to respond to conservative measures. Friedman and Nashold [65] also reported 17 DREZ-treated cases of PHN in a separate article, with good results achieved in ten of these at 6–25 months of follow-up.

CONCLUSIONS

Postherpetic pain persisting for 1 month or longer occurs in only a small percentage of all patients with herpes zoster [1–3] and in most patients PHN tends to diminish with time [1]. The incidence is, however, directly related to age [1–4]. Any therapeutic claim for prophylaxis or treatment of PHN has to be evaluated with this in mind. There is some information about the pathologic features [7–9] and a concept of the pathogenesis can be suggested. There is evidence for an imbalance in fiber input (reduced large inhibitory fibers and intact or increased small excitatory fibers) to an abnormal dorsal horn which may contain hypersensitive neurones.

Prevention of PHN remains difficult. There is evidence that systemic steroids exert a preventative effect when employed in the treatment of herpes zoster in the immunocompetent patient without the risk of generalized zoster [15,16]. A reasonable regimen would be 60 mg prednisone with reduction over 10–14 days. One double-blind controlled study supports the use of amantadine in this situation [21]. This would be an option in patients with a contraindication to steroids, such as those with peptic ulcer or diabetes mellitus or those who are immunocompromised. The dosage of amantadine used in this study was 100 mg twice daily for a month.

Although a number of other therapies have been suggested, these remedies remain in need of further, more scientific, study.

For established PHN there is firm support for the reduction of pain from severe to mild in two-thirds of patients by the use of low doses of amitriptyline with gradual, small increments [10]. In the age group > 65 years one may use as small a dose as 10 mg with an increase of 10 mg every 5–7 days. In those younger than 65 a dose of 25 mg to start is reasonable, with increments of 25 mg. Although unproven, the addition of a phenothiazine such as fluphenazine may provide further pain relief [39,40]. Preliminary studies indicate that topical capsaicin may be a useful new treatment [51,52]. Although widely used, there is no good evidence of the use of anticonvulsants alone in this disorder [42–45]. Studies of local anesthetic sprays with vibration [53–55] and continuous TENS [58] are uncontrolled but these modalities may be of some merit. One uncontrolled study reports the benefit of epidural steroids [56]. Dorsal root entry zone (DREZ) lesions are a possibility in failed medical cases [62–65], but other surgical procedures appear to be of little or no use.

Although the measures described above will be of benefit to a number of patients, the management of PHN remains, in some cases, an intractable problem. Therapies such as amantadine and epidural steroids bear corroboration, and some of the older approaches such as local anesthetic sprays, vibration and TENS, need further, more scientific, study. Newer approaches are necessary and one useful avenue may be the exploration of drugs related to or mimicking the action of tricyclic antidepressants. Topical capsaicin is a novel approach which shows promise in preliminary open-label trials and now requires a controlled study.

References

1. Ragozzino, M. W., Melton, L. J., Kirland, L. T. *et al.* Population based study of herpes zoster and its sequelae. *Medicine*, **21**, 310–316 (1982)
2. Burgoon, C. F., Burgoon, J. S. and Baldridge, G. D. The natural history of herpes zoster. *Journal of the American Medical Association*, **164**, 265–269 (1957)
3. Hope-Simpson, R. E. Postherpetic neuralgia. *Journal of the Royal College of General Practitioners*, **25**, 571–575 (1975)
4. Demoragas, J. M. and Kierland, R. R. The outcome of patients with herpes zoster. *Archives of Dermatology*, **75**, 193–196 (1957)
5. Hope-Simpson, R. E. The nature of herpes zoster: a long-term study and a new hypothesis. *Proceedings of the Royal Society of Medicine*, **58**, 9–20 (1965)
6. Noordenbos, W. *Problems Pertaining to the Transmission of Nerve Impulses which give rise to Pain: Preliminary Statement*, Elsevier Science Publishers, Amsterdam, p. 182 (1959)
7. Head, H. and Campbell, A. W. The pathology of herpes zoster and its bearing on sensory localization. *Brain*, **23**, 353–523 (1900)
8. Zacks, S. I., Langfitt, T. W. and Elliott, F. A. Herpetic neuritis: a light and electron microscopic study. *Neurology*, **14**, 744–750 (1964)
9. Watson, C. P. N., Morsehead, C., Vanderkooy, D. and Deck, J. Postherpetic neuralgia postmortem. *Pain*, **34**, 129–138 (1988)
10. Watson, C. P., Evans, R. J., Reed, K. *et al.* Amitriptyline versus placebo in postherpetic neuralgia. *Neurology*, **32**, 670–673 (1982)
11. Eaglstein, W. H., Katz, R. and Brown, J. A. The effects of corticosteroid therapy on the skin eruption and pain of herpes zoster. *Journal of the American Medical Association*, **211**, 1681–1683 (1970)
12. Sauer, G. C. Herpes zoster: Treatment of postherpetic neuralgia with cortisone, corticotropin and placebos. *Archives of Dermatology*, **71**, 488–489 (1955)
13. Elliott, F. A. Treatment of herpes zoster with high doses of prednisone. *Lancet*, **ii**, 610–611 (1964)
14. Pearce, J. Postherpetic neuralgia. *British Medical Journal*, **1**, 679–681 (1973)

15. Eaglstein, W. H., Katz, R. and Brown, J. A. The effects of early corticosteroid therapy on the skin eruption and pain of herpes zoster. *Journal of the American Medical Association*, **211**, 1681–1683 (1970)
16. Keczkes, K. and Basheer, A. M. Do corticosteroids prevent postherpetic neuralgia? *British Journal of Dermatology*, **102**, 551–555 (1980)
17. Merselis, J. G., Kaye, D. and Hook, E. W. Disseminated herpes zoster. *Archives of Internal Medicine*, **113**, 679–686 (1964)
18. Esmann, V., Kroon, S., Peterslund, N. A. *et al*. Prednisolone does not prevent postherpetic neuralgia. *Lancet*, **8551**, 126–129 (1987)
19. Colding, A. The effect of sympathetic blocks on herpes zoster. *Acta anaesthesiologica scandinavica*, **13**, 113–141 (1969)
20. Colding, A. Treatment of pain: Organization of a pain clinic, treatment of herpes zoster. *Proceedings of the Royal Society of Medicine*, **66**, 541–543 (1973)
21. Galbraith, A. W. Treatment of acute herpes zoster with amantadine hydrochloride (Symmetrel). *British Medical Journal*, **4**, 693–695 (1983)
22. Kernbaum, S. and Hauchecorne, J. Administration of levodopa for relief of herpes zoster pain. *Journal of the American Medical Association*, **246**, 132–134 (1981)
23. Merigan, T. C., Gallagher, J. G., Pollard, R. B. *et al*. Short course human leukocyte interferon in treatment of herpes zoster in patients with cancer. *Antimicrobial Agents and Chemotherapy*, **19**, 193–195 (1981)
24. Merigan, T. C., Rand, K. H., Pollard, R. B. *et al*. Human leukocyte interferon for the treatment of herpes zoster in patients with cancer. *New England of Medicine*, **298**, 981–987 (1978)
25. Whitley, R. J., Soong, S. J., Dolin, R. *et al*. Early vidarabine therapy to control the complications of herpes zoster in immunosuppressed patients. *New England Journal of Medicine*, **307**, 971–975 (1982)
26. Bean, B., Aeppli, D. and Balfour, H. H. Acyclovir in shingles. *Journal of Antimicrobial Chemotherapy*, **12**, (Suppl.B), 123–127 (1983)
27. Peterslund, N. A., Seyer-Hansen, K., Ipsen, J. *et al*. Acyclovir in herpes zoster. *Lancet*, **ii**, 827–831 (1981)
28. Esmann, V., Ipsen, J., Peterslund, N. A. *et al*. Therapy of acute herpes zoster with acyclovir in the nonimmunocompromised host. *American Journal of Medicine*, **73**, 320–325 (1982)
29. Bean, B., Braun, C. and Balfour, H. H. Acyclovir therapy for acute herpes zoster. *Lancet*, **ii**, 118–121 (1982)
30. Balfour, H. Acyclovir therapy for herpes zoster: advantages and adverse effects. *Journal of the American Medical Association*, **255**, 387–388 (1986)
31. Balfour, H., Bean, B., Laskin, O. L. *et al*. Acyclovir halts progression of herpes zoster in immunocompromised patients. *New England Journal of Medicine*, **308**, 1453 (1983)
32. Shepp, D. H., Dandliker, P. S. and Meyers, J. D. Treatment of varicella zoster virus infection in severely immunocompromised patients: a randomized comparison of acyclovir and vidarabine. *New England Journal of Medicine*, **314**, 208–212 (1986)
33. Sklar, S. H., Blue, W. T., Alexander, E. J. *et al*. Herpes zoster, the treatment and prevention of neuralgia by adenosine monophosphate. *Journal of the American Medical Association*, **253**, 1427–1430 (1985)
34. Sherlock, C. H. and Corey, L. Adenosine monophosphate for the treatment of varicella zoster infections, a large dose of caution. *Journal of the American Medical Association*, **253**, 1444–1445 (1985)
35. Farber, G. A. and Burks, J. W. Chlorprothixene therapy for herpes zoster neuralgia. *Southern Medical Journal*, **67**, 808–812 (1974)
36. Nathan, P. W. Chlorprothixene (Taractan) in postherpetic neuralgia and other severe chronic pains. *Pain*, **5**, 367–371 (1978)
37. Woodforde, J. M., Dwyer, B., McEwan, B. W. *et al*. The treatment of postherpetic neuralgia. *Medical Journal of Australia*, **2**, 869–872 (1965)
38. Merskey, H. and Hester, R. A. Treatment of chronic pain with psychotropic drugs. *Postgraduate Medical Journal*, **48**, 594–598 (1982)
39. Taub, A. Relief of postherpetic neuralgia with psychotropic drugs. *Journal of Neurosurgery*, **39**, 235–239 (1973)
40. Taub, A. and Collins, W. F. Observations on the treatment of denervation dysesthesia with psychotropic drugs. *Advanced Neurology*, **4**, 309–315 (1974)
41. Watson, C. P. Therapeutic window effect for amitriptyline analgesia. *Canadian Medical Association Journal*, **130**, 105 (1984)
42. Killian, J. M. and Fromm, G. H. Carbamazepine in the treatment of neuralgia. *Archives of Neurology*, **19**, 129–136 (1968)

43. Hatangdi, V. S., Boad, R. A. and Richards, E. G. Postherpetic neuralgia: management with anti-epileptic and tricyclic drugs. In *Advances in Pain Research and Therapy, Vol. 1* (ed. J. J. Bonica and D. Albe-Fessard), Raven Press, New York, pp. 583–587 (1976)
44. Gerson, G. R., Jones, R. B. and Luscombe, D. K. Studies on the concomitant use of carbamazepine and clomipramine for the relief of postherpetic neuralgia. *Postgraduate Medical Journal*, **54**, (Suppl. 4), 104–109 (1977)
45. Raftery, H. The management of postherpetic pain using sodium valproate and amitriptyline. *Irish Medical Journal*, **72**, 399–401 (1979)
46. Jansco, N., Jansco-Gabor, A. and Szolcsanyi, J. Direct evidence for neurogenic inflammation and its prevention by denervation and by pretreatment with capsaicin. *British Journal of Pharmacology*. **31**, 138–151 (1967)
47. Jansco, G., Kiraly, E. and Jansco-Gabor, A. Pharmacologically induced selective degeneration of chemosensitive primary sensory neurons. *Nature*, **270**, 741–743 (1977)
48. Jessell, T. M., Iversen, L. L. and Cuello, A. C. Capsaicin-induced depletion of substance P from primary sensory neurones. *Brain Research*, **152**, 132–188 (1978)
49. Otsuka, M. and Konski, S. Release of substance P-like immunoreactivity from isolated spinal cord of newborn rat. *Nature*, **164**, 83 (1976)
50. Yaksh, T. L., Farb, D. H., Leeman, S. E. and Jessell, T. M. Intrathecal capsaicin depletes substance P in the rat spinal cord and produces prolonged thermal analgesia. *Science*, **206**, 481–483 (1979)
51. Bernstein, J. E., Bickers, D. R., Dahl, M. V. *et al.* Treatment of chronic postherpetic neuralgia with topical capsaicin. *Journal of the American Academy of Dermatology*, **17**, 93–96 (1987)
52. Watson, C. P. N., Evans, R. J. and Watt, V. R. Postherpetic neuralgia and topical capsaicin. *Pain*, **33**, 333–340 (1988)
53. Russell, W. R., Espir, M. L. E. and Morganstern, F. S. Treatment of postherpetic neuralgia. *Lancet*, **i**, 242–245 (1957)
54. Taverner, D. Alleviation of postherpetic neuralgia. *Lancet*, **ii**, 671–673 (1960)
55. Todd, E. M., Crue, B. L., Jr and Vergadamo, M. Conservative treatment of postherpetic neuralgia. *Bulletin of the Los Angeles Neurological Society*, **30**, 148–152 (1965)
56. Forrest, J. B. The response to epidural steroid injections in chronic dorsal root pain. *Canadian Anaesthetists' Society Journal*, **27**, 40–46 (1980)
57. Perkins, H. M. and Hanlon, P. R. Epidural injection of local anesthetic and steroids for relief of pain secondary to herpes zoster. *Archives of Surgery*, **113**, 253–254 (1978)
58. Nathan, P. W. and Wall, P. D. Treatment of postherpetic neuralgia by prolonged electrical stimulation. *British Medical Journal*, **3**, 645–647 (1974)
59. Haas, L. F. Postherpetic neuralgia. *Transactions of the Ophthalmological Society of New Zealand*, **29**, 133–136 (1977)
60. Lewith, G. T., Field, F. and Machin, D. Acupuncture versus placebo in postherpetic pain. *Pain*, **17**, 361–368 (1983)
61. White, J. C. and Sweet, W. H. *Pain and the Neurosurgeon: A 40-Year Experience*, Charles C. Thomas, Springfield, Illinois (1969)
62. Hitchcock, E. R. and Schvarcz, J. R. Stereotaxic trigeminal tractotomy for postherpetic facial pain. *Journal of Neurosurgery*, **37**, 412–417 (1972)
63. Nashold, B. S., Jr, Ostdahl, R. H., Bullitt, E. *et al.* Dorsal root entry zone lesions: A new neurosurgical therapy for deafferentation pain. In *Advances in Pain Research and Therapy, Vol. 5* (ed. J. J. Bonica and D. Albe-Fessard), Raven Press, New York, pp. 738–750 (1983)
64. Friedman, A. H., Nashold, B. S. and Overlmann-Levitt, J. DREZ lesions for postherpetic neuralgia. *Journal of Neurosurgery*, **60**, 1258–1262 (1984)
65. Friedman, A. H. and Nashold, B. S. DREZ lesions for postherpetic neuralgia. *Neurosurgery*, **15**, 969–970 (1984)

10
Diagnosis of cancer pain syndromes
Russell K. Portenoy

INTRODUCTION

Pain is a commonly anticipated and universally feared consequence of cancer [1]. Twenty per cent to 50% of patients at the time of diagnosis and approximately one-third undergoing active treatment report pain; this prevalence rises to almost three-quarters of those who progress to an advanced phase of disease [2–5]. Pain is moderate to severe in about one-half of these patients [5] and most experience pain in multiple sites [4]. A worldwide prevalence of cancer pain of more than 3.5×10^6 patients daily has been estimated by the World Health Organization [6].

Compounding this prevalence are other data indicating that cancer pain is often inadequately treated. Despite evidence that approximately three-quarters of cancer pain can be controlled with simple pharmacologic techniques [7], and the additional suggestion that most of the remaining patients can be managed with one or more of a variety of other approaches [8], most surveys agree that the proportion of patients successfully treated is substantially less [5,9–13]. This can be attributed to several factors, the most troubling of which are inappropriate application of pain management techniques by treating clinicians [5,11,14–17] and the lack of availability of effective oral opioids [18–20]. The disheartening picture emerging from these data indicates that pain is an extremely common symptom for which the available, potentially efficacious therapies are commonly misapprehended or inappropriately used.

The tragedy of these statistics, of course, can only be appreciated at the level of the individual. Pain is a compelling symptom, enervating to the patient and capable of impeding all efforts to retain normal function. Chronic pain is often accompanied by depression with vegetative signs [21–24]. As a harbinger of recurrent cancer or a signal of progressive disease, pain may fuel the anxiety, anger, hopelessness, and isolation so often experienced by the cancer patient. Pain in a loved one is also extremely stressful to the family. Witnesses to unrelieved pain may experience a pervasive sense of impotence; anger and despair often follow. Members of the family may react by subtle distancing, exacerbating the patient's sense of isolation, or paradoxically, by such overconcern with the patient's medical condition that rumination about illness is reinforced and function further compromised.

Uncontrolled pain thus intrudes into virtually every sphere of the patient's life. It renders cure an empty victory, denies quality of life to those successfully palliated, and immeasurably augments the suffering imminent in the dying experience. It is evident that the evaluation and treatment of pain in the cancer patient must receive the highest priority.

EVALUATION OF THE CANCER PAIN PATIENT

Pain evaluation in the patient with cancer is a complex process from which is derived a specific therapeutic strategy. The goal of the assessment process can be conceptualized as the development of the 'pain diagnosis' (Figure 10.1). The 'pain

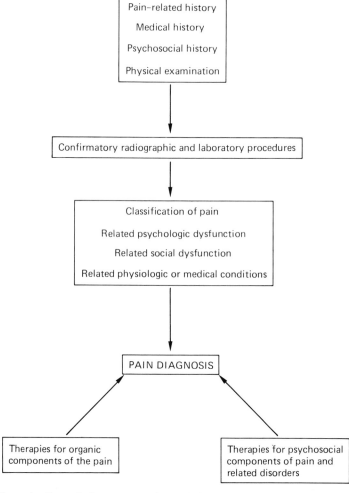

Figure 10.1 The pain diagnosis incorporates the multifactorial nature of pain and its associated symptoms and signs, and is a guide to targeting interventions appropriately and efficiently. See text for the various classifications of pain

diagnosis' is drawn from the construct of 'total pain' advocated by proponents of the hospice movement [25,26] and represents a synopsis of salient features of the pain complaint (*see below*) and the medical, psychologic, social, and spiritual factors with which it interacts. Additionally, this construct attempts to provide practical guidance in identifying and ordering problems amenable to specific interventions. It may be useful in determining the most appropriate group of laboratory and radiographic procedures needed to evaluate the pain complaint, and may suggest a combination of therapies more likely to succeed than any one applied in isolation.

Elaboration of the 'pain diagnosis' presupposes recognition of the distinctions among nociception, pain and suffering. Although it was applied originally to patients with non-malignant pain syndromes [27], this terminology has special relevance to those with cancer pain. Nociception describes the activity in somato-sensory pathways responsive to potentially tissue-damaging stimuli. Nociception is only loosely related to pain, which can be viewed as a perception incorporating both actual or potential injury and the psychologic reactions that occur as a consequence. It is a common clinical observation that pain can be experienced out of proportion to the degree of injury or, indeed, in its absence, and conversely, that substantial nociception, such as that accompanying wounds incurred during times of stress (e.g. battle or sporting injury), may be painless.

Distinct from nociception and pain, suffering can be defined as an unpleasant emotional state related to all aversive perceptions, one of which may be pain, but which may include physical disability, inability to work, financial concerns, loss of role within the family, fear of death and many others. Just as pain may not be effectively addressed if all clinical interventions are limited to the attempted eradication of the nociceptive focus without concern for the associated psychologic issues, the patient's suffering, and hence quality of life, may not be improved if therapy addresses only the experience of pain.

The 'pain diagnosis' attempts to encompass all these concepts, beginning with identification of the nociceptive focus that underlies most of cancer pain. The medical history and physical examination provide the initial data in this process. The pain complaint should be characterized by its onset, course, duration, severity, quality, location, radiation, temporal relationships, and provocative and palliative factors. Specific queries should address previous experience with analgesic drugs, past history of chronic non-malignant pain or significant psychiatric disease, and the experience of pain in the family. The presumed extent of disease should be noted, as well as the patient's psychologic and social status at the time of presentation.

Dysphoria and vegetative signs, such as sleep disturbance, are not normal accompaniments of cancer and should be independently assessed as potentially remediable problems. Although pain in the absence of an organic contribution is exceedingly rare in the cancer patient, psychologic factors commonly influence the expression of the pain and may underlie the clinical observation of pain out of proportion to the presumed organic lesion. Similarly, the existence of maladaptive behaviors not enforced by the rigors of the disease or its therapy, such as the inability to work, loss of interest in avocations, unnecessary dependence on others for activities of daily living, social withdrawal, or overuse of non-essential medications of medical resources, should be assessed for their contribution to the pain, suffering and level of disability. Astute clinical evaluation of organic factors and the psychosocial processes with which they interact provides the means to distinguish and assess the priorities of a series of distinct problems, each potentially amenable to clinical intervention – the 'pain diagnosis'.

The physical examination, which may include a neurologic assessment, should attempt to establish the extent of disease and identify nociceptive lesions. The painful area must always be observed and palpated; functional testing should be performed if possible.

The data obtained through the history and physical examination should be used to develop a series of clinical hypotheses about the potential organic etiologies for the pain. These provide the basis for the ordering of appropriate tests to confirm or refute these suspicions. Tests should be limited as much as possible; they are exhausting to the patient and divert attention from efforts to regain normal life. When tests are necessary, adequate analgesic medication should be offered to reduce their aversive quality, enhance cooperation, and increase diagnostic yield by providing the opportunity for the best study possible. Finally, all studies should be personally reviewed by the clinician caring for the patient, who is best able to provide the necessary clinical correlation.

CLASSIFICATION OF PAIN

This process of assessment provides the data necessary to classify the pain complaint and the patient, a fundamental element in the development of the 'pain diagnosis' (Figure 10.1). Given the complexity of the clinical situation, the use of pain-related classifications is extremely helpful in guiding therapy and determining prognosis. Although efforts have been made to create a comprehensive taxonomy of pain which incorporates temporal, topographic, etiologic and other facets of the pain experience [28], the differences among cancer pain patients are so great that a process of independent classification within one or more specific classificatory schema often has greater clinical relevance. The most salient taxonomies can be termed *temporal, topographic, etiologic, pathophysiologic, and syndromic.*

Temporal classification

The fundamental temporal distinction is between acute and chronic pain. Although pain duration *per se* (typically 6 months) has been used to define chronicity, particularly in the literature of non-malignant pain, these labels have greater clinical relevance when defined by the symptoms and signs that typify each.

Acute pain usually has a clear-cut proximate cause and a well-defined onset. The pain complaint is accompanied by signs of sympathetic hyperactivity, including tachycardia, tachypnea, hypertension, diaphoresis and mydriasis, and often by overt behaviors, such as grimacing, moaning and splinting, that are recognized and linked to pain by the clinician. The associated affect is anxiety.

In contrast, chronic pain usually has an ill-defined onset. The behavioral and autonomic signs that characterize acute pain gradually wane, and may be super-seded in some patients by vegetative signs, including anorexia and loss of taste for food, weight loss, lassitude, loss of libido and constipation. The associated mood disturbance, if one exists, is usually depression [22–24]. In some patients, the pain experience disrupts every aspect of life, impairing the ability to work or enjoy recreation and compromising social relationships inside and outside the family.

A third temporal pattern common in the cancer patient is chronic pain punctuated by acute exacerbations. When brief and precipitated by movement or change in position, the latter are termed 'incident pains'. This type of pain is often highly disturbing to the patient and very difficult to treat.

Recurrent acute pain, with pain-free intervals, can also be identified in the cancer patient. The pains may be brief, either spontaneous or incident pains, or may take the form of prolonged episodes. The substrate for the latter may be related to the tumor, for example intermittent bowel obstruction, or to anti-neoplastic therapy, such as recurrent mucositis following chemotherapy.

Recognition of the acute component to the pain syndrome, superimposed or not on a chronic pain, is clinically important, often indicating the need for intermittent changes in therapy to address the exacerbations specifically. Furthermore, the appearance of an acute pain, similar to progression of a previously stable chronic pain, is suggestive of a change in the underlying organic lesion and often impels clinical re-evaluation. Finally, different temporal courses greatly influence the psychologic reaction to the pain, and in turn alter the direction of therapy. For example, recognition that a pain syndrome, such as that accompanying mucositis, will probably be monophasic and short-lived, can be extremely salutary to the patient, who may fear that all pain represents progressive disease.

Topographic classification

Topographic classification, or that based on the location of the pain, can have useful diagnostic and therapeutic implications. Although pain is often experienced superficial to the causative lesion, so-called focal pain, it is exceedingly common for pain to appear at a distant site; recognition of these patterns is essential for accurate diagnosis. Pain can be referred from involvement of both neural and non-neural tissues [29–31], and these referral patterns act as a guide to the physical examination and radiographic evaluation of the patient. For example, the complaint of pain in the inguinal crease may relate to a lesion affecting peripheral nerve, lumbosacral plexus, upper lumbar nerve roots, iliopsoas or paraspinal muscles, hip joint, femoral head or pelvic bones. An appropriate assessment for this complaint encompasses all these regions.

Therapeutically, the distinction between localized and generalized pains is most salient [32]. Although both may be effectively treated with pharmacotherapy in most cases, second-line approaches diverge (*see below*). For example, a large number of neuro-ablative surgical procedures have been developed for the treatment of localized pains, while hypophysectomy has been employed in the management of refractory generalized pains.

Etiologic classification

Cancer pain has been divided into three broad etiologic categories. In more than two-thirds of patients, the cause of the pain is a direct result of the tumor [4,33,34]. Most commonly, this is due to invasion of bone or neural structures. Pain may also follow obstruction of hollow viscus, distortion or occlusion of blood vessels or disruption of soft tissues. Most patients with advanced cancer have multiple pains related to tumor involvement or some combination of these structures [4].

The etiology of the pain in up to one-quarter of patients relates to the effects of antineoplastic therapy [33,34]. Specific pain syndromes have been defined following a variety of surgical procedures, radiation therapy protocols, and chemotherapeutic approaches (*see below*). Finally, > 90% of cancer patients with pain have an etiology of the symptom related to the neoplasm or its treatment.

Pathophysiologic classification

An empirical classification which has proved to be useful in clinical decision-making is based on presumed pain mechanisms. Most broad is the distinction between pain that is predominantly somatogenic, better termed organic, and that which is psychogenic. As stated, cancer pain almost always has an important organic component, although psychologic factors influence its expression and may require primary treatment in some patients.

Several mechanisms may operate in the production of organic pain. Nociceptive pain is pain that appears clinically to be proportionate to the degree of ongoing activation of afferent nerve fibers sensitive to noxious mechanical, thermal or chemical stimuli. Somatic or visceral, the nociceptive focus often involves the chemical mediators of inflammation, which may activate or sensitize these primary afferents [35,36]. Most cancer pain is nociceptive, which is generally the most responsive to therapy; primary treatment directed at a causative lesion, such as radiotherapy, often exists, and if the usual, non-invasive measures of pain control fail, neurolytic anesthetic and surgical approaches can be very effective in relieving pain. It can also be speculated that certain nerve injuries produce chronic pain that can also be termed nociceptive, in that pain originates from ongoing activation of normal or aberrant nociceptive primary nerve fibers that are derived themselves from nerves (e.g. neuroma formation). Clinical experience suggests that these putative neuropathic nociceptive pains are more difficult to treat than nociceptive pains arising in visceral or somatic structures.

Other pains that follow injury to peripheral or central afferent neural pathways persist in the absence of peripheral stimuli of the intensity required to activate these nociceptive primary afferent neurons. Instead, these neuropathic pains presumably result from alterations of central and/or peripheral somatosensory function through one or more of a variety of pathophysiologic processes that may be set in motion by nerve injury. Such processes include denervation hypersensitivity of central pain-transmission neurons, loss of inhibitory controls and ephaptic transmission between axons in peripheral nerve [35–38]. For some neuropathic pains, the primary site of aberrant activity is in the central nervous system and relates to the process of deafferentation. Other pains are maintained by activity in the sympathetic nervous system and may be substantially ameliorated by sympathetic nerve blocks. Primary antineoplastic therapy is usually ineffective in these neuropathic pains and clinical observation suggests that the usual analgesic drugs are less efficacious than for the more common pains that are due to an obvious focus of ongoing tissue damage (e.g. arthritis, fractured bone, abscess). In contrast, the so-called adjuvant analgesics may be more effective and have an important role in the clinical management of neuropathic pains.

Syndromic classification

Like the pathophysiologic classification, the attempt to identify discrete pain syndromes is founded on the principle that recognition and treatment of underlying organic causes is the most effective means of achieving analgesia. Additionally, syndrome identification may provide insight into the status of the underlying disease and prognosis of the pain.

As noted, pain in the cancer patient may be due to direct tumor involvement, an antineoplastic therapy, or unrelated factors. Common cancer pain syndromes can be divided similarly (Table 10.2).

Syndromes related to direct tumor involvement

The best-characterized pain syndromes related directly to the neoplasm are those due to involvement of bony and neural structures [4,33,39,40].

Pain due to bony involvement
Tumor may involve bone at one or multiple sites. Although metastatic body deposits are often asymptomatic, bone destruction is the most common cause of pain in patients with metastatic disease [33]. The specific factors – mechanical, humoral and neural – that convert a painless metastasis into a painful one are unknown, but may in part involve local release of prostaglandins [41,42]. Several specific syndromes can be identified:

Base of skull syndromes [43,44]   The location of the lesion determines the presentation in these syndromes. Orbital tumors may cause frontal, periorbital or retro-orbital headache associated with proptosis and diplopia. Parasellar lesions may produce similar pain and diplopia with or without proptosis. Tumor invasion of the sphenoid sinus may be characterized by bifrontal, bitemporal or retro-orbital headache, associated with a sense of fullness in the head or nasal stuffiness and, ultimately, diplopia, usually due to an abducens nerve palsy. Neoplasms in the middle cranial fossa may cause facial pain (paroxysmal or constant) and numbness, while midline lesions that invade the clivus may refer pain to the vertex, which worsens with neck flexion. Tumors in the region of the foramen magnum refer pain to the occiput or neck. Those involving the jugular foramen often produce occipital pain radiating to the vertex or ipsilateral shoulder, which is associated with dysfunction of one or more of cranial nerves IX, X and XI. Encroachment of the tumor on structures adjacent to this location may also result in a hypoglossal or oculosympathetic palsy. Destruction of the occipital condyle may cause severe ipsilateral occipital pain, which flares on movement of the head and may be accompanied by a hypoglossal palsy.

All of these lesions are often poorly visualized by plain radiography. Computerized tomography (CT) is generally the procedure of choice, although some patients will require plain tomograms. Magnetic resonance imaging (MRI) may be helpful in outlining the relationship of the tumor to adjacent soft tissues.

Vertebral syndromes [33,39,40]   Destruction of the atlas or fracture of the odontoid with secondary subluxation may cause severe pain in the neck, which radiates to the occiput and worsens with neck flexion. Compression of the spinal

Table 10.1 Cancer pain syndromes

Pain associated with direct tumor involvement
  Due to invasion of bone
    Base of skull
      Orbital syndrome
      Parasellar syndrome
      Sphenoid sinus syndrome
      Middle cranial fossa syndrome
      Clivus syndrome
      Jugular foramen syndrome
      Occipital condyle syndrome
    Vertebral body
      Atlanto-axial syndrome
      C7–T1 syndrome
      L1 syndrome
      Sacral syndrome
    Generalized bone pain
  Due to invasion of nerves
    Peripheral nerve syndromes
      Paraspinal mass
      Chest wall mass
      Retroperitoneal mass
    Painful polyneuropathy
    Brachial, lumbar, sacral plexopathies
    Leptomeningeal metastases
    Epidural spinal cord compression
  Due to invasion of viscera
  Due to invasion of blood vessels
  Due to invasion of mucous membranes
Pain associated with cancer therapy
  Postoperative pain syndromes
    Post-thoracotomy syndrome
    Post-mastectomy syndrome
    Post-radical neck syndrome
    Post-amputation syndromes
  Post-chemotherapy pain syndromes
    Painful polyneuropathy
    Aseptic necrosis of bone
    Steroid pseudorheumatism
    Mucositis
  Post-radiation pain syndromes
    Radiation fibrosis of brachial or lumbosacral plexus
    Radiation myelopathy
    Radiation-induced peripheral nerve tumors
    Mucositis
Pain indirectly related or unrelated to cancer
  Myofascial pains
  Postherpetic neuralgia
  Chronic headache syndromes

cord and roots may lead to motor, sensory and autonomic dysfunction, which often begins in the arms and progresses. Untreated, patients are at significant risk of quadriplegia or death.

Other specific syndromes are similarly important to recognize. Damage to C7 or T1 may cause interscapular pain and may escape detection when radiographic evaluation is targeted more inferiorly than the etiologic lesion or the region is poorly visualized due to overlying clavicular heads and shoulders. Similarly, damage to T12 or L1 may refer pain to the iliac crest or sacroiliac joints. Sacral lesions often produce focal pain that may radiate to the perineum or posterior aspect of the legs and worsens with lying or sitting. Sphincteric dysfunction occurs early and is followed by S1 sensory loss, weakness in toe flexors and loss of ankle jerks. The pubic bone often obscures the sacrum on routine radiographs and specific sacral radiographs are often necessary to identify the damage. In all of these vertebral syndromes, the failure of plain radiography to identify a lesion should not preclude the use of more sensitive techniques if the clinical suspicion remains. CT scanning is often very effective and is empirically the second-line procedure of choice at present. Plain tomography, bone scintigraphy and MRI are alternative procedures that may be useful in selected patients.

Diffuse or multifocal bone pain   A more generalized pain syndrome may occur in patients with multiple bony metastases. More rarely, a similar pain syndrome follows marrow replacement by malignant cells. This has been observed both in patients with hematologic malignancies and solid tumors, and can occur in the absence of abnormalities on scintigraphy or radiography. Its pathogenesis is not clear.

Pain due to neural involvement
Tumor infiltration of peripheral nerve, plexus and root may produce well-defined pain syndromes, identification of which may assist in diagnosis and management.

Peripheral nerve syndromes Pain due to peripheral nerve involvement most commonly occurs as a consequence of a paravertebral, retroperitoneal or chest wall/rib lesion. A paravertebral mass may damage one or more spinal nerves and result in a pain syndrome that mimics radicular pain. Discomfort, which may be aching or dysesthetic, is often experienced along the distal course of the nerve, and may thereby pose a diagnostic problem. Back pain may also be due to a paravertebral lesion, and must be distinguished from that due to invasion of the vertebral body or of the spinal canal. Indeed, paravertebral lesions commonly infiltrate into the spinal canal, often without producing bony damage [45,46] and evaluation of the epidural space with myelography is usually indicated in patients with lesions abutting the spine, even in the absence of scintigraphic or radiographic changes [47] (*see* Figure 10.2).

Retroperitoneal tumor may also produce back pain, or pain localized to the flank, abdomen, buttocks or legs. The latter pains are similar to those caused by paravertebral masses and may mimic radiculopathy. In addition, a deep boring epigastric discomfort related to infiltration of the celiac plexus may also complicate retroperitoneal masses. Finally, chest wall or rib metastases may infiltrate intercostal nerves and produce local discomfort and a neuropathic pain that radiates around the chest wall.

CT or MRI is usually required to evaluate the clinical suspicion of a peripheral nerve lesion. Electrophysiologic studies may also be useful in localizing the lesion.

Brachial and lumbosacral plexopathy [48–51]   Pain is the most common symptom in the malignant plexopathies. Patients with Pancoast syndrome and tumor infiltration of the brachial plexus usually present with some combination of aching shoulder and paraspinal pain, pain in the elbow and dysesthesias in the medial hand and two fingers. In addition to the pain and the sensorimotor dysfunction that ultimately affects the arm, epidural spinal cord compression occurs as a complication in up to 50% of these patients [52]. Progressive pain, evidence of panplexopathy on neurologic examination, and a Horner's syndrome are all associated with the development of epidural cord compression [50].

Malignant lumbosacral plexopathy is similarly typified by the occurrence of pain followed by sensory changes and ultimately weakness in the affected extremity. Pain may occur in the back, usually in a paraspinal distribution, or may be referred down the leg in either a radicular or non-segmental distribution. As in patients with brachial plexopathy, those with lumbosacral plexus lesions are at risk for epidural extension of the tumor. Although the lack of spinal tenderness and failure to flare with spinal movements or Valsalva maneuvers suggests plexopathy in the absence of epidural extension, this determination is not reliable. The risk of epidural disease, as high as 35% in one study [49], indicates that evaluation of the epidural space with myelography must be strongly considered in those patients with plexopathy and either a clinical indication of coexistent radiculopathy or radiographic evidence of a paraspinal lesion [47].

A common clinical dilemma with profound prognostic and therapeutic implications is the distinction between recurrent tumor and radiation fibrosis of the plexus in patients with symptoms following radiation therapy to a known plexus lesion [48–51]. Pain is more severe and prevalent in the malignant plexopathies than those caused by radiotherapy. Radiation injury is commonly associated with skin changes and lymphedema in the affected extremity, and with the finding of myokymia on electromyography [50,51]. Patients with radiation fibrosis of the brachial plexus typically have symptoms and signs indicative of upper plexus involvement, in contrast to those with tumor, in whom damage in the distribution of the C8 and T1 roots is typical [50]. Two-dimensional imaging with CT and, although experience is limited as yet, probably with MRI as well, is the procedure of choice in the evaluation of patients with progressive plexopathy following radiotherapy to a malignant lesion. Rarely, the failure of the clinical evaluation, and the importance of accurate diagnosis, combine to indicate the need for surgical exploration of the plexus [53].

Leptomeningeal metastases   This syndrome with protean neurological manifestations is accompanied by pain in less than half of patients [54,55]. Headache, back pain and unifocal or multifocal radicular pain can all occur in these patients.

Epidural spinal cord compression   Pain is the presenting symptom in over 95% of patients with this lesion [56–59]. The pain may be focal, radicular, or referred. Whereas the neurological concomitants of spinal cord, conus medullaris or cauda equina compression are well appreciated, and patients presenting with these signs generally receive prompt evaluation and treatment, the association between back pain without neurologic deficit and early epidural extension of tumor is less well recognized. As neurologic outcome is inversely related to the degree of dysfunction at the time that treatment is instituted [58,59] and, at present, definitive treatment is generally delayed until neurologic signs appear, it is evident that the overall management of these patients could be improved. To this end, a systematic approach to the evaluation of back pain in the cancer patient has been proposed [47] (Figure 10.2). This algorithm suggests immediate myelography for patients with emerging cord or cauda signs, urgent myelography for those with mild and stable signs of myelopathy or radiculopathy, and a systematic radiographic and scintigraphic evaluation of those with back pain alone to identify those at risk of epidural lesions.

Radiation myelopathy is an uncommon entity complicated by pain in < 20% of afflicted patients [60]. The clinical distinction between this entity and recurrent tumor is therefore rarely a problem and, when posed, can usually be resolved by the combination of myelography and CT scanning.

Peripheral neuropathy   Peripheral neuropathy is a common remote effect of cancer [61]. Pain is a relatively rare symptom, however, with the important exception of a subgroup of patients with plasma cell dyscrasias, particularly multiple myeloma. It is important to note that the painful polyneuropathy accompanying these hematologic malignancies can precede clinical evidence of the neoplasm by months or years. These observations have led to the clinical axiom that the occurrence of a painful neuropathy in a middle-aged individual should impel an assiduous search for one of the myelomatous disorders; if unrevealing and no alternative diagnosis is demonstrable, this evaluation should be repeated at regular intervals [62].

Syndromes related to antineoplastic therapy

Pain syndromes have been described following chemotherapy, selected surgical procedures and some radiation therapy protocols. Implicit in the diagnosis is the recognition that pain represents neither recurrence nor progression of tumor. This has important therapeutic and prognostic impact and may profoundly alter the patient's psychologic reaction to the pain. Although some patients appear to draw support from the reassurances that the tumor has been eradicated, others demonstrate the type of pervasive disturbances in mood and functioning usually associated with chronic non-malignant pain syndromes. In the latter group, treatment of these disturbances is often as therapeutically relevant as pain management itself.

Post-chemotherapy pain syndromes
Polyneuropathy is extremely common following treatment with several chemotherapeutic agents, particularly vincristine (much less common with other vinca alkaloids) and *cis*-platinum [62]. Paresthesias occur uniformly in patients who develop clinical neuropathy; some patients experience discomfort from these sensations and some report more disabling dysesthesias. Treatment is symptomatic and relies primarily on the adjuvant analgesics. The pain often improves gradually after discontinuation of chemotherapy.

Corticosteroid-induced pain syndromes include both aseptic necrosis of the femoral or humoral head [63] and steroid pseudorheumatism [64]. The latter is an under-recognized syndrome in which dose reduction or withdrawal of steroid therapy is accompanied by myalgias, arthralgias and constitutional symptoms.

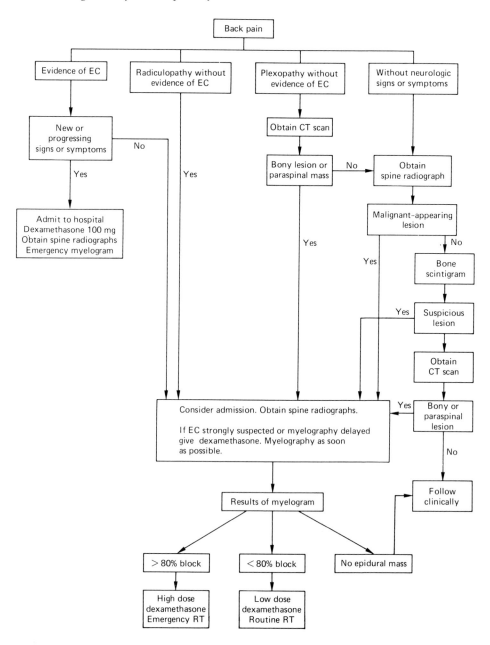

Figure 10.2 Algorithm for the management of back pain in the cancer patient. CT computerized tomography; RT, radiotherapy; EC, epidural spinal cord compression (Adapted from Portenoy *et al.*, (47))

Post-radiotherapy pain syndromes
Radiation fibrosis of the brachial and lumbosacral plexus commonly causes discomfort in the affected extremity, often described as some combination of heaviness, numbness or tingling, but seldom as the severe aching and dysesthesias accompanying tumor infiltration [50,51]. Radiation is more likely to be the cause in those patients with lymphedema, radiation skin changes, local induration, electromyographic myokymia, and the lack of a defined soft-tissue mass on CT of the region.

Radiation fibrosis of the plexus may become clinically manifest from 6 months to 20 years after treatment. With those neoplasms in which late recurrence is rare, a long period between treatment and symptoms may also aid the distinction between radiation and malignant plexopathy. However, an alternative possibility in this setting is a radiation-induced primary neoplasm. These can originate from peripheral nerve itself [65] or from surrounding tissues, may also produce local pain and neurologic dysfunction and can become a challenge in differential diagnosis. Ultimately, however, this entity declares itself through the discovery of a enlarging mass.

Pain is an uncommon symptom in delayed post-radiation myelopathy [60]. As in other myelopathies, the pain in this syndrome may be local, referred in a radicular or funicular pattern, or have no clear somatotopic distribution below the level of the damage. The distinction from recurrent intramedullary or epidural tumor is again of paramount importance. There is no effective treatment for the progressive neurologic dysfunction in radiation myelopathy, although the pain, if present, should be viewed as a primary problem for which one or more of a variety of approaches may be appropriate (*See Chapter 11*).

Postoperative pain syndromes
For a small group of patients, refractory pain becomes a sequela of cancer surgery. As in the post-radiation syndromes, recurrent tumor is prominent in the differential diagnosis at presentation and often remains a concern throughout the patient's course, particularly at times of pain exacerbation. The best-described postoperative pain syndromes in the cancer population are those following thoracotomy, mastectomy, limb amputation and radical neck dissection. It must be recognized, however, that a surgical incision at any location can occasionally lead to a chronic pain disorder, and patients with refractory pain after inguinal dissection, nephrectomy and sternotomy, as well as others, are occasionally encountered.

Post-thoracotomy pain is related to damage to an intercostal nerve. As such, there is a common misapprehension that intra-operative nerve section or traction is the usual etiology for the persistent pains that may follow this procedure. Rather, the two most common pain patterns – early improvement of pain followed by later recurrence and progressive pain from the time of surgery – are highly associated with tumor recurrence, usually in the chest wall but at times in the lung parenchyma [66]. Only a pattern of stable or decreasing pain in the absence of radiographic and laboratory evidence of tumor recurrence can be attributed with any confidence to a benign cause.

In contrast, post-mastectomy pain, which is usually experienced as uncomfortable squeezing and burning dysesthesias along the anterior chest wall, axilla and medial aspect of the upper arm, appears to be related to the development of a traumatic neuroma of the intercostobrachial nerve, a cutaneous branch of T1–T2 [67,68]. The syndrome can follow any surgical procedure on the breast and may develop at any point from the immediate postoperative period until a year or more later. Treatment relies on adjuvant analgesics and other approaches to ameliorate the discomfort and prevent secondary complications, such as frozen shoulder and contractures due to voluntary immobility and psychologic disturbances that may become as compelling as the pain itself.

Following amputation of a limb, virtually all patients experience phantom sensations. Some degree of pain after the immediate postoperative period occurs in nearly all patients [69,70], but the incidence of clinically significant persistent pain is controversial, ranging in different surveys from < 5% to 85% [70,71]. Two distinct types of pain syndromes can be distinguished. Stump pain, due to neuroma formation, is localized to the distal stump, is often related to trigger points in the scar, typically has continuous and lancinating components, and can often be relieved for prolonged periods through local injection of anesthetic drugs. This pain, therefore, is a form of neuropathic pain related to persistent activity in abnormal afferent fibers within the neuroma; removal of this focus through resection of the neuroma may provide effective relief of pain.

Phantom pain, which occurs with greater incidence in those patients with local pain before surgery and in those who later develop concurrent stump pain [69,71], is, in contrast, a deafferentation pain, the pathogenesis of which relates to ill-defined central reorganization of somatosensory pathways. The pain is experienced in the phantom, which is often telescoped or distorted, and is also usually characterized by continuous and paroxysmal components. A huge number of different treatments have been applied, with pharmacotherapy with adjuvant analgesics the current mainstay, but the outcome is usually inadequate [69,71].

Stereotyped patterns of pain may also follow radical neck dissection, or the combination of this procedure and subsequent radiotherapy. Continuous tightness or burning in the anterolateral neck, jaw, ear and surrounding area, usually accompanied by lancinating pains often shooting to the ear or angle of the jaw, presumably relate to damaged cervical cutaneous nerves. Pain in the shoulder, anterior chest and scapula may also occur, and in some cases may be due to an evident droopy shoulder. This pain is probably myofascial in most patients. Treatment for these pains varies and must be targeted to the specific pain experienced.

CONCLUSIONS

Great advances have been made in the diagnosis, classification and treatment of cancer pain. Systematic assessment, followed by the vigorous application of one or more therapeutic modalities, holds the promise of successful analgesia and improved quality of life for the great majority of patients so afflicted. Clinical recognition of pain management as an achievable goal of highest priority is the foundation for future progress.

References

1. Levin, D. N. Cleeland, C. S. and Dar, R. Public attitudes toward cancer pain. *Cancer*, **56**, 2337–2339 (1985)

2. Daut, R. L. and Cleeland, C. S. The prevalence and severity of pain in cancer. *Cancer*, **50**, 1913–1918 (1982)
3. Foley, K. M. and Sundaresan, N. The management of cancer pain. In *Cancer Principles and Practice of Oncology*, 2nd edn (ed. V. T. DeVita, S. Hellman, and S. A. Rosenberg), J. L. Lippincott, New York, pp. 1940–1962 (1984)
4. Twycross, R. G. and Fairfield, S. Pain in far-advanced cancer. *Pain*, **14**, 303–310 (1982)
5. Bonica, J. J. Treatment of cancer pain: current status and future needs. In *Advances in Pain Research and Therapy, Vol. 9* (ed. H. L. Fields, R. Dubner and F. Cervero), Raven Press, New York, pp. 589–616 (1985)
6. World Health Organization. *Cancer Pain Relief*, World Health Organization, Geneva (1986)
7. Ventafridda, V., Tamburini, M., Caraceni, A. *et al.* A validation study of the WHO method for cancer pain relief. *Cancer*, **59**, 850–856 (1987)
8. Ventafridda, V., Tamburini, M. and DeConno, F. Comprehensive treatment in cancer pain. In *Advances in Pain Research and Therapy, Vol. 9* (ed. H. L. Fields, R. Dubner and F. Cervero), Raven Press, New York, pp. 617–628 (1985)
9. Aitken-Swan, J. Nursing the late cancer patient at home. *Practitioner*, **183**, 64–69 (1959)
10. Parkes, C. M. Home or hospital: terminal care as seen by surviving spouse. *Journal of the Royal College of General Practitioners*, **28**, 19–30 (1978)
11. Marks, R. M. and Sachar, E. J. Undertreatment of medical inpatients with narcotic analgesics. *Annals of Internal Medicine*, **78**, 173–181 (1973)
12. Turnbull, F. The nature of pain that may accompany cancer of the lung. *Pain*, **7**, 371–375 (1979)
13. Pannuti, E., Rossi, A. P. and Marraro, D. Natural history of cancer pain. In *The Continuing Care of Terminal Cancer Patients* (ed. R. G. Twycross and V. Ventafridda), Pergamon Press, New York, pp. 75–89 (1980)
14. Charap, A. D. The knowledge, attitudes and experience of medical personnel treating pain in the terminally ill. *Mount Sinai Journal of Medicine, New York*, **45**, 561–580 (1978)
15. Weis, O., Sriwatanakul, K., Alloza, J. L. *et al.* Attitudes of patients, housestaff, and nurses toward postoperative analgesic care. *Anesthesia and Analgesia*, **62**, 70–74 (1983)
16. Watt-Watson, J. H. Nurses' knowledge of pain issues: a survey. *Journal of Pain and Symptom Management*, **2**, 207–211 (1987)
17. Rankin, M. Use of drugs for pain with cancer patients. *Cancer Nursing*, **5**, 181–190 (1982)
18. Kanner, R. M. and Portenoy, R. K. Unavailability of narcotic analgesics for ambulatory cancer patients in New York City. *Journal of Pain Symptom Management*, **1**, 87–90 (1986)
19. Wenk, R. Availability of analgesics in Argentina. *Journal of Pain Symptom Management*, **2**, 191–192 (1987)
20. Caraceni, A. Availability and use of opioids for cancer pain patients in Italy. *Journal of Pain Symptom Management*, **2**, 127–128 (1987)
21. Massie, M. J. and Holland, J. C. The cancer patient with pain: psychiatric complications and their management. *Medical Clinics of North America*, **71**, 243–258 (1987)
22. Silberfarb, P. M. and Greer, S. Psychological concomitants of cancer: clinical aspects. *American Journal of Psychotherapy*, **36**, 470–478 (1982)
23. Bukberg, J., Penman, D. and Holland, J. Depression in hospitalized cancer patients. *Psychosomatic Medicine*, **46**, 199–212 (1984)
24. Ahles, T. A., Blanchard, E. B. and Ruckdeschel, J. C. The multidimensional nature of cancer-related pain. *Pain*, **17**, 277–288 (1983)
25. Saunders, C. The philosophy of terminal care. In *The Management of Terminal Malignant Disease* (ed. C. Saunders), Edward Arnold, London, pp. 232–241 (1984)
26. Twycross, R. G. and Lack, S. A. *Symptom Control in Far Advanced Cancer: Pain Relief*, Pitman, London (1983)
27. Loeser, J. D. Perspectives on pain. In *Proceedings of First World Conference on Clinical Pharmacology and Therapeutics*, Macmillan, London, pp. 313–316 (1980)
28. Subcommittee on Taxonomy, International Association for the Study of Pain. Classification of chronic pain. *Pain*, Suppl. 3, S1–S225 (1986)
29. Kellgren, J. H. On the distribution of pain arising from deep somatic structures with charts of segmental pain areas. *Clinical Science*, **4**, 35–46 (1939)
30. Torebjork, H. E., Ochoa, J. L. and Schady, W. Referred pain from intraneural stimulation of muscle fascicles in the median nerve. *Pain*, **18**, 145–156 (1984)
31. Inman, V. T. and Saunders, J. B. Referred pain from skeletal structures. *Journal of Nervous and Mental Disease*, **99**, 660–667 (1944)
32. Cleeland, C. S., Rotondi, A., Brechner, T. *et al.* A model for the treatment of cancer pain. *Journal of Pain Symptom Management*, **1**, 209–216 (1986)

33. Foley, K. M. Pain syndromes in patients with cancer. In *Advances in Pain Research and Therapy, Vol. 2* (ed. J. J. Bonica and V. Ventafridda), Raven Press, New York, pp. 59–75 (1979)
34. Kanner, R. M. and Foley, K. M. Patterns of narcotic drug use in a cancer pain clinic. *Annals of the New York Academy of Sciences*, **362**, 161–172 (1981)
35. Janig, W. Neurophysiological mechanisms of cancer pain. *Recent Results in Cancer Research*, **89**, 45–58 (1984)
36. Payne, R. Anatomy, physiology and neuropharmacology of cancer pain. *Medical Clinics of North America*, **71**, 153–168 (1987)
37. Tasker, R. R. Deafferentation. In *Textbook of Pain* (ed. P. D. Wall and R. Melzack), Churchill Livingstone, New York, pp. 119–132 (1984)
38. Wall, P. D. Mechanisms of acute and chronic pain. In *Advances in Pain Research and Therapy, Vol. 5* (ed. J. J. Bonica, U. Lindblom and A. Iggo), Raven Press, New York, pp. 95–104 (1984)
39. Foley, K. M. Pain syndromes in patients with cancer. *Medical Clinics of North America*, **71**, 169–184 (1987)
40. Coyle, N. and Foley, K. M. Pain in patients with cancer: profile of patients and common pain syndromes. *Seminars in Oncology Nursing*, **1**, 93–99 (1985)
41. Foley, K. M. Analgesic management of bone pain. In *Bone Metastasis* (ed. L. Weiss and H. A. Gilbert), GK Hall Medical Publishers, Boston, pp. 348–368 (1981)
42. Galasko, C. S. B. Mechanism of bone destruction in the development of skeletal metastasis. *Nature*, **263**, 507–510 (1976)
43. Greenberg, J. S., Deck, M. D. F., Vikram, B. *et al.* Metastasis to the base of the skull: clinical findings in 43 patients. *Neurology*, **31**, 530–537 (1981)
44. Bingas, B. Tumors of the base of the skull. In *Handbook of Clinical Neurology, Vol. 17* (ed. P. J. Vinken and G. W. Bruyn), North Holland Publishing Co, Amsterdam, pp. 136–233 (1974)
45. Graus, F., Krol, G. and Foley, K. M. Early diagnosis of spinal epidural metastasis: correlation with clinical and radiological findings. *Proceedings or the American Society of Clinical Oncology*, 4, 269 (1985)
46. Haddad, P., Thaell, J. F., Kiely, J. M. *et al.* Lymphoma of the spinal extradural space. *Cancer*, **38**, 1862–1866 (1976)
47. Portenoy, R. K., Lipton, R. B. and Foley, K. M. Back pain in the cancer patient: an algorithm for evaluation and management. *Neurology*, **37**, 134–138 (1987)
48. Cascino, T. L., Kori, S., Krol, G. *et al.* CT scanning of the brachial plexus in patients with cancer. *Neurology*, **33**, 1553–1557 (1983)
49. Jaeckle, K. A., Young, D. F. and Foley, K. M. The natural history of lumbosacral plexopathy in cancer. *Neurology*, **35**, 8–15 (1985)
50. Kori, S., Foley, K. M. and Posner, J. B. Brachial plexus lesions in patients with cancer: clinical findings in 100 cases. *Neurology*, **31**, 45–50 (1981)
51. Thomas, J. E., Cascino, T. E. and Earle, J. D. Differential diagnosis between radiation and tumor plexopathy of the pelvis. *Neurology*, **35**, 1–7 (1985)
52. Kanner, R., Martini, N. and Foley, K. M. Incidence of pain and other clinical manifestations of superior pulmonary sulcus tumor (Pancoast's tumors). In *Advances in Pain Research and Therapy, Vol. 4*, (ed. J. J. Bonica, V. Ventafridda and C. A. Pagni), Raven Press, New York, pp. 27–38 (1982)
53. Payne, R. and Foley, K. M. Exploration of the brachial plexus in patients with cancer. *Neurology*, **36** (Suppl. 1) 329 (1986)
54. Wasserstrom, W. R., Glass, J. P. and Posner, J. B. Diagnosis and treatment of leptomeningeal metastasis from solid tumors: experience with 90 patients. *Cancer*, **49**, 759–772 (1982)
55. Olson, M. E., Chernik, N. L. and Posner, J. B. Infiltration of the leptomeninges by systemic cancer: a clinical and pathological study. *Archives of Neurology*, **30**, 122–137 (1978)
56. Gilbert, R. W., Kin, J-H and Posner, J. B. Epidural spinal cord compression from metastatic tumor: diagnosis and treatment. *Annals of Neurology*, **5**, 40–51 (1978)
57. Posner, J. B. Back pain and epidural spinal cord compression. *Medical Clinics of North America*, **71**, 185–206 (1987)
58. Findlay, G. F. G. Adverse effects of the management of malignant spinal cord compression. *Journal of Neurology, Neurosurgery and Psychiatry*, **47**, 761–768 (1984)
59. Barcena, A., Lobato, R. D., Rivas, J. J. *et al.* Spinal metastatic disease: analysis of factors determining functional prognosis and choice of treatment. *Neurosurgery*, **15**, 820–827 (1984)
60. Jellinger, K. and Sturm, K. W. Delayed radiation myelopathy in man. *Journal of the Neurological Sciences*, **14**, 389–408 (1971)
61. McLeod, J. G. Carcinomatous neuropathy. In *Peripheral Neuropathy* (ed P. J. Dyck, P. K. Thomas, E. H. Lambert and R. Bunge), W. B. Saunders, Philadelphia, pp. 2180–2191 (1984)

62. Lequesne, P. M. Neuropathy due to drugs. In *Peripheral Neuropathy* (ed. P. J. Dyck, P. K. Thomas, E. H. Lambert and R. Bunge), W. B. Saunders, Philadelphia, pp. 2126–2179 (1984)
63. Ihde, D. C. and DeVita, V. T. Osteonecrosis of the femoral head in patients with lymphoma treated with intermittent combination chemotherapy (including corticosteroids). *Cancer*, **36**, 1585–1588 (1975)
64. Rotstein, J. and Good, R. A. Steroid pseudorheumatism. *Archives of Internal Medicine*, **99**, 545–555 (1957)
65. Foley, K. M., Woodruff, J., Elis, F. *et al*. Radiation-induced malignant and atypical peripheral nerve sheath tumors. *Annals of Neurology*, **7**, 311–318 (1980)
66. Kanner, R. M., Martini, N. and Foley, K. M. Nature and incidence of postthoracotomy pain. *Proceedings of the American Society of Clinical Oncology*, **1**, 152 (1982)
67. Assa, J. The intercostobrachial nerve in radical mastectomy. *Journal of Surgical Oncology*, **6**, 123–126 (1974)
68. Granek, I., Ashikari, R. and Foley, K. M. Postmastectomy pain syndrome: clinical and anatomic correlates, *Proceedings of the American Society of Clinical Oncology*, **3**, 122 (1984)
69. Sherman, R. A., Sherman, C. J. and Parker, L. Chronic phantom and stump pain among American veterans: results of a survey. *Pain*, **18**, 83–95 (1984)
70. Weis, A. The phantom limb. **44**, 668–677 (1956)
71. Sherman, R. A. and Sherman, C. J. Prevalence and characteristics of chronic phantom limb pain among American veterans: results of a trial survey. *American Journal of Physical Medicine*, **62**, 227–238 (1983)

11
Pharmacologic management of chronic pain

Russell K. Portenoy

INTRODUCTION

Recent advances in understanding the basic mechanisms of pain transmission and modulation, combined with acceptance of more sophisticated methodology in clinical trials with analgesic drugs, have spurred extraordinary changes in the pharmacologic armamentarium for the management of chronic pain. An abundance of different drug classes, each with its own diverse set of specific agents, is now available, and this has proved both a boon and a burden to the practising clinician. A great deal can now be offered to the patient with persistent pain, and it is very likely that a larger proportion of patients can obtain relief than could before this era began. None the less, the rapid changes in available therapies and the extremely diverse group of pharmacologic interventions place great demands on the clinician, who must maintain a current and critical understanding of the medical literature to offer the best care to patients. This need is particularly compelling as the disorder in question is chronic pain, where the traditional availability of nostrums and the variable quality and general applicability of clinical investigation complicates all efforts to maintain a rational foundation for the selection and administration of drugs.

This chapter summarizes and critically evaluates the data relevant to the use of three broad categories of drugs in the management of chronic pain: the non-steroidal anti-inflammatory drugs (NSAIDs), adjuvant analgesics and opioid analgesics. Adjuvant analgesics represent a diverse group of distinct drug classes, all of which have other primary therapeutic indications but may be analgesic in selected circumstances (e.g. antidepressants, anticonvulsants, neuroleptics, etc.). The focus throughout this discussion is on the management of chronic non-malignant pain, the greatest challenge for the typical practitioner; the pharmacotherapy of cancer pain has been recently reviewed elsewhere [1–3].

GENERAL CONSIDERATIONS

The following principles guide the clinical application of analgesic therapy in patients with chronic pain.

1. The great variability in drug response, punctuated by the ever-present specter of the placebo effect, requires that the prospective randomized double-blind controlled clinical assay be accepted as the gold standard against which drug trials are compared. The value of a therapy remains unproved until tested in such a model. Moreover, given the broad interindividual variability in drug response, the extrapolation of positive results to other populations, symptoms or diseases must again relegate the drug to the status of an unproved entity. This, of course, is not to say that treatments based solely on survey data or on extrapolations of controlled studies may not be appropriate and acceptable in the absence of such data. The need for confirmatory studies should be recognized, however, and the clinician should both maintain an open mind about the validity of an unproved therapy and exercise caution in adopting such an approach before a clinical consensus builds about its utility.

2. It should be recognized that pharmacotherapy represents one of many diverse approaches that may be explored in the clinical management of chronic pain. Other approaches include neurostimulatory procedures, anesthetic techniques, surgical interventions, physiatric modalities and psychologically orientated interventions. A description of these approaches is beyond the scope of this discussion, but it is incumbent on the clinician to be aware of the existence of these other modalities and to determine the proper role of pharmacologic therapy at the time of the initial assessment and periodically throughout the patient's course. Multimodal therapy should be considered in all patients with chronic pain and, in some, pharmacotherapy should be superseded by other approaches.

3. The selection of one or more therapeutic modalities should be based on a comprehensive understanding of the factors that may be contributing to the patient's experience of pain and associated functional impairment. This is accomplished through a process of pain assessment, the goal of which can be usefully conceptualized as the development of a 'pain diagnosis'. The pain diagnosis summarizes the relevant features of the pain complaint in terms of its major organic and psychologic contributions, and clarifies the role of the pain in the medical, psychologic, social and cultural condition of the patient. This understanding depends on a comprehensive history and physical examination, supplemented with appropriate radiographic and laboratory tests. Classification of the pain by its temporal relations, associated syndrome, known etiologies and presumed pathophysiology provides a needed framework. The outcome of this process, or pain diagnosis, can be viewed as a summary statement in which the types and presumptive causes of the patient's major problems are listed and thereby targeted for therapy (*see* Chapter 10 for a further discussion of pain assessment and a description of classificatory schema for pain).

   The potential value of such assessment and conceptualization is clear, given the great variability among patients with a complaint of chronic pain. For example, should this process yield a judgement that the major contribution to the patient's disability is pain, and that the major contribution to the pain is an organic disturbance for which no primary therapy exists, then aggressive therapeutic trials with analgesic drugs alone may be the appropriate intervention. In contrast, should the assessment process conclude that the patient experiences disability that appears to be out of proportion to the pain complaint, or that the pain complaint is far in excess of what is typical for the underlying organic dysfunction, then pharmacologic therapies may best be viewed as adjunctive to primary psychologic and physiatric interventions designed to enhance function and reduce suffering, as well as to ameliorate pain.

4. The dosing regimens recommended for most of the drug therapies described below share several features. Most important is the requirement for an understanding of the pharmacologic properties of the drug class and specific agent. These pharmacologic characteristics include approved indications, unapproved indications accepted in medical practice, spectrum of side-effects, potential for more serious adverse effects, usual time–action relationships, and pharmacokinetic profile.

   Of the variety of measurable pharmacokinetic parameters, half-life is usually most relevant in the clinical setting. Four to five half-lives are required for steady-state plasma levels to be approached and an equal time is needed after discontinuation of dosing to remove almost all drug from the body. Although the relationship between plasma levels and effects may be variable in an individual, both generally continue to increase until steady state is approached. This may require days or weeks with drugs of long half-life. A large initial dose that rapidly raises plasma levels is preferred with drugs of long half-life, if such a loading dose would not produce intolerable side-effects when its plasma level peaks. Unfortunately, most analgesics cannot be safely loaded and both patient and clinician have no recourse but to wait until steady state is approached to determine the dosing schedule required for adequate analgesia.

5. Dosing titration is needed with virtually all analgesic medications. For chronic pain, relatively low doses should be administered initially (with the exception of those few drugs in which loading doses can be used), followed by gradual upward dose titration. This approach is somewhat counterintuitive, given the usual approach to medical therapeutics in which an effective dose range is defined a priori and failure to achieve the desired response at a certain quantity is interpreted as inefficacy of the agent, rather than inadequacy of the dose. Initial low doses are especially recommended in the treatment of chronic pain because some patients respond to these quantities and the likelihood of side-effects is reduced. Side-effects may be particularly troublesome in patients with pre-existent and excessive somatic concerns, and their avoidance often allows an adequate drug trial to ensue that would otherwise be discontinued by the patient. The desire to avoid untoward side-effects also justifies the recommendation that only one drug be added or titrated at a time.

   Although a poor response to a dose should lead to consideration of upward dose titration in all analgesic classes, the guidelines vary greatly from class to class. For the opioid drugs in the treatment of cancer pain, doses should be increased until analgesia occurs or intolerable side-effects supervene. For the other classes, clinically appropriate dosing limits are set, based on the presumption of a ceiling effect (a dose above which additional increments in dose fail to achieve more analgesia), a concern with toxicity, and recognition of customary use. These limits are discussed below.

6. A final principle based on the pharmacology of the specific agent is the need to continue a drug trial for an adequate duration. For virtually all analgesic drugs, some time is required after a dose is reached to evaluate drug efficacy. This interval is only partly determined by the half-life of the drug and the resultant time to approach steady state. With classes such as the NSAIDs and tricyclic antidepressants, it is commonly observed that the analgesic efficacy of a dose can accrue for days or weeks beyond the period required for steady-state plasma

drug levels. In the administration of most of these classes, therefore, it is recommended that at least 2 weeks elapse at what is presumed by the clinician to be a likely therapeutic dose before further dose titration or drug discontinuation occur. It should be recognized that patients require encouragement to continue taking an agent that yields little initial benefit, especially when it is causing side-effects. A clear description, at the outset of therapy, of the titration process and the anticipated side-effects often increases compliance with this demanding regimen, allowing adequate therapeutic trials to ensue.

NON-STEROIDAL ANTI-INFLAMMATORY DRUGS

The NSAIDs (here including acetaminophen) are believed to provide analgesia through a peripheral mechanism related to inhibition of the enzyme cyclo-oxygenase and consequent reduction of inflammatory mediators known to sensitize or activate peripheral nociceptors [4,5]. However, the marked disproportion between anti-inflammation and analgesia observed with some of these drugs, such as acetaminophen and zomepirac, suggest than other, as yet unknown, mechanisms may also be important.

A variety of subclasses comprise the NSAIDs [6]. Although anecdotal evidence suggests that efficacy and side-effect liability cluster within each group, the inter-individual variability in the response to different agents, even those within a sub-class, often appears more clinically compelling. NSAID analgesia is characterized by a ceiling dose, beyond which additional increments fail to yield greater pain relief, and by a lack of demonstrable physical dependence or tolerance. The ceiling dose limits the utility of the NSAIDs to the treatment of relatively mild to moderate pain. It is important to recognize that the ceiling dose may not be that recommended as the standard dose for the individual drug. The latter is derived from studies typically conducted in relatively young patients with an inflammatory disease and no other significant medical problems, a population very different from some of the patients with chronic pain, who may be elderly, have coexistent organ failure, or may be receiving multiple other drugs. This variability must be considered in the development of rational dosing guidelines.

The currently available classes of NSAIDs, the specific agents within each class and important pharmacologic details are summarized in Table 11.1. The differential toxicity of some agents and the great variability in pharmacokinetics also influence clinical decision-making in the selection and management of these drugs.

Drug selection

The NSAIDs are often effective when used alone for mild to moderate pain and provide additive analgesia when combined with opioid drugs in the treatment of more severe pain [7,8]. Relatively few agents have been specifically approved as analgesics, but clinical experience suggests that any can potentially be useful for this indication. NSAIDs appear to be especially useful in patients with malignant bone pain and pain related to grossly inflammatory lesions; their efficacy in neuropathic pain is minimal.

The profile of toxic effects associated with NSAIDs as a class, with each of the sub-classes and with specific agents, influences the process of drug selection. For example, the pyrazole sub-class, specifically phenylbutazone, carries a greater risk of adverse effects than the other NSAIDs and has been supplanted by newer drugs. All NSAIDs should be used cautiously in patients with renal insufficiency; if indicated in this setting, sulindac is the preferred drug and acetaminophen can be used safely. Most agents are relatively contraindicated in patients with a diathesis for bleeding or peptic ulcer disease. Appropriate first-line drugs in this setting are acetaminophen and two non-acetylated salicylates, choline magnesium salicylate and salsalate. These salicylates have far less ulcer potential than other NSAIDs and, at usual clinical doses, do not impair platelet aggregation [9]. All NSAIDs, except acetaminophen, may cause or exacerbate encephalopathy and may be problematic in patients at risk from volume overload; they must therefore be administered cautiously to patients with pre-existing encephalopathy and those with congestive heart failure, peripheral edema or ascites. Finally, it should be noted that significant hepatopathy mandates prudence in the administration of acetaminophen.

Several other factors should be considered in the selection of an NSAID. First, the great inter-individual variability in the response to different drugs suggests that a favorable previous exposure to a particular agent is an indication to use the same drug again. Second, concern about compliance with a prescribed regimen may be lessened by the use of an NSAID with once-daily (piroxicam) or twice-daily dosing (e.g. choline magnesium trisalicylate, diflunisal, naproxen, and others). Finally, the cost of the different NSAIDs varies widely and, when this is an important issue, pharmacies can be screened for a schedule of charges so that this factor may be taken into consideration.

Exploration of the dose–response relationship

In light of the pharmacologic considerations discussed earlier, it is reasonable to begin with a relatively low dose, then to increase it gradually every several days or less often in an attempt to identify the ceiling dose (or maximum pain relief) in the individual patient. Should no additional analgesia accrue from an increase in dose, the ceiling has presumably been reached and the dose should be lowered to the minimum level that provides optimal relief or, if the relief is insignificant, the drug should be discontinued. In recognition of the dose-related toxicities observed with the NSAIDs and the paucity of information available about the safety of long-term administration of high doses, it is recommended on clinical grounds that doses should not exceed 1.5–2 times the standard dose. Below this maximum, the dose–response function can be explored to find the lowest dose that yields the greatest degree of analgesia attainable.

Duration of trials

Several weeks are needed to judge the efficacy of a dose when NSAIDs are used in the treatment of grossly inflammatory lesions, such as arthritis. Clinical experience suggests that a briefer period, such as a week, is adequate for the same purpose in pain patients without a grossly inflammatory lesion.

Table 11.1 Non-steroidal anti-inflammatory drugs

Chemical class	Generic name	Approximate half-life (h)	Dosing schedule	Recommended starting dose (mg/day)	Maximum recommended dose (mg/day)	Comment
p-Aminophenol derivatives	Acetaminophen	2–4	q.4–6 h	1400	6000	Overdosage produces hepatic toxicity. Not anti-inflammatory and therefore not preferred as first-line analgesic or co-analgesic in patients with inflammatory lesions. Lack of GI or platelet toxicity, however, may be important in some patients
Salicylates	Aspirin	3–5	q.4–6 h	1400	6000	Standard for comparison. May not be tolerated as well as some of the newer NSAIDs
	Diflunisal	8–12	q.12 h	1000 × 1 then 500 q.12 h	1500	Less GI toxicity than aspirin
	Choline magnesium trisalicylate	8–12	q.12 h	1500 × 1 then 1000 q.12 h	4000	Unlike other NSAIDs, choline Mg trisalicylate and salsalate have minimal GI toxicity and no effect on platelet aggregation, despite potent anti-inflammatory effects
	Salsalate	8–12	q.12 h	1500 × 1 then 1000 q.12 h	4000	
Proprionic acids	Ibuprofen	3–4	q.6–8 h	1200	3200	Available over the counter
	Naproxen	13	q.12 h	500	1000	
	Naproxen sodium	13	q.12 h	550	1100	
	Fenoprofen	2–3	q.6 h	800	3200	

						Comments
Acetic acids	Indomethacin	4–5	q.8–12 h	75	200	Available in sustained-release and rectal formulation. Higher incidence of side-effects, particularly GI and CNS, than proprionic acids
	Tolmetin	5	q.6–8 h	600	2000	Less renal toxicity than other NSAIDs
	Sulindac	18	q.12 h	300	400	Experience limited
	Suprofen	2–4	q.6 h	600	800	
Oxicams	Piroxicam	45	q.24 h	20	40	Generally more toxic than proprionic acids
Fenamates	Mefenamic acid	2	q.6 h	500 × 1 then 250 q.6 h	1000	Not recommended for use > 1 week
	Meclofenamic acid	2–4	q.6–8 h	150	400	
Pyrazoles	Phenylbutazone	50–100	q.6–8 h	300	400	Not a first-line drug due to risk

Switching drugs

Given the inter-individual variability in drug response and the anecdotal evidence that drugs within a sub-class may yield similar effects, it is reasonable to follow failure with one of the NSAIDs by a trial with a drug in an alternative sub-class.

ADJUVANT ANALGESICS

The adjuvant analgesics can be divided into the antidepressants, anticonvulsants, neuroleptics, oral local anesthetics, muscle relaxants, antihistamines, sympatholytic agents, and several miscellaneous agents.

Antidepressants

There is a great deal of evidence in support of a primary analgesic effect of the tricyclic antidepressants (TCAs) in a large number of chronic pain states (for reviews, *see* [10–12]). The analgesic effects of these drugs were first believed to be related solely to the reversal of depression [13]. This notion has been negated by a number of clinical observations. For example, pain relief usually occurs earlier than mood change in chronic pain patients [14] and analgesia can develop in the absence of mood changes in depressed patients with pain [14,15], as well as in chronic pain patients without depression [14,16,17]. Analgesic effects have also been demonstrated in animals [18], further confirmation that mood alteration is not prerequisite to pain relief.

Current hypotheses for the mode of action of TCA drugs focuses on their relationship to endogenous monoamine-dependent pain-modulating systems. It is assumed that TCAs increase the availability of central monamines in these pathways through blockade of re-uptake mechanisms. The best-characterized of these monoamine-dependent pain-modulating systems is a serotonergic tract that originates in the rostroventral medulla, descends to the dorsal horn of the spinal cord and functions through an enkephalinergic interneuron to inhibit transmission of nociceptive information at the first central synapse [19–22]. It is interesting to note that the specific tricyclics most widely accepted as analgesics are the tertiary amine compounds, such as amitriptyline (Table 11.2), the activity of which is relatively greatest on serotonin re-uptake. Other monoaminergic pain-modulating systems exist, however, including one that uses norepinephrine as a transmitter [23]. The importance of these pathways in the mode of action of the TCAs remains ill defined. Indeed, it is important to recognize both that TCAs bind to a large variety of different receptors [24] and that a diverse group of neurotransmitters and neuromodulators have now been implicated in the process of pain modulation [19]. The potential interactions of the TCAs are thus extremely complex and have prevented the clear elucidation of the analgesic mechanism of these drugs.

In addition to a large number of uncontrolled studies suggesting the analgesic efficacy of TCA compounds (*see* [10–12]), many controlled studies have been performed. These studies have established the efficacy of amitriptyline in diabetic neuropathy [16], postherpetic neuralgia [14], tension and migraine headache [17,25], myofascial pain [26] and psychogenic pain [27]. Imipramine has been found to be effective in arthritic pain [28] and painful diabetic neuropathy [29] and

Table 11.2 Commonly used adjuvant analgesics

Class	Rationale for use	Indication	Preferred drugs	Dosing schedule	Starting dose (mg/day)	Usual daily dose (mg/day)	Comment
Tricyclic antidepressants	Proven analgesics in a variety of non-malignant pain states	Numerous chronic pains. Pain complicated by depression or insomnia	Amitriptyline Doxepin Imipramine	q.h.s. q.h.s. q.h.s.	10–25 10–25 10–25	50–150 (pain); up to 300 (depression)	If side effects, trial of nortriptyline or desipramine
Anticonvulsants	Extensive survey data suggesting efficacy in lancinating neuropathic pain	Lancinating neuropathic pain	Carbamazepine Phenytoin Valproate Clonazepam Baclofen	q. 6–8 h q.h.s. q. 8 h q. 12 h q. 8 h	200 300 500 0.5 15	600–1600 300 750–2250 2–7 30–60	Baclofen is not an anticonvulsant, but has potential efficacy in lancinating pain
Oral local anesthetics	Controlled trials of tocainide in trigeminal neuralgia and mexiletine in diabetic neuropathy	Neuropathic pain	Mexiletine Tocainide	q. 8 h q. 8 h	300 600	450–900 1200–1800	Mexiletine is safer than tocainide and should be tried first
Neuroleptics	Anecdotal experience in continuous neuropathic pain	Pain complicated by delirium or nausea; refractory neuropathic pain	Fluphenazine Haloperidol Methotrimeprazine	q.8 h q. 6–12 h q.6 h	2 2 20	3–6 2–10 20–60	Not first line. Has lack of supporting documentation and potential toxicity. Methotrimeprazine is proven analgesic, but no oral form; appears useful for terminal pain and agitation
Muscle relaxants	Analgesia greater than placebo in controlled trials	Acute musculoskeletal pain	Orphenadrine Carisoprodol Chlorzoxazone Methocarbamol Cyclobenzaprine	q. 6–8 h q. 6 h q. 6–8 h q. 6 h q. 8 h	100 800 750 4000 30	100–200 800–1200 750–1000 4000 30	Mechanism of action unknown; analgesia may be due to non-specific sedative effects. Should not be used chronically

doxepin has been determined to be analgesic in psychogenic headache [30] and coexistent chronic pain and depression [31]. Two drugs not available in the United States – clomipramine and zimelidine – have also been noted to be analgesic in several pain syndromes [32–34].

Monoamine oxidase inhibitors also increase central monoamines, but do so through a mechanism which differs from that of the TCAs. The inherent toxicity of these drugs, specifically the potential for hypertensive crisis after ingestion of tyramine-containing foodstuffs, severely compromises the utility of these agents in the management of chronic pain. They have achieved some measure of acceptance in refractory migraine [35] and their analgesic potential has been supported by a controlled trial in patients with atypical facial pain [15]. Given their toxicity, however, their routine use cannot be recommended.

Dosing guidelines

With efficacy proven in a broad group of chronic pain states, a trial of a TCA should be considered in virtually all chronic pain syndromes, unless contraindicated by significant cardiac arrhythmias, symptomatic prostatic hypertrophy or narrow-angle glaucoma. Clinical experience suggests that the indication is strongest in patients with chronic neuropathic pain characterized by continuous dysesthesias and in those individuals with pain of any type complicated by depression.

The choice of TCA is empiric. Given the data from controlled studies, a tertiary amine TCA, specifically amitriptyline, doxepin or imipramine, is preferred. In patients unable to tolerate these agents because of their anticholinergic or hypotensive effects, a trial with a secondary amine TCA, specifically nortriptyline or desipramine, is warranted.

Initial doses of one of the tertiary amine TCAs should be low, 10–25 mg at night. Doses should be increased gradually over 1–2 weeks to 50–75 mg at night, then held for a week or so, before resuming upward titration. Analgesic effects usually occur within 4–7 days and typically require a dose of 50–150 mg per night [14,16]. Twice-daily dosing should be considered should effects wane before the evening dose. If neither analgesia nor intolerable side-effects occur at a dose of 150 mg at night, or if pain is complicated by depression, a trial of higher doses is indicated. At some point, a plasma level can be determined to assure that non-compliance, poor absorption or unusually rapid catabolism is not compromising efforts to achieve therapeutic levels; there are no data relating a specific plasma level to analgesia. Finally, clinical experience suggests that the analgesic response to the different TCA drugs varies within the same patient; hence, failure to respond to adequate doses of one should be followed by a trial with another.

Anticonvulsants

Despite a paucity of controlled clinical trials, anticonvulsant medications (Table 11.2) have become widely accepted in the management of chronic neuropathic pain, particularly those characterized as lancinating pains [36]. Their mode of analgesic action in these syndromes is not known, but presumably relates to the variety of mechanisms underlying their anticonvulsant effects, such as suppression of paroxysmal discharges, neuronal hyperexcitability or spread of abnormal discharges [37].

Phenytoin was the first anticonvulsant employed in the treatment of pain. Efficacy in trigeminal neuralgia was suggested in uncontrolled series [38,39], and favorable effects were reported in isolated cases or small groups of patients with glossopharyngeal neuralgia [40], tabetic lightning pains [41], paroxysmal pain in postherpetic neuralgia [42], thalamic pain [43], post-sympathectomy pain [44], and post-traumatic neuralgia [45]. A similar outcome was noted in controlled trials of painful neuropathy in Fabry's disease [46] and painful diabetic neuropathy [47]. Most of the neuropathic pains in these syndromes were characterized by a prominent lancinating component.

Controlled trials have established the efficacy of carbamazepine in trigeminal neuralgia [48–50]. A controlled trial in postherpetic neuralgia demonstrated efficacy against the lancinating, but not continuous, pains of this disorder [50] and another controlled trial noted a favorable outcome in painful diabetic neuropathy [51]. Published case series and anecdotal reports have also suggested efficacy in glossopharyngeal neuralgia, tabetic lightning pains, paroxysmal pain in multiple sclerosis, post-sympathectomy pain, lancinating pains due to cancer and post-traumatic neuralgia [40,44,45,52,55].

Uncontrolled clinical trials and anecdotal reports have similarly suggested that clonazepam and valproate may be effective in these neuropathic pains. Clonazepam has been reported to be useful in the treatment of trigeminal neuralgia, paroxysmal post-laminectomy pain and post-traumatic neuralgia [45,56,57] while valproate has been suggested in the management of trigeminal neuralgia, postherpetic neuralgia and other similar pains [45,58,59].

Although not themselves anticonvulsant, two other drugs have been demonstrated in controlled trials to be efficacious in trigeminal neuralgia and are thus often classified with these anticonvulsant medications. Clinical experience suggests that these agents, too, can be considered in the management of lancinating neuropathic pains of other types. The first, baclofen, is a GABA agonist primarily indicated in the treatment of spasticity [60], and the second is tocainide, an oral local anesthetic chemically related to lidocaine [61].

Guidelines

In trigeminal neuralgia, controlled studies support the use of carbamazepine, baclofen and tocainide. Carbamazepine is usually considered to be the first-line drug. The combined evidence in controlled and uncontrolled studies suggests that lancinating pains in other neuropathic pain states may respond to any of the agents described. The use of these drugs in non-neuropathic pains is not supported, and there are only meager data suggesting potential efficacy in the continuous dysesthesias that often characterize neuropathic disorders. Clinical experience suggests that one or more of these drugs can occasionally be useful for the latter type of pain, and a trial in refractory cases is reasonable. Surveys [45] and clinical experience likewise indicate that patients may have markedly different analgesic responses to the various drugs described. Should one fail, a trial of another is in order. Combination therapy) (e.g. baclofen and carbamazepine or diphenylhydantoin plus carbamazepine) may also be worth trying if monotherapy is suboptimal.

There have been no studies to determine the relationship between plasma level and pain relief with any of these drugs. The anticonvulsants are typically prescribed in a manner and dose identical to that employed in the treatment of seizures. A conservative oral loading dose of phenytoin is reasonable, but the other drugs should be initiated at low doses, then gradually titrated upward to limit side-effects. Doses should generally be increased until favorable effects or side-effects occur, although clinical experience suggests that patients who fail to respond as plasma levels rise to the upper limits of the usual therapeutic range, and then above, are unlikely to respond, and it may be reasonable in this setting to discontinue the drug and institute another.

Neuroleptics

The data in support of the use of neuroleptic drugs (Table 11.2) in the treatment of chronic pain is largely anecdotal. Controlled studies have established the analgesic efficacy of methotrimeprazine and determined its analgesic potency to be near that of morphine [62–64]. This drug, however, is available in a parenteral formulation only and has prominent sedative effects. Although clinical experience suggests that it may be extremely useful in the management of cancer pain, particularly in those with concurrent anxiety or nausea, or gastrointestinal or pulmonary disease sufficient to impede opioid dosing, it cannot be recommended in the treatment of non-malignant pain syndromes. Oddly, a controlled trial of another phenothiazine, chlorpromazine, in cancer pain failed to demonstrate analgesic effects [65].

The remainder of the evidence in support of the analgesic potential of this class of drugs comprises anecdotal reports and case series. These have suggested the value of haloperidol, fluphenazine, perphenazine, thioridazine, chlorprothixene and chlorpromazine in the management of patients with a variety of painful disorders, the majority of which are neuropathic. These include postherpetic neuralgia, painful polyneuropathy, plexopathy, thalamic pain and arthritis [66–71]. Despite the dramatic benefit sometimes observed after the addition of a neuroleptic drug, the analgesic efficacy of this class, with the exception of methotrimeprazine, remains unconfirmed (even doubtful).

Guidelines

Neuroleptics should be viewed as second-line agents potentially of value in the management of refractory neuropathic pain states. This conclusion attempts to balance the well-known risks of these drugs, including the possibility of irreversible movement disorders, with the relatively meager evidence of analgesic efficacy. Clinical experience is greatest with fluphenazine and haloperidol. Doses reported to be effective are generally low and, in contrast to the drugs described previously, there are no clinical data to support the concept of upward dose titration beyond this range (Table 11.2).

Oral local anesthetics

The recent introduction of oral local anesthetic drugs for the management of cardiac arrhythmias has spurred interest in the analgesic potential of this class, particularly in neuropathic pain states (Table 11.2). This potential has been suggested by the reported efficacy of brief intravenous infusions of lidocaine in patients with painful diabetic neuropathy and chronic pain from Dercum's disease

[72–74]. Two oral analogs of lidocaine have been tested in well-controlled clinical trials. The efficacy of tocainide in the lancinating pain of trigeminal neuralgia has been confirmed [61] and, more recently, a carefully controlled trial established the analgesic efficacy of mexiletine in patients with painful diabetic polyneuropathy [75]. Interestingly, these data suggest that these two similar drugs may be effective in both the lancinating and continuous dysesthesias of neuropathic pain states.

Guidelines

Many more controlled investigations will be needed to clarify the analgesic potential of these and other local anesthetics but, at present, it is reasonable to view them as second-line agents for the treatment of refractory neuropathic pain syndromes of any type. Of the two available drugs, mexiletine appears to be the safer compound [76] and should be attempted first. Dosing is empiric at present and should mimic that appropriate for the treatment of chronic arrhythmias [76].

Muscle relaxants

Muscle-relaxant drugs are commonly employed in the treatment of musculoskeletal pains. This clinical acceptability, however, does not indicate either a clear understanding of their mechanisms of action or an abundance of data establishing their analgesic efficacy. Problems with nomenclature further complicate an understanding of the pharmacology of these drugs and impede efforts to develop rational dosing guidelines.

The muscle-relaxant drugs must be distinguished from those agents useful in the treatment of spasticity. Stiffness, cramps and painful flexor or extensor spasms may occur in this setting. This phenomenon is clearly different from the muscle 'spasms' that occur in the setting of nerve or myofascial injury. The latter represent focal areas of increased muscle activity associated with tenderness and splinting of the painful part. Drugs useful in the treatment of true spasticity, such as baclofen and dantrolene, are not indicated for the far more common myofascial pains due to local spasm. Likewise, the muscle-relaxant drugs are not indicated in the treatment of true spasticity. The exception to this notion is diazepam, which is commonly used in both settings.

The muscle-relaxant drugs used in the United States include orphenadrine, carisoprodol, chlorzoxazone, methocarbamol and cyclobenzaprine (Table 11.2). All but cyclobenzaprine are similar in pharmacologic effects and are believed to exert muscle-relaxant effects through the suppression of polysynaptic spinal reflexes [72,78]. This phenomenon, however, is observed in experimental preparations and there is no evidence that the clinical effects of these drugs is related to relaxation of striated muscle. Cyclobenzaprine is pharmacologically related to the tricyclic antidepressants. Its mechanism of action is also unknown; like the other compounds in this class, it has no direct effect on muscle and there is no evidence that muscle relaxation *per se* underlies the effects observed clinically.

Controlled studies have, in general, demonstrated efficacy greater than placebo for each of these agents in the treatment of musculoskeletal pain of one type or another [79,80]. Some studies have demonstrated analgesia above that provided by aspirin or acetaminophen, or analgesia from the combination of a muscle relaxant and either aspirin or acetaminophen above that provided by the analgesic alone

[81]. Available data are inadequate to determine whether these favorable responses are due to a non-specific sedative action shared by all these drugs, a primary analgesic effect, a partial lessening of local muscle tension, or some combination of these effects. There are no data comparing the efficacy or side-effect liability of different drugs within this class, nor have studies been performed that compare any of the drugs of this class to an NSAID other than aspirin, an opioid or a sedative/hypnotic drug. Moreover, no study has adequately assessed the long-term consequences of chronic administration of any of these compounds to patients with persistent pain.

Guidelines

The data available suggest that there may be value in the administration of one of these drugs to patients with acute musculoskeletal pain. No drug can be recommended over any other. There is no support at present for long-term administration and therapy should generally be limited to no more than 2 weeks. Dosing also remains empiric and there is no evidence to suggest that upward dose titration beyond usually recommended doses produces any other effect than progressive sedation, with an unknown degree of accruing risk. For this group of drugs, therefore, the concept of dose escalation cannot be recommended.

Antihistamines

A large number of controlled and uncontrolled studies have demonstrated the analgesic efficacy of antihistamine drugs [82]. In addition to orphenadrine, which is classified both as a centrally acting muscle relaxant and an antihistamine, controlled trials of diphenhydramine and hydroxyzine have established the analgesic potential of these drugs [80–84]. The mechanism of action of these drugs is not known, although it is interesting to speculate about the role of specific histamine receptors in the endogenous pathways for pain modulation [82]. In the clinical setting, it is difficult to distinguish observed analgesic effects from the often prominent sedative effects of these drugs. Moreover, it remains uncertain that the doses typically employed clinically, which are often less than those studied in analgesic trials, are themselves analgesic. For example, a small controlled trial comparing repetitive doses of hydroxyzine 25 mg orally failed to demonstrate an analgesic effect [85].

On the basis of clinical experience, hydroxyzine is commonly used as a co-analgesic in the management of cancer pain patients with concurrent anxiety or nausea [1,2]. With the exception of orphenadrine compounds, which are used as a muscle relaxant in acute musculoskeletal pains, the clinical use of antihistamine drugs for analgesia has otherwise not achieved wide acceptance. Given the limited clinical experience, the routine use of these drugs in the long-term management of chronic pain cannot be recommended.

Sympatholytic drugs

Although sympathetic nerve blocks remain the first-line approach in the management of sympathetic-maintained neuropathic pain, such as reflex sympathetic dystrophy (86), oral sympatholytic therapy can be considered for those unable to tolerate these techniques or who fail to benefit adequately. There have been no controlled trials assessing the efficacy of any of these drugs in this type of neuropathic pain. A controlled study of propranolol in patients with post-traumatic neuralgia failed to demonstrate any therapeutic benefit, but no effort was made to distinguish patients with a sympathetic-maintained pain syndrome from those with neuropathic pain of other pathophysiologies [87]. Efficacy of this drug was claimed, however, in an anecdotal report of two patients with reflex sympathetic dystrophy [88]. Oral guanethidine and prazosin have also been reported to be of benefit in small series of patients with this disorder [89–91]. Phenoxybenzamine was reported to be uniformly successful in treating the pain of 40 patients with causalgia [92]. All the patients in this report, however, had pain of relatively short duration and the efficacy of this drug in more established cases of sympathetic-maintained pain remains unknown.

On both theoretical and clinical grounds, a trial of sympatholytic therapy can be recommended only for those neuropathic pain syndromes for which the presumption of a sympathetically mediated pathophysiology can be adduced (e.g. causalgia and reflex sympathetic dystrophy). This is best determined by at least a partial response to sympathetic blockade but, in the absence of this, includes pain syndromes characterized by the association of neuropathic pain and local signs of autonomic dysregulation, with or without the development of trophic changes [86]. In addition to oral sympatholytic therapy, corticosteroids [93] and oral nifedipine [94] have been suggested in anecdotal reports to be potentially useful in these syndromes. Other drugs, including TCAs, anticonvulsants and neuroleptics, are also commonly administered as more non-specific agents sometimes useful for chronic neuropathic pain.

Miscellaneous drugs

Studies in the postoperative setting have suggested analgesic potential for some of the benzodiazepine drugs, including diazepam and midazolam [95,96]. A recent survey similarly suggested the potential value of alprazolam in patients with chronic neuropathic pain [97]. On the other hand, a small controlled study of repeated doses of chordiazepoxide in chronic pain failed to demonstrate any benefit [85]. A study of experimental pain, which used sophisticated analytical methods designed to distinguish a change in sensory function from psychologic effects, suggested that the reduction of pain intensity following an injection of diazepam results from psychologic influences alone [98]. In the light of concerns about the induction of physical dependence to the benzodiazepine drugs and the long-term cognitive effects of these compounds [99], these data do not provide adequate support for the administration of these agents as analgesics in patients with chronic pain. Given abundant clinical experience, there may be a role for diazepam in the short-term management of acute musculoskeletal pain, and the use of the other drugs should rely on primary psychotropic indications.

L-Tryptophan, a precursor of serotonin, has also been demonstrated to have analgesic effects in patients with chronic non-malignant pain [100]. Clinical experience with this drug has not been very favorable, but side-effects other than mild sedation or nausea are uncommon, and a trial in chronic pain syndromes of varying types is reasonable. The combination of L-tryptophan and a TCA is theoretically sensible, but additive analgesia has never been confirmed experimentally. As with the TCAs, it is useful to begin at a relatively low dose, then increase to the range of 3–5 g daily.

Drugs with sympathomimetic effects, specifically dextroamphetamine, methylphenidate and caffeine, are also analgesic [101–103]. Caffeine is employed in combination products used in the treatment of headache, and both dextroamphetamine and methylphenidate are accepted as co-analgesics useful in the management of opioid-induced sedation in those with cancer pain [1,2]. Given the potential for tachyphylaxis and toxicity with the latter two drugs, use in patients with chronic non-malignant pain should be avoided.

Clonidine, an α_2-adrenergic agonist, has been suggested as an analgesic in an anecdotal report describing the successful treatment of nocturnal leg pains in several diabetics [104], a single-dose study in postherpetic neuralgia [105] and controlled studies of migraine [106]. The efficacy in migraine has been disputed [107] and, in the light of the limited favorable data and the potential for side-effects, a trial of this drug should be viewed as a second-line approach in those with refractory neuropathic pain.

Finally, cannabinoid drugs also have analgesic potential [108]. This benefit, however, is compromised by a significant incidence of side-effects. At present they cannot be recommended for patients with chronic pain.

OPIOID ANALGESICS

The most controversial pharmacologic approach to the management of chronic non-malignant pain is opioid maintenance therapy. It is generally taken as a clinical axiom that the long-term administration of these drugs is contraindicated in patients without malignant disease, because of the potential for loss of efficacy over time (i.e. the development of tolerance), side-effects and serious toxicity and, most importantly, the development of drug addiction. Recently, however, series of cases have been reported in which patients with a wide variety of painful disorders refractory to usual therapies were maintained for long periods on opioid drugs [109–114]. Although improvement in physical and psychologic functioning as a consequence of this therapy cannot be reliably adduced from these surveys, persistent partial analgesia was a commonly observed outcome. Opioid toxicity was never viewed as a problem and management difficulties compatible with the development of addictive behaviors occurred in a very small number of patients. On the basis of this clinical experience, guidelines for management have been suggested (Table 11.3).

Exhaustive reviews [110,115] do not support concerns about loss of efficacy. Furthermore, there are considerable data suggesting that addiction, defined as a syndrome characterized by drug craving, efforts to secure a supply, recidivism and unsanctioned use, is an extraordinarily uncommon outcome in patients with no previous history of substance abuse and a clear-cut medical indication for analgesic drugs [110,115–119].

It is thus conceivable that opioid maintenance therapy is an alternative approach capable of providing some relief to selected patients with refractory pain who are motivated and responsible enough to adhere to the strict guidelines necessary for the management of this therapy (Table 11.3). The available surveys cannot exclude the possibility, however, that the success of these patients represents more the intense and stable involvement of concerned and knowledgeable practitioners than

Table 11.3 Proposed guidelines in the management of opioid maintenance therapy for non-malignant pain

---

1. Should be considered only after all other reasonable attempts at analgesia have failed
2. A history of substance abuse should be viewed as a relative contraindication
3. A single practitioner should take primary responsibility for treatment
4. Patients should give informed consent before the start of therapy; points to be covered include recognition of the low risk of psychologic dependence as an outcome, potential for cognitive impairment with the drug alone and in combination with sedative/hypnotics, and understanding by female patients that children born when the mother is on opioid maintenance therapy will be likely to be physically dependent at birth
5. After drug selection, doses should be given on an around-the-clock basis; several weeks should be agreed upon as the period of initial dose titration, and although improvement in function should be continually stressed, all should agree to at least partial analgesia as the appropriate goal of therapy
6. Failure to achieve at least partial analgesia at relatively low initial doses in the non-tolerant patient raises questions about the potential treatability of the pain syndrome with opioids
7. Emphasis should be given to attempts to capitalize on improved analgesia by gains in physical and social function
8. In addition to the daily dose determined initially, patients should be permitted to escalate dose transiently on days of increased pain; two methods are acceptable:
    (a) Prescription of an additional 4–6 'rescue doses' to be taken as needed during the month
    (b) Instruction that one or two extra doses may be taken on any day, but must be followed by an equal reduction of dose on subsequent days
9. Patients must be seen and drugs prescribed at least monthly
10. Exacerbations of pain not effectively treated by transient, small increases in dose are best managed in the hospital, where dose escalation, if appropriate, can be observed closely and a return to baseline doses can be accomplished in a controlled environment
11. Evidence of drug hoarding, acquisition of drugs from other physicians, uncontrolled dose escalation, or other aberrant behaviors should be followed by tapering and discontinuation of opioid maintenance therapy

---

the pharmacotherapy itself. Controlled prospective studies are needed to evaluate this proposition and determine the general applicability of therapy and the risks and benefits for patients with chronic non-malignant pain. Given the enormous political and social pressures surrounding the issue of drug use, there is a compelling need for professionals engaged in the treatment of these challenging patients to undertake an ongoing, dispassionate and scientifically grounded discussion about the medical role of opioid drugs.

References

1. Foley, K. M. The treatment of cancer pain. *New England Journal of Medicine*, **313**, 84–95 (1985)
2. Portenoy, R. K. and Foley, K. M. The management of cancer pain. In *Handbook of Psycho-oncology* (ed. J. Holland and L. Rowland), Oxford University Press, New York, in press
3. Twycross, R. G. and Lack, S. A. *Symptom Control in Far Advanced Cancer: Pain Relief*, Pitman, London, pp. 100–293 (1983)
4. Vane, J. R. Inhibition of prostaglandin synthesis as a mechanism of action for aspirin-like drugs. *Nature New Biology*, **234**, 231–238 (1971)
5. Higgs, G. A. and Moncada, S. Interactions of arachidonate products with other pain mediators. In *Advances in Pain Research and Therapy, Vol. 5*, (ed. J. J. Bonica, U. Lindblom and A. Iggo), Raven Press, New York, pp. 617–626 (1983)

6. Kantor, T. G. Peripherally-acting analgesics. In *Analgesics: Neurochemical, Behavioral, and Clinical Perspectives* (ed. M. Kuhar and G. Pasternak), Raven Press, New York, pp. 289–313 (1984)
7. Ventafridda, V., Fochi, C., DeConno, F. and Sganzerla, E. Use of nonsteroidal anti-inflammatory drugs in the treatment of pain in cancer. *British Journal of Clinical Pharmacology*, **10**, 343–346 (1980)
8. Ferrer-Brechner, T. and Ganz, P. Combination therapy with ibuprofen and methadone for chronic cancer pain. *American Journal of Medicine*, **77**, 78–83 (1984)
9. Cohen, A., Thomas, G. B. and Coen, E. E. Serum concentration, safety and tolerance of oral doses of choline magnesium trisalicylate. *Current Therapeutic Research*, **23**, 358–364 (1978)
10. Walsh, T. D. Antidepressants in chronic pain. *Clinical Neuropharmacology*, **6**, 271–295 (1983)
11. Butler, S. Present status of tricyclic antidepressants in chronic pain. In *Advances in Pain Research and Therapy, Vol. 7* (ed. C. Benedetti, C. R. Chapman and G. Moricca), Raven Press, New York, 173–198 (1984)
12. Getto, C. J., Sorkness, C. A. and Howell, T. Antidepressants and chronic nonmalignant pain: a review. *Journal of Pain Symptom Management*, **2**, 9–18 (1987)
13. Evans, W., Gensler, F., Blackwell, B. and Galbrecht, C. The effects of antidepressant drugs on pain relief and mood in the chronically ill. *Psychosomatics*, **14**, 214–219 (1973)
14. Watson, C. P. N., Evans, R. J., Reed, K. *et al.* Amitriptyline versus placebo in postherpetic neuralgia. *Neurology*, **32**, 671–673 (1982)
15. Lascelles, R. G. Atypical facial pain and depression. *British Journal of Psychology*, **122**, 651–659 (1966)
16. Max, M. B., Culnane, M., Schafer, S. C. *et al.* Amitriptyline relieves diabetic neuropathy pain in patients with normal or depressed mood. *Neurology*, **37**, 589–594 (1987)
17. Couch, J. R., Ziegler, D. K. and Hassanein, R. Amitriptyline in the prophylaxis of migraine: effectiveness and relationship of antimigraine and antidepressant effects. *Neurology*, **26**, 121–127 (1976)
18. Spiegel, K., Kalb, R. and Pasternak, G. W. Analgesic activity of tricyclic antidepressants. *Annals of Neurology*, **13**, 462–465 (1983)
19. Hammond, D. L. Pharmacology of central pain-modulating networks (biogenic amines and nonopioid analgesics). In *Advances in Pain Research and Therapy, Vol. 9* (ed. H. L. Fields, R. Dubner and F. Cervero), Raven Press, New York, pp. 499–513 (1985)
20. Basbaum, A. I. and Fields, H. L. Endogenous pain control systems: brainstem spinal pathways and endorphin circuitry. *Annual Review of Neuroscience*, **7**, 309–338 (1984)
21. Yaksh, T. L. Direct evidence that spinal serotonin and noradrenaline terminals mediate the spinal antinociceptive effects of morphine in the periaqueductal gray. *Brain Research*, **160**, 180–185 (1979)
22. Yaksh, T. L. and Tyce, G. M. Microinjection of morphine into the periaqueductal gray evokes the release of serotonin from the spinal cord. *Brain Research*, **171**, 176–181 (1979)
23. Howe, J. R., Wang, J.-R. and Yaksh, T. L. Selective antagonism of the antinociceptive effect of intrathecally applied alpha adrenergic agonists by intrathecal prazocin and intrathecal yohimbe. *Journal of Pharmacology and Experimental Therapeutics*, **224**, 552–558 (1983)
24. Richelson, E. Tricyclic antidepressants and neurotransmitter receptors. *Psychiatric Annals*, **9**, 186–194 (1979)
25. Diamond, S. and Baltes, B. J. Chronic tension headache – treatment with amitriptyline – a double-blind study. *Headache*, **11**, 110–116 (1971)
26. Carette, S., McCain, G. A., Bell, D. A. and Fam, A. G. Evaluation of amitriptyline in primary fibrositis. *Arthritis and Rheumatism*, **29**, 655–659 (1986)
27. Pilowsky, I., Hallet, E. C., Bassett, K. L. *et al.* A controlled study of amitriptyline in the treatment of chronic pain. *Pain*, **14**, 169–179 (1982)
28. Gingras, M. A clinical trial of Tofranil in rheumatic pain in general practice. *Journal of International Medical Research*, **4**, 41–49 (1976)
29. Kvinsdahl, B., Molin, J., Froland, A. and Gram, L. F. Imipramine treatment of painful diabetic neuropathy. *Journals of the American Medical Association*, **251**, 1727–1730 (1984)
30. Okasha, A., Ghaleb, H. A. and Sadek, A. A double-blind trial for the clinical management of psychogenic headache. *British Journal of Psychology*, **122**, 181–183 (1973)
31. Hameroff, S. R., Cork, R. C., Scherer, K. *et al.* Doxepin effects on chronic pain, depression and plasma opioids. *Journal of Clinical Psychology*, **43**, 22–27 (1982)
32. Langohr, H. D., Stohr, M. and Petruch, F. An open and double-blind cross-over study on the efficacy of clomipramine (Anafranil) in patients with painful mono- and polyneuropathies. *European Neurology*, **21**, 309–317 (1982)

33. Sternbach, R. A., Janowsky, D. S., Huey, I. Y. and Segal, D. S. Effects of altering brain serotonin activity on human chronic pain. In *Advances in Pain Research and Therapy, Vol. 1* (ed. J. J. Bonica *et al.*), Raven Press, New York, pp. 601–606 (1976)

34. Johansson, F. and Von Knorring, L. A double-blind controlled study of a serotonin uptake inhibitor (zimelidine) versus placebo in chronic pain patients. *Pain*, **7**, 69–78 (1979)

35. Anthony, M. and Lance, J. W. MAO inhibition in the treatment of migraine. *Archives of Neurology*, **21**, 263–268 (1969)

36. Swerdlow, M. Anticonvulsant drugs and chronic pain. *Clinical Neuropharmacology*, **7**, 51–82 (1984)

37. Weinberger, J., Nicklas, W. J. and Berl, S. Mechanism of action of anticonvulsants. *Neurology*, **26**, 162–173 (1976)

38. Braham, J. and Saia, A. Phenytoin in the treatment of trigeminal and other neuralgias. *Lancet*, **ii**, 892–893 (1960)

39. Blom, S. Tic douloureux treated with new anticonvulsant. *Archives of Neurology*, **9**, 285–290 (1963)

40. Taylor, P. H., Gray, K., Bicknell, R. G. and Rees, J. R. Glossopharyngeal neuralgia with syncope. *Journal of Laryngology and Otology*, **91**, 859–868 (1977)

41. Green, J. B. Dilantin in the treatment of lightning pains. *Neurology*, **11**, 257–258 (1961)

42. Hatangdi, V. S., Boas, R. A. and Richards, E. G. Postherpetic neuralgia: management with antiepileptic and tricyclic drugs. In *Advances in Pain Research and Therapy, Vol. 1* (ed. J. J. Bonica *et al.*), Raven Press, New York, pp. 583–587 (1976)

43. Cantor, F. K. Phenytoin treatment of thalamic pain. *British Medical Journal*, **2**, 590 (1972)

44. Raskin, N. H., Levinson, S. A., Hoffman, P. M., Pickett, J. B. E. and Fields, H. L. Postsympathectomy neuralgia: amelioration with diphenylhydantoin and carbamazepine. *American Journal of Surgery*, **128**, 75–78 (1974)

45. Swerdlow, M. and Cundill, J. G. Anticonvulsant drugs used in the treatment of lancinating pains: a comparison. *Anesthesia*, **36**, 1129–1132 (1981)

46. Lockman, L. A., Hunninghake, D. B., Drivit, W. and Desnick, R. J. Relief of pain of Fabry's disease by diphenylhydantoin. *Neurology*, **23**, 871–875 (1973)

47. Chadda, V. S. and Mathur, M. S. Double blind study of the effects of diphenylhydantoin sodium in diabetic neuropathy. *Journal of the Association of Physicians of India*, **26**, 403–406 (1978)

48. Campbell, F. G., Graham, J. G. and Zilkha, K. J. Clinical trial of carbamazepine (Tegretol) in trigeminal neuralgia. *Journal of Neurology, Neurosurgery and Psychiatry*, **29**, 265–267 (1966)

49. Rockliff, B. W. and Davis, E. H. Controlled sequential trials of carbamazepine in trigeminal neuralgia. *Archives of Neurology*, **15**, 129–136 (1966)

50. Killian, J. M. and Fromm, G. H. Carbamazepine in the treatment of neuralgia: use and side effects. *Archives of Neurology*, **19**, 129–136 (1968)

51. Rull, J. A., Quibrera, R., Gonzalez-Milan, H. and Castaneda, O. L. Symptomatic treatment of peripheral diabetic neuropathy with carbamazepine (Tegretol): double blind cross-over trial. *Diabetologia*, **5**, 215–218 (1969)

52. Ekbom, K. Carbamazepine in the treatment of tabetic lightning pains. *Archives of Neurology*, **26**, 374–378 (1972)

53. Elliot, F., Little, A. and Milbrandt, W. Carbamazepine for phantom limb phenomena. *New England Journal of Medicine*, **295**, 678 (1976)

54. Espir, M. L. E. and Millac, P. Treatment of paroxysmal disorders in multiple sclerosis with carbamazepine (Tegretol). *Journal of Neurology, Neurosurgery and Psychiatry*, **33**, 528–531 (1970)

55. Mullan, S. Surgical management of pain in cancer of the head and neck. *Surgical Clinics of North America*, **53**, 203–210 (1973)

56. Caccia, M. R. Clonazepam in facial neuralgia and cluster headache: clinical and electrophysiological study. *European Neurology*, **13**, 560–563 (1975)

57. Martin, G. The management of pain following laminectomy for lumbar disc lesions. *Annals of the Royal College of Surgeons of England*, **63**, 244–252 (1981)

58. Peiris, J. B., Perera, G. L. S., Devendra, S. V. and Lionel, N. D. W. Sodium valproate in trigeminal neuralgia. *Medical Journal of Australia*, **2**, 278 (1980)

59. Raftery, H. The management of postherpetic pain using sodium valproate and amitriptyline. *Journal of the Irish Medical Association*, **72**, 399–401 (1979)

60. Fromm, G. H., Terence, C. F. and Chatta, A. S. Baclofen in the treatment of trigeminal neuralgia. *Annals of Neurology*, **15**, 240–247 (1984)

61. Lindstrom, P. and Lindblom, U. The analgesic effect of tocainide in trigeminal neuralgia. *Pain*, **28**, 45–50 (1987)

62. Bloomfield, S., Simard-Savoie, S., Bernier, J. and Tetreault, L. Comparative analgesic activity of levomepromazine and morphine in patients with chronic pain. *Canadian Medical Association Journal*, **90**, 1156–1159 (1964)

63. Beaver, W. T., Wallenstein, S. M., Houde, R. W. and Rogers, A. A comparison of the analgesic effects of methotrimeprazine and morphine in patients with cancer. *Clinical Pharmacology and Therapeutics*, **7**, 436–446 (1966)

64. Lasagna, L. and Dekornfeld, T. J. Methotrimeprazine – a new phenothiazine derivative with analgesic properties. *Journal of the American Medical Association*, **178**, 119–122 (1961)

65. Houde, R. W. and Wallenstein, S. L. Analgesic power of chlorpromazine alone and in combination with morphine (abstr). *Federal Proceedings*, **14**, 353 (1966)

66. Margolis, L. H. and Gianascol, A. J. Chlorpromazine in thalamic pain syndrome. *Neurology*, **6**, 302–304 (1956)

67. Weis, O., Sriwatanakul, K. and Weintraub, M. Treatment of postherpetic neuralgia and acute herpetic pain with amitriptyline and perphenazine. *South African Medical Journal*, **62**, 274–275 (1982)

68. Nathan, P. W. Chlorprothixene (Taractan) in postherpetic neuralgia and other severe pains. *Pain*, **5**, 367–371 (1978)

69. Kocher, R. Use of psychotrophic drugs for the treatment of chronic severe pain. In *Advances in Pain Research and Therapy, Vol. 1* (ed. J. J. Bonica *et al.*), Raven Press, New York, pp. 279–282 (1976)

70. Taub, A. Relief of postherpetic neuralgia with psychotropic drugs. *Journal of Neurosurgery*, **39**, 235–239 (1973)

71. Bourhis, A., Boudouresque, G., Pellet, W. *et al.* Pain infirmity and psychotropic drugs in oncology. *Pain*, **5**, 263–274 (1978)

72. Kastrup, J., Peterson, P., Dejgard, A. *et al.* Treatment of chronic painful diabetic neuropathy with intravenous lidocaine infusion. *British Medical Journal*, **292**, 173 (1986)

73. Kastrup, J. Petersen, P., Dejgard, A. *et al.* Intravenous lidocaine infusion – a new treatment of chronic painful diabetic neuropathy. *Pain*, **28**, 69–75 (1987)

74. Peterson, P. and Kastrup, J. Dercum's disease (adiposis dolorosa). Treatment of the severe pain with intravenous lidocaine. *Pain*, **28**, 77–80 (1987)

75. Dejgard, A., Petersen, P. and Kastrup, J. Mexiletine for treatment of chronic painful diabetic neuropathy. *Lancet*, **i**, 9–11 (1988)

76. Kreeger, W. and Hammill, S. C. New antiarrhythmic drugs: tocainide, mexiletine, flecainide, encainide, and amiodarone. *Mayo Clinic Proceedings*, **62**, 1033–1050 (1987)

77. Davidoff, R. A. Pharmacology of spasticity. *Neurology*, **28**, 46–51 (1978)

78. Smith, C. M. Relaxants of skeletal muscle. In *Physiological Pharmacology, Vol. 2* (ed. W. S. Root and F. G. Hoffmann), Academic Press, New York, pp. 2–96 (1965)

79. Bercel, N. A. Cyclobenzaprine in the treatment of skeletal muscle spasm in osteoarthritis of the cervical and lumbar spine. *Current Therapeutic Research*, **22**, 462–468 (1977)

80. Gold, R. H. Treatment of low back syndrome with oral orphenadrine citrate. *Current Therapeutic Research*, **23**, 271–276 (1978)

81. Birkeland, I. W. and Clawson, D. K. Drug combinations with orphenadrine for pain relief associated with muscle spasm. *Clinical Pharmacology and Therapeutics*, **9**, 639–646 (1968)

82. Rumore, M. M. and Schlichting, D. A. Clinical efficacy of antihistamines as analgesics. *Pain*, **25**, 7–22 (1986)

83. Stambaugh, J. E. and Lance, C. Analgesic efficacy and pharmacokinetic evaluation of meperidine and hydroxyzine, alone and in combination. *Cancer Investigation*, **1**, 111–117 (1983)

84. Bellville, J. W., Dorey, F., Capparell, D. *et al.* Analgesic effects of hydroxyzine compared to morphine in man. *Journal of Clinical Pharmacology and Therapeutics*, **19**, 290–296 (1979)

85. Yosselson-Superstine, S., Lipman, A. G. and Sanders, S. H. Adjunctive antianxiety agents in the management of chronic pain. *Israel Journal of Medical Sciences*, **21**, 113–117 (1985)

86. Payne, R. Neuropathic pain syndromes with special reference to causalgia and reflex sympathetic dystrophy. *Clinical Journal of Pain*, **2**, 59–73 (1986)

87. Scadding, J. W., Wall, P. D., Parry, C. B. W. and Brooks, D. M. Clinical trial of propranolol in post-traumatic neuralgia. *Pain*, **14**, 283–292 (1982)

88. Simson, G. Propranolol for causalgia and Sudek's atrophy. *Journal of the American Medical Association*, **227**, 327 (1974)

89. Abram, S. E. and Lightfoot, R. W. Treatment of longstanding causalgia with prazosin. *Regional Anesthesia*, **6**, 79–81 (1981)

90. Tabira, T., Shibasaki, H. and Kuroiwa, Y. Reflex sympathetic dystrophy (causalgia) treatment with guanethidine. *Archives of Neurology*, **40**, 430–432 (1983)

91. Loh, L. and Nathan, P. W. Painful peripheral states and sympathetic blocks. *Journal of Neurology, Neurosurgery and Psychiatry*, **41**, 664–671 (1978)
92. Ghostine, S. Y., Comair, Y. G., Turner, D. M. *et al*. Phenoxybenzamine in the treatment of causalgia. *Journal of Neurosurgery*, **60**, 1263–1268 (1984)
93. Kozin, F., Ryan, L. M., Carerra, G. F. *et al*. The reflex sympathetic dystrophy syndrome (RSDS). III. Scintigraphic studies, further evidence for the therapeutic efficacy of systemic corticosteroids, and proposed diagnostic criteria. *American Journal of Medicine*, **70**, 23–29 (1981)
94. Prough, D. S., McLeskey, C. H., Borshy, G. G. *et al*. Efficacy of oral nifedipine in the treatment of reflex sympathetic dystrophy. *Anesthesiology*, **62**, 796–799 (1985)
95. Singh, P. N., Sharma, P., Gupta, P. K. and Pandey, K. Clinical evaluation of diazepam for relief of postoperative pain. *British Journal of Anaesthesia*, **53**, 831–836 (1981)
96. Miller, R., Eisenkraft, J. B., Cohen, M. *et al*. Midazolam as an adjunct to meperidine analgesia for postoperative pain. *Clinical Journal of Pain*, **2**, 37–43 (1986)
97. Fernadez, F., Adams, F. and Holmes, V. F. Analgesic effect of alprazolam in patients with chronic organic pain of malignant origin. *Journal of Clinical Psychopharmacology*, **7**, 167–169 (1987)
98. Yang, J. C., Clark, W. C., Ngai, S. H. *et al*. Analgesic action and pharmacokinetics of morphine and diazepam in man: an evaluation by sensory decision theory. *Anesthesiology*, **51**, 495–502 (1979)
99. Hendler, N., Cimini, C., Ma, T. and Long, D. A comparison of cognitive impairment due to benzodiazepines and to narcotics. *American Journal of Psychology*, **137**, 828–830 (1980)
100. Seltzer, J., Dewar, T., Pollack, R. L. and Jackson, E. The effects of dietary tryptophan on chronic maxillofacial pain and experimental pain tolerance. *Journal of Psychiatric Research*, **17**, 181–186 (1983)
101. Bruera, E., Chadwick, S., Brenneis, C. *et al*. Methylphenidate associated with narcotics for the treatment of cancer pain. *Cancer Treatment Reports*, **71**, 67–70 (1987)
102. Forrest, W. H., Brown, B., Brown, C. *et al*. Dextroamphetamine with morphine for the treatment of postoperative pain. *New England Journal of Medicine*, **296**, 712–715 (1977)
103. Laska, E. M., Sunshine, A., Mueller, F. *et al*. Caffeine as an analgesic adjuvant. *Journal of the American Medical Association*, **251**, 1711–1718 (1984)
104. Tan, Y.-M. and Croese, J. Clonidine and diabetic patients with leg pains. *Annals of Internal Medicine*, **105**, 633 (1986)
105. Max, M. B., Schafer, S. C., Culnane, M. *et al*. Association of pain relief with drug side effects in post-herpetic neuralgia: a single-dose study of clonidine, codeine, ibuprofen, and placebo. *Clinical Pharmacology and Therapeutics*, **43**, 363–371 (1988)
106. Shafar, J., Tallet, E. R. and Knowlson, P. A. Evaluation of clonidine in prophylaxis of migraine. *Lancet*, **i**, 403–407 (1972)
107. Boisen, E., Deth, S., Hubbe, P. *et al*. Clonidine in the prophylaxis of migraine. *Acta neurologica scandinavica*, **58**, 288–295 (1978)
108. Noyes, R., Brunk, S. F., Avery, D. H. and Canter, A. The analgesic properties of delta-9-tetrahydrocannabinol and codeine. *Clinical Pharmacology and Therapeutics*, **18**, 84–89 (1975)
109. Portenoy, R. K. and Foley, K. M. Chronic use of opioid analgesics in non-malignant pain: report of 38 cases. *Pain*, **25**, 171–186 (1986)
110. Portenoy, R. K. Opioid therapy in the management of chronic back pain. In *Interdisciplinary Rehabilitation of Low Back Pain* (ed. C. D. Tollinson), Williams and Wilkins, Baltimore (1989), in press
111. France, R. D., Urban, B. J. and Keefe, F. J. Long-term use of narcotic analgesics in chronic pain. *Social Science and Medicine*, **19**, 1379–1382 (1984)
112. Urban, B. J., France, R. D., Steinberger, D. L. *et al*. Long-term use of narcotic/antidepressant medication in the management of phantom limb pain. *Pain*, **24**, 191–197 (1986)
113. Taub, A. Opioid analgesics in the treatment of chronic intractable pain of non-neoplastic origin. In *Narcotic Analgesics in Anesthesiology* (ed. L. M. Kitahata and D. Collins), Williams and Wilkins, Baltimore, pp. 199–208 (1982)
114. Tennant, F. S. and Uelman, G. F. Narcotic maintenance for chronic pain: medical and legal guidelines. *Postgraduate Medicine*, **73**, 81–94 (1983)
115. Halpern, L. M. and Robinson, J. Prescribing practices for pain in drug dependence: a lesson in ignorance. *Advances in Alcohol and Substance Abuse*, **5**, 184–197 (1985 Fall–1986 Winter)
116. Neuman, R. G. The need to redefine addiction. *New England Journal of Medicine*, **18**, 1096–1098 (1983)
117. Porter, J. and Jick, H. Addiction rare in patients treated with narcotics. *New England Journal of Medicine*, **302**, 123 (1980)

118. Perry, S. and Heidrich, G. Management of pain during debridement: a survey of US burn units. *Pain*, **13**, 267–280 (1982)
119. Medina, J. L. and Diamond, S. Drug dependency in patients with chronic headache. *Headache*, **17**, 12–14 (1977)

Index